AF813767

Surgical Inflammation

Edited By

Jaime Arias

Department of Surgery, Medical School
Complutense University of Madrid
Madrid
Spain

Maria-Angeles Aller

Department of Surgery, Medical School
Complutense University of Madrid
Madrid
Spain

&

Jose-Ignacio Arias

General and Digestive Surgery Unit
Monte Naranco Hospital
Oviedo, Asturias
Spain

CONTENTS

Foreword *i*

Preface *ii*

List of Contributors *iii*

CHATPERS

1. **A Brief History of Surgical Inflammation** **3**
   J. Arias, M.A. Aller and J.I. Arias

2. **Surgical Inflammation: From Molecule to Clinic** **18**
   J.I. Arias, M.A. Aller, G. Rodríguez-Boto, M. Giner and J. Arias

3. **The Embryological Bases of Surgical Inflammation** **51**
   M.A. Aller, J.I. Arias, C. Gilsanz, V. Martínez, P. Vergara and J. Arias

4. **Phases of the Acute Inflammatory Response to the Injury** **99**
   M.A. Aller, J.I. Arias, I. Prieto, C. Gilsanz, J.L. Arias, H. Yang and J. Arias

5. **The Wound Healing Reaction** **129**
   M.A. Aller, I. Prieto, J.Blanco-Rivero, J.I. Arias, G.Balfagon and J. Arias

6. **The Polytraumatized Patient** **154**
   M.A. Aller, J.I. Arias, L. Lorente, I. Prieto, A. Alonso-Poza and J. Arias

7. **Inflammation Related with Surgical Infections** **180**
   M.A. Aller, M. Giner, G. Rodríguez-Boto, M. Losada, A.Alonso-Poza, J.I. Arias and J. Arias

8. Cancer: Using the Inflammatory Way to Invade the Host **214**

J.I. Arias, M.A.Aller, l. Prieto, A. Arias, H. Yang and J. Arias

9. Mesenchymal Stem Cells: Advances and Surgical Applications **250**

M.A. Aller, M.P. de Miguel, C. Jiménez, S. Fuentes-Julián, A. Manrique, A. Blázquez- Martínez, J. Calvo, C.Y. Pascual, F. Arnalich-Montiel and J. Arias

10. Inflammation Meets Evo-Devo **277**

M.A. Aller, N. Arias, S. Fuentes-Julián, A. Blázquez-Martínez, S. Argudo, M.P. de Miguel, J.L. Arias and J. Arias

11. Experimental Models of Surgical Inflammation **309**

M.A. Aller, N. de las Heras, N. Arias, I. Prieto, L. Lorente, M.P. Nava, L. Santamaría, J.L.Arias, V. Lahera and J. Arias

Index **344**

FOREWORD

I am delighted to write an introduction to this new volume "Inflammation-related Surgery" which covers information in all its forms including new developments in the exciting area of stem cells. The healing of surgical wounds has always been of central importance to surgeons and even more especially to their patients.

There have been many advances in our understanding of various forms of inflammation and many of these features are relevant to surgical research and clinical surgery. This volume discusses the basic science relating to wound care and injury and should be of interest to all academic surgeons. I wish the authors every success with this *magnum opus.*

Sir Roy York Calne

University of Cambridge

Cambridge

UK

PREFACE

This eBook aims at offering an integrated point-of-view about the inflammatory response related to injuries, infections and tumors. This integration is made by considering that the multiple pathophysiological mechanisms making up inflammation represent the re-expression of ontogenic mechanisms during early embryo development as well as the recapitulation of ancestral phylogenetic mechanisms.

The many publications about inflammation have made it difficult for us to reference all of them in detail, even though some could be considered fundamental for our paper. We would like to apologize to the authors for this limitation.

We would like to thank all those people whose talents and time made this eBook a reality. We would like to thank Maria Elena Vicente for preparing the manuscript, Elizabeth Mascola for translating it into English, Pedro Cuesta and Santiago Cano, from the Complutense University Computer Unit for Teaching and Research Supporting and the librarians of the Complutense University Medical School particularly the Director Javier de Jorge, Sub-director Manuela Crego and Maria Jose Valdemoro. This eBook was supported, in part, by grants from Mutua Madrileña Research Foundation (Ref. nº PA 3077/2008 and AP5966/2009), MICINN PSI2010-19348 and with the special collaboration of the INEUROPA (Instituto de Neurociencias del Principado de Asturias).

Jaime Arias

Maria-Angeles Aller

Department of Surgery, Medical School
Complutense University of Madrid
Madrid
Spain

&

Jose-Ignacio Arias

General and Digestive Surgery Unit
Monte Naranco Hospital
Oviedo. Asturias
Spain

List of Contributors

Alejandro Blazquez-Martinez

Cell Engineering Laboratory, idiPaz, La Paz Hospital Research Institute, Madrid, Spain

Alejandro Manrique

Abdominal Organ Transplantation and General and Digestive Surgery Department, 12 de Octubre University Hospital, Madrid, Spain

Alfredo Alonso-Poza

General and Digestive Surgery Unit, Sudeste Hospital, Arganda del Rey, Madrid, Spain

Ana Arias

Internal Medicine Department, Puerta de Hierro Hospital, Autónoma University of Madrid, Madrid, Spain

Carlos Gilsanz

General and Digestive Surgery Unit, Sudeste Hospital, Arganda del Rey, Madrid, Spain

Carlos Jiménez

Abdominal Organ Transplantation and General and Digestive Surgery Department, 12 de Octubre University Hospital, Madrid, Spain

Cristina Y, Pascual

Allergology Department, Infanta Sofia Hospital, Madrid, Spain

Francisco Arnalich-Montiel

Ophthalmology Department, Ramon y Cajal Hospital, Autonoma University of Madrid, Madrid, Spain

Gloria Balfagon

Department of Physiology, School of Medicine, Autonoma University of Madrid, Madrid, Spain

Gregorio Rodriguez-Boto

Department of Surgery, Medical School, Complutense University of Madrid, Madrid, Spain

Heping Yang

Division of Gastroenterology and Liver Diseases, USC Research Center for Liver Diseases, Keck School of Medicine USC, Los Angeles, California, USA

Isabel Prieto

Department of Surgery, La Paz Hospital, Autonoma University of Madrid, Madrid, Spain

Jaime Arias

Department of Surgery, Medical School, Complutense University of Madrid, Madrid, Spain

Javier Blanco-Rivero

Department of Physiology, School of Medicine, Autonoma University of Madrid, Madrid, Spain

Jorge Calvo

Abdominal Organ Transplantation and General and Digestive Surgery Department, 12 de Octubre University Hospital, Madrid, Spain

Jorge-Luis Arias

Neurosciences Laboratory. Psychobiology Department. School of Psychology. University of Oviedo, Asturias. Spain

Jose-Ignacio Arias

General and Digestive Surgery Unit, Monte Naranco Hospital, Oviedo, Asturias, Spain

Laureano Lorente

Department of Surgery, Medical School, Complutense University of Madrid, Madrid, Spain

Luis Santamaria

Cellular Biology and Morphological Sciences Department, School of Medicine, Autonoma University of Madrid, Madrid, Spain

Manuel Giner

Department of Surgery, Medical School, Complutense University of Madrid, Madrid, Spain

Manuel Losada

General and Digestive Surgery, Unit of General and Digestive Surgery, Sudeste Hospital, Arganda del Rey, Madrid, Spain

Maria-Angeles Aller

Department of Surgery, Medical School, Complutense University of Madrid, Madrid, Spain

Maria-Paz de Miguel

Cell Engineering Laboratory, idiPaz, La Paz Hospital Research Institute, Madrid, Spain

Maria-Paz Nava

Department of Animal Physiology (Physiology II), Biology School, Complutense University of Madrid, Madrid, Spain

Natalia Arias

Neurosciences Unit, Deparment of Psychobiology, School of Psychology, University of Oviedo, Asturias, Spain

Natalia de las Heras

Department of Physiology, School of Medicine, Complutense University of Madrid, Madrid, Spain

Patri Vergara

Department of Cell Biology, Physiology and Immunology, School of Veterinary, Autonoma University of Barcelona, Bellaterra, Barcelona, Spain

Salvador Argudo

Unit of General and Digestive Surgery, Sudeste Hospital, Arganda del Rey, Madrid, Spain

Sherezade Fuentes-Julian

Cell Engineering Laboratory, idiPaz, La Paz Hospital Research Institute, Madrid, Spain

Vicente Lahera

Department of Physiology, School of Medicine, Complutense University of Madrid, Madrid, Spain

Vicente Martinez

Department of Cell Biology, Physiology and Immunology, School of Veterinary, Autonoma University of Barcelona, Bellaterra, Barcelona, Spain

ACKNOWLEDGEMENTS

We would like to thank Maria Elena Vicente for preparing the manuscript, Elizabeth Mascola for translating it into English and librarians of Complutense University Medical School, particularly the Director, Francisco Javier Jorge García-Reyes, and Manuela Crego and María José Valdemoro and B. Braun Surgical S.A. for their technical assistance.

This study was carried out in part with grants from Mutua Madrileña Research Foundation (Ref. nº PA 3077/2008 and AP5966/2009), MICINN PSI2010-19348 and with the special collaboration of the INEUROPA (Instituto de Neurociencias del Principado de Asturias).

CHAPTER 1

A Brief History of Surgical Inflammation

Jaime Arias[1,*], Maria-Angeles Aller[1] and Jose-Ignacio Arias[2]

[1]Department of Surgery, School of Medicine, Complutense University of Madrid, Madrid, Spain and [2]General Surgery Unit, Monte Naranco Hospital, Oviedo, Asturias, Spain

Abstract. The concept of inflammation throughout its history has become exceedingly enhanced by the discovery that inflammation does not just participate in conditions that produce redness, swelling, heat, pain and loss of function. Nowadays, inflammation is associated with numerous and diverse diseases, including arterial hypertension, atherosclerosis, type 2 diabetes, neurodegeneration and cancer. In addition, inflammation is a process also involved in many physiological processes like embryogenesis, regeneration, aging and animal development. Understanding the great versatility of the inflammatory response is very useful for surgeons given its application potential during pre-, intra- and postoperative management of their patients.

Keywords: Inflammation, surgery, surgical history, injury, elective surgery, accidental surgery, surgical treatment, transplantation, vessels anastomosis, para-inflammation, meta-organism.

INTRODUCTION

Inflammation is a surgical-related pathology mainly because it is related to traumatisms. Many inflammatory processes of infectious origin also require surgery. Consequently, surgery is considered a curative or palliative treatment in diseases closely linked with inflammation, such as tumors [1, 2]. In turn, the inflammatory response related to elective or accidental surgery could be considered as "surgical inflammation" [3]. Inflammation can be caused or may be the consequence of a surgical treatment. For this reason fully understanding the inflammatory response is crucial for the surgeon.

***Address correspondence to Jaime Arias:** Cátedra de Cirugía, Facultad de Medicina, Universidad Complutense, Pza. de Ramón y Cajal s.n., 28040 MADRID, Spain; Tel: +34 91 394 1389; Fax: +34 91 3947115; E-mail: jariasp@med.ucm.es

HISTORY

Inflammation is a disease that was already described in the Egyptian medical papyri (c. 2500 BC) and the clay tablets of Mesopotamia (c. 600 BC) [4]. These pictographs were derived from verbs meaning "to blow" and in these cultures, the association between blowing, fire and inflammation was common [4].

Local acute inflammation has been studied since ancient times. Aulus Cornelius Celsus (Fig. **1**) described the four cardinal signs of acute inflammation as "rubor et tumor cum calorc ct dolore" [5]. Thus the tissue response to injury gave rise to rubor (redness, due to hyperemia), tumor (swelling, caused by increased permeability of the microvasculature and leakage of protein into the interstitial space), calor (heat, associated with the increased blood flow and the metabolic activity of the cellular mediators of inflammation) and dolor (pain, in part due to changes in the perivasculature and associated nerve endings) [6]. Galen (130-200 AD) identified this condition as a body response to injury and named it "phlogosis" and added the fifth clinical sign, "functio laesa" (loss of function) to inflammation [4]. The word inflammation itself comes from the Latin inflammare: "to set on fire" [7].

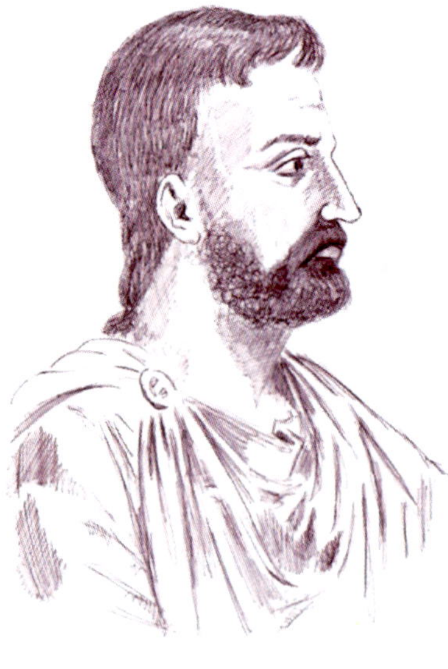

Figure 1: Aulus Cornelius Celsus (ca 25BC-ca50AD) was a Roman doctor and encyclopedist, author of "De Medicina", an encyclopedia that included information about diet, pharmacy, surgery and related fields.

However, John Hunter (Fig. **2**) was the first surgeon in making a scientific study of inflammation. Hunter made a broad research on inflammation and its role in surgical diseases, including studies of wound healing, transplantation, angiogenesis and abscess formation [4]. He recognized the prominence of inflammation in surgical conditions and explained its concept as "the first principle of surgery" [4, 8]. John Hunter was keenly devoted in science, as well as in the influence of the experimental method on surgery. This Hunter´s amazing attitude has lasted far beyond his own time [9, 10].

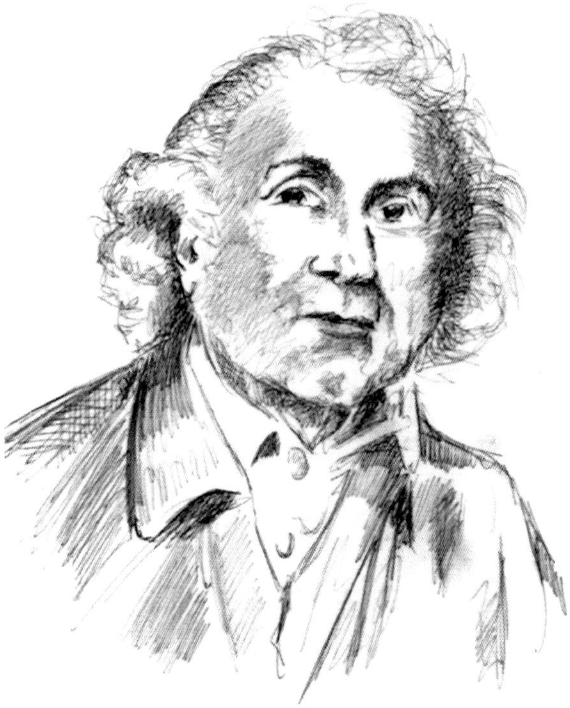

Figure 2: John Hunter (1728-1793) was one of the first investigators to perform a scientific study of inflammation describing it as erythema, edema, heat and pain.

The contemporary understanding of the inflammatory process is owed to 19th century milestone discoveries by Rudolph Virchow, Friedrich Daniel von Recklinghausen, Julius Friedrich Cohnheim and Elie Metschnikoff [11-13].

Rudolph Virchow (Fig. **3**) completed the cellular theory set forth by Theodor Schwann. He established that the cell is the fundamental unit of life. He also ascertained that cells are only derived from another cells. Consequently, Virchow´s main thesis is the cellular concept used for both the organism and its pathology. His important book and medical masterpiece known as "Die Cellularpathologie", was a great success, requiring multiple reprints and translations. Recklinghausen and Cohnheim stand out among Virchow disciples [12]. Friedrich Daniel von Recklinghausen (Fig. **4**) is one of the most important classical authors on bone diseases and his works related to corneal inflammation highly influenced Cohnheim master studies [12]. Von Recklinghausen was the first to describe wandering leukocytes, which were demonstrated in experimental keratitis. He also showed that "pus" cells could migrate from the places of their origin in the interstitium to other tissues. He also contributed to the concept of phagocytosis [13]. Julius Friedrich Cohnheim (Fig. **5**) described the mechanisms involved in the extravasations of leukocytes through the capillaries and venules into the interstitial space of the inflamed tissue, known as diapedesis [13, 14]. He showed that in the inflamed mesentery of the rat, "pus cells" did not have a local origin, but were leukocytes coming from the blood. He described the time-dependent alterations in the inflammatory process, with dilatation of vessels, adhesion of leukocytes to the endothelial cells and the subsequent transmigration into the interstitium [13]. Cohnheim had a leading role in driving the pathophysiological mind. Consequently, pathology relies on physiological research and on pathological experiment, which John Hunter began to perform in England and Magendie in France [12]. Elie Metschnikoff (Fig. **6**) discovered the phagocytosis phenomenon and its key role as one of the body's defense mechanisms against microorganisms [15]. In 1891, he wrote: "The broad fact that the invasion of the organism by microbes most often induces, on the one hand, an inflammatory reaction with its associated emigration of leucocytes, and that, on the other hand, the phagocytes are capable of including and destroying the invaders, lead us to admit that the afflux of phagocytes to the invaded region, and their bactericidal properties, are mechanisms which serve to ward off bacterial attack and to maintain the integrity of the organism" [15]. Owing to this discovery, Metschnikoff was awarded in 1908 the Nobel Prize for Physiology of Medicine that was shared with Paul Ehrlich (Fig. **7**), a pioneer on the study on humoral immunity, a key component of adaptive immunity [6].

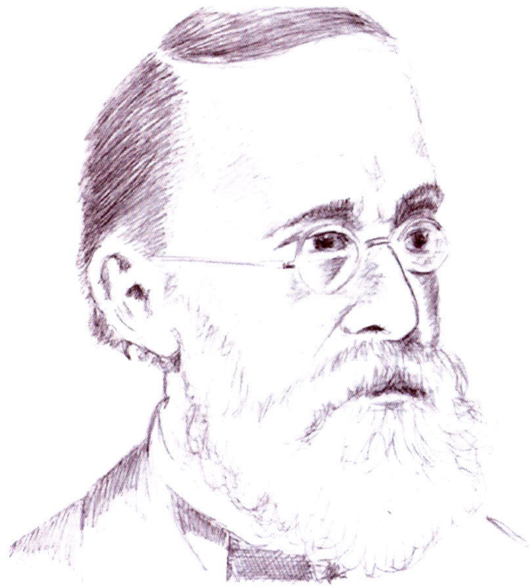

Figure 3: Rudolph Carl Virchow (1821-1902) was a German doctor, disciple of Johannes Peter Müller (1801-1858), and is considered the father of modern pathology. Function *laesa*, or dysfunction of the injured tissues or organs was marked as a fifth characteristic of inflammation, a proposition attributed by some authors to Virchow.

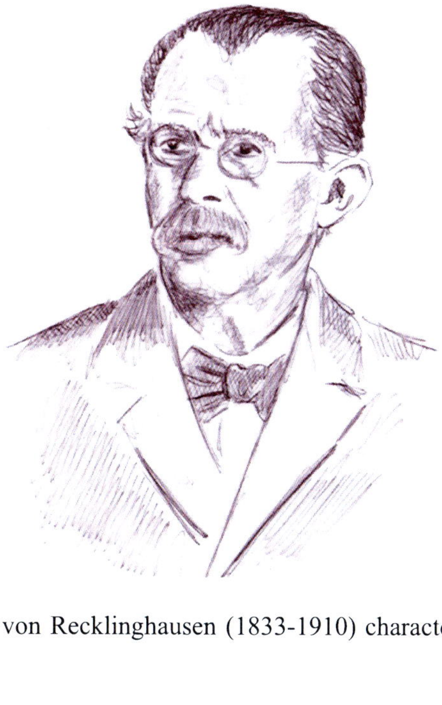

Figure 4: Friedrich Daniel von Recklinghausen (1833-1910) characterized the pus cells in acute inflammation.

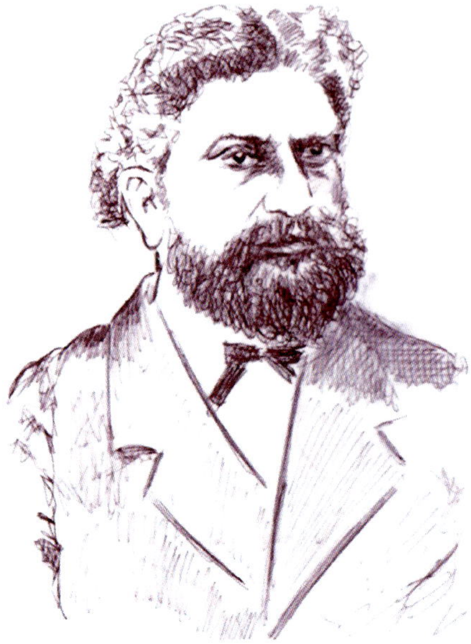

Figure 5: Julius Friedrich Cohnheim (1839-1884) discovered the "pus cells" that do not have local origin as considered by Virchow, but were leukocytes from the blood. Consequently, Cohnheim based his thesis on the aphorism "without blood vessels, there is no inflammation" [9].

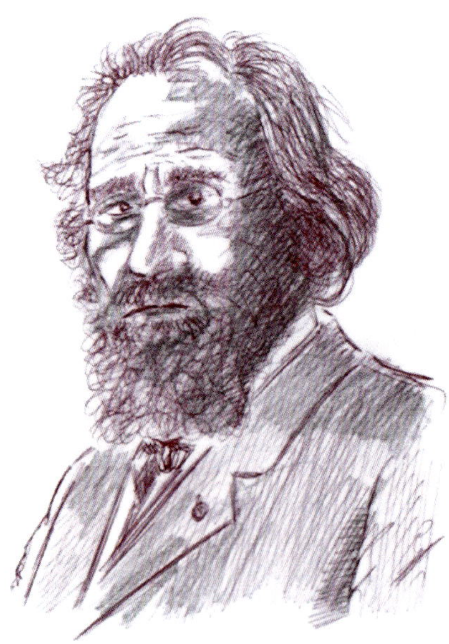

Figure 6: Elie Metschnikoff (1845-1916) wrote his thesis on compared embryology in his native country Russia as a professor of Zoology in Odesa. His research in marine zoology led to the discovery of phagocytosis. At Pasteur Institute (Paris) he continued his research by developing his phagocytosis theory, as a defense mechanism of the body.

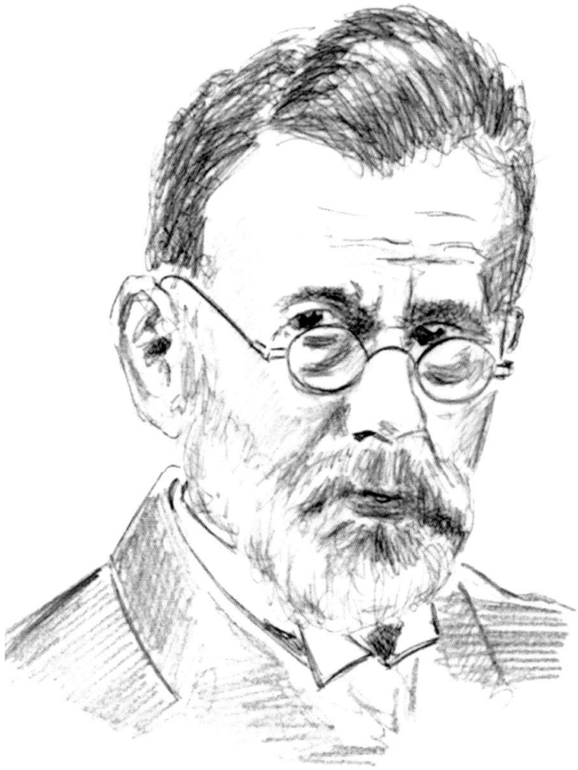

Figure 7: Paul Ehrlich (1854-1915), German doctor and bacteriologist, made important contributions to humoral immunity and important advances with his clinical application in the production of specific anti-bodies.

From ancient times nutritional impairments have been associated with inflammation. Santiago Ramón y Cajal (Fig. **8**), in order to obtain his doctor's degree, presented in 1877 a manuscript titled "Pathogeny of the Inflammation". In this ahead work the future Spanish Nobel Prize winner cited the existence of disorders or perturbations of the nutritional activity in the organic territory suffering irritation, thus seconding Virchow and Jacoud [16]. These authors proposed that irritation of the cell, which would be expressed by feeding the cell itself most actively while enlarging upon function and by cell genesis, was indeed the key phenomenon of the inflammatory process. Thus, Ramón y Cajal suggested the existence of cellular hypergenesis, with the presence of embryonic cells in the diseased tissue. When the embryonic cells mix with the migrated leukocytes, many of the repair processes developed for inflammation resolution are produced

[16]. Ramón y Cajal also exposed that, according to this idea, the physiological hyperplastic process characteristic of growing is very similar to the inflammatory process. Indeed, the hyperplastic tumors that occur without inflammation and the own inflammation are almost identical since there is a transient excess of the nutrition activity in the injured area in all of these phenomena [16]. Lastly, in the above mentioned thesis, Ramon y Cajal proposed that the end of the inflammatory response can be obtained by resolution or by organization. The former is the best way for finishing inflammation since normal tissue integrity is restored, while through organization, connective tissue and fibrosis are produced [16]. A more active role than those which Virchow proposed is attributed to the vessels in this Review on inflammation made by Ramón y Cajal. This author also reports the existence of cells with embryonic characteristics as well as, the similarity between apparently different processes like hyperplasia, neoplasia and inflammation, which seem to share a similar disorder of nutrition [16].

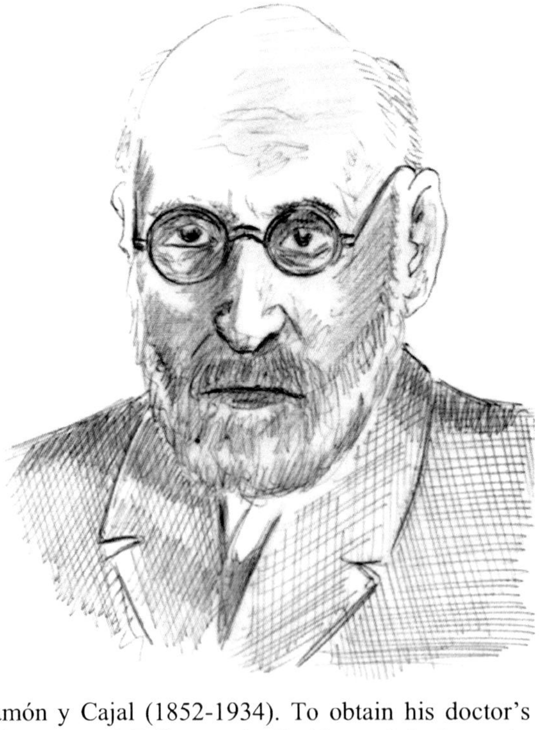

Figure 8: Santiago Ramón y Cajal (1852-1934). To obtain his doctor's degree, he presented a manuscript titled "Pathogeny of Inflammation". The original version can be read at the Complutense University Medical School Library, although it has also been published in a facsimile edition.

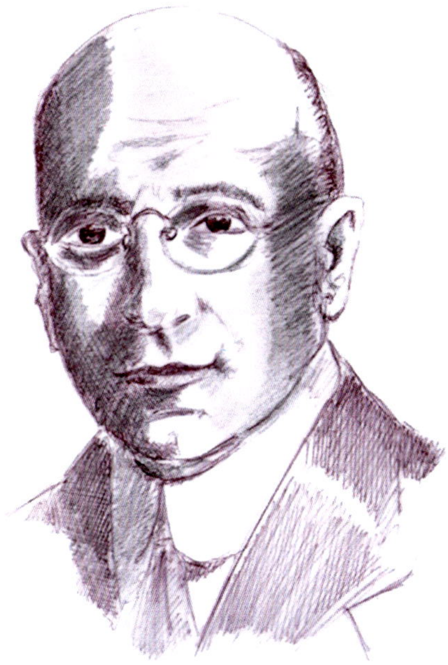

Figure 9: Alexis Carrel (1873-1944) described the technique for vascular anastomosis using manual sutures and later applied them to organ transplantation.

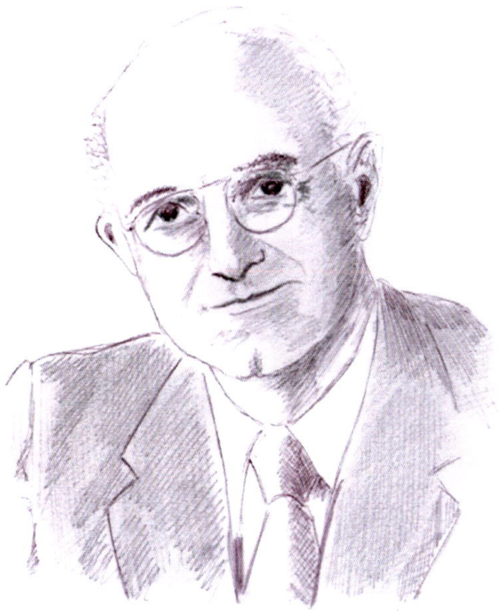

Figure 10: Joseph Murray (1919). After years of experimental work and as surgeon at the Peter Bent Brigham Hospital (Boston), he undertook organ transplantation in humans. Murray headed the team that performed the first successful organ transplant in 1954.

Research about the inflammatory mechanisms was promoted during the 20th century since organ and tissue transplantations, validated by their previous experimental study as therapeutical choice, became widespread [17-19]. Organ transplantation is based on the vessel anastomosis technique, described by the French surgeon Alexis Carrel, who won the Nobel Prize in 1912 [20] (Fig. **9**). Joseph Murray, in turn, received the Nobel Prize in 1990 for his pioneering works on kidney transplantation [21] (Fig. **10**). Surgeons are also indebted to Thomas E. Starzl (Fig. **11**) and Sir Roy York Calne (Fig. **12**), pioneers in liver transplantation.

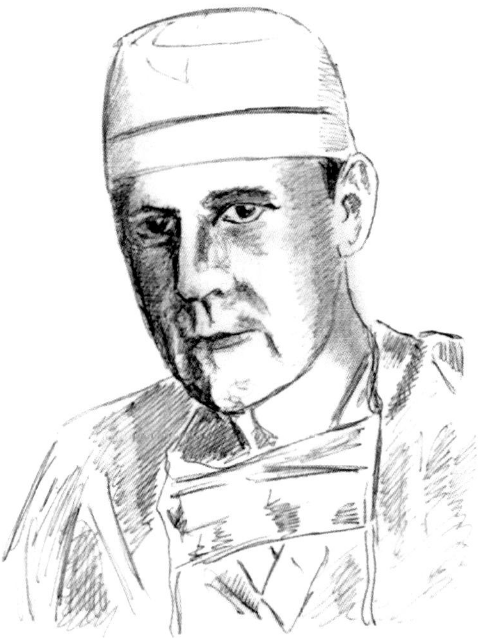

Figure 11: Thomas E. Starzl performed the first successful liver transplant in 1963.

Nowadays, inflammation is considered a highly beneficial and adaptive response triggered by noxious injuries and conditions, such as tissue traumatisms, infection and neoplasia [1, 2, 22]. However, this accepted point of view of inflammation as a response triggered by injury, infection or tumor might need to be expanded for including those inflammatory processes induced by other types of adverse conditions [22]. In this way, human diseases associated with these conditions, like atherosclerosis, asthma, type 2 diabetes and neurodegenerative diseases, are all defined by chronic low-grade inflammation. Since these chronic pathological processes are intermediate between basal and inflammatory states, they have been named "para-inflammation" [22]. Therefore, in basal conditions, tissues are supported in a homeostatic state, but in noxious conditions, tissues can suffer stress and can malfunction. It has been proposed that the function of the stressed tissues is derived by macrophages and mast cells, and is intermediate between the normal cell autonomous function, a condition that results in cell-autonomous inflammatory response, which can be referred to as para-inflammation [22, 23].

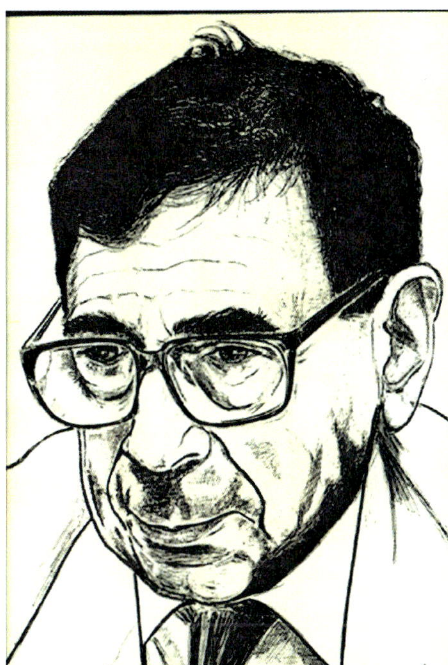

Figure 12: Sir Roy York Calne was the European pioneer in liver transplant and established immunosupression with Cyclosporine A.

Furthermore, human aging can be explained by the novel concept of para-inflammation-driven inflammaging, *i.e.* an association of inflammation and aging [24]. Inflammaging seems to favor the onset of typical age-related diseases, like atherosclerosis, osteoporosis, dementia and cancer [25, 26]. Therefore, inflammation underlies a wide variety not only of pathological, but also physiological, processes. However, the physiological functions of the inflammatory mechanisms are mostly unknown [22]. The relationship existing between the human organism and the microbiota indeed represents an attractive area of research because in particular the gut-microbiota balance plays a fundamental role in preserving human homeostasis [27, 28]. Human beings have been newly defined as "meta-organisms" because of their close symbiotic linking with the gut microbiota [29]. The expression "metaorganisms" was first used to relate organisms that are between two levels of organization [30]. This concept is also based on the "Biocenosis" concept, created by Karl Möbius, in 1877, in order to describe a community of living beings belonging to different species and linked by way of inter-species relationship [31]. Karl Möbius biocenosis theory is now accepted as the basis of ecology [31]. In the light of the metaorganisms, hypothesis has been suggested the involvement in the ageing process [32].

Surgical inflammation could recapitulate ontogeny through the re-expression of two hypothetical extraembryonic trophic axes, namely coelomic-amniotic- and trophoblastic-yolk sac-related, in the interstitial space of the injured tissues [33]. If so, surgical inflammation could mean the expression during postnatal life of ancestral biochemical mechanisms that were also used for embryonic development. However, the re-expression of these embryonic functions in a different environment could be inappropriate and this is the reason why their results are not the same during the adult life [33, 34].

However, tissue repair in embryos is made by regeneration and does not leave a scar [35]. Thus, the correct repair achieved by embryos as they heal wounds demonstrates how perfect tissue regeneration is possible. It also provides a very useful target for improving healing by creating treatments to modify the inflammatory post-natal response [34, 35]. On the other hand, the benefits of studying the mechanisms of embryonic repair are the demonstration that repair and morphogenesis mirror one another in many regards [14, 35]. In particular, regeneration, considered as the replacement of body parts lost by injury, is most certainly not a masked figure emerging only after trauma, but it is always present and characterizes everyday adult biology [36].

In essence, inflammation could represent a group of basic mechanisms that work in an array of micro-environmental situations throughout both the vertebrate and invertebrate animal life cycles [14, 36-38]. In summary, it is worth answering whether the different types of the inflammatory responses marking the life of living beings integrate ancestral evolutionary mechanisms. Through careful and intentional research, we could indeed trace the biochemical origins of life [38]. Ecological, medical and evolutionary biology are becoming integrated through evolutionary developmental of biology (evo-devo). In the case of this new integrated idea (eco-evo-devo) is successful, it would represent a fascinating revolution in our way of thinking about the origins of biodiversity [39]. On the contrary, we could also ask ourselves in terms of the role that the mechanisms of inflammation could play regarding our future evolution as an animal species [38]. In conclusion, the concept of inflammation has extensively been enhanced because of the progressive incorporation of pathological and physiological processes. This amazing versatility of the inflammatory response suggests that its seminal mechanisms take root closely to the origin of life on Earth. Maybe this is the reason why the inflammatory response incorporates so easily all the new knowledge in Medicine and in addition is today becoming a useful tool for understanding many aspects of Biology. For the surgeon, it is especially crucial to understand this great adaptive ability of inflammation, given its application potential during pre-, intra- and postoperative management of patients.

ACKNOWLEDGEMENTS

We would like to thank Maria Elena Vicente for preparing the manuscript, Elizabeth Mascola for translating it into English and librarians of Complutense University Medical School, particularly the Director, Francisco Javier Jorge García-Reyes, and Manuela Crego and María José Valdemoro and *B Braun Surgical S.A.* for their technical assistance.

This study was carried out in part with grants from Mutua Madrileña Research Foundation (Ref. nº PA 3077/2008 and AP5966/2009), MICINN PSI2010-19348 and with the special collaboration of the INEUROPA (Instituto de Neurociencias del Principado de Asturias).

CONFLICT OF INTEREST

The author(s) confirm that this chapter content has no conflict of interest.

REFERENCES

[1] Arias JI, Aller MA, Arias J. Surgical inflammation: a pathophysiological rainbow. J Transl Med 2009; 7: 19.

[2] Arias JI, Aller MA, Arias J. The use of inflammation by tumor cells. Cancer 2005; 104: 223-228.

[3] Kohl BA, Deutschman CS. The inflammatory response to surgery and trauma. Curr Opin Crit Care 2006; 12: 325-332.

[4] Cone JB. Inflammation. Am J Surg 2001; 182: 558-562.

[5] Aller MA, Arias JI, Nava MP, Arias J. Post-traumatic inflammation is a complex response based n the pathological expression of the nervous, immune and endocrine functional systems. Exp Biol Med 2004; 229: 170-181.

[6] Libby P. Inflammatory mechanisms: The molecular basis of inflammation and disease. Nutr Rev 2007; 65: S140-S146.

[7] Rivas F. In this issue: Inflammation. Cell 2010; 140: 755-757.

[8] Turk JL. Inflammation: John Hunter's treatise on the blood, inflammation and gun-shot wounds. Int J Exp Pathol 1994; 75: 385-395.

[9] Wangensteen OH. Great opportunity: A binding summons to achieve. Musings upon surgical history. Am J Surg 1981; 142: 605-614.

[10] DeBakey ME. A surgical perspective. Ann Surg 1991; 213: 499-531.

[11] Plytycz B, Seljelid R. From inflammation to sickness: historial perspective. Arch Immunol Ther Exp (Warsz) 2003; 51: 105-109.

[12] Lain P. Ed. "Positivismo". In: Historia Universal de la Medicina. 1st Edition. Barcelona, Spain: Salvat Editores S.A. 1974 pp: 1-380.

[13] Heidland A, Klassen A, Sebekova K, Bahner U. Beginning of modern concept of inflammation: the work of Friedrich Daniel von Recklinhausen and Julius Friedrich Cohnheim. J Nephrol 2009; 14: 71-79.

[14] Campos Ramos G. Inflammation as an animal development phenomenon. Clin Dev Immunol 2012; 2012: 983203.

[15] Metschnikoff E. Lecture on phagocytosis and immunity. Br Med J 1891; 1: 213-217.

[16] Ramon y Cajal S. Patogenia de la inflamación. In: Discurso de Doctorado. Edición Facsimil. Universidad de Zaragoza y Gobierno de Aragón. INO. Reproducciones S.A. Zaragoza 2007 pp: 1-109.

[17] Murray JE, Merrill JP, Harrison JH. Renal homotransplantation in identical twins. Surg Forum 1955; 6: 432-436.

[18] Calne RY. Liver transplantation. The Cambridge-King College Hospital Experience. London: Grun and Stratton. 1983 pp: 3-399.

[19] Roberts AJ, Painvin GA. Organ transplantation. Surg Clin North America 1986; 66: 425-657.

[20] Carrel A. La technique operatoire des anastomoses vascularies *et al* transplantation des visceres. Lyon Med 1902; 98: 859-862

[21] Vacanti JP. Beyond transplantation. Third Annual Samuel Jason Mixter Lecture. Arch Surg 1988; 123: 545-549.

[22] Medzhitov R. Origin and physiological roles of inflammation. Nature 2008; 454: 428-435.

[23] Medzhitov R. Inflammation 2010: New adventures of an old flame. Cell 2010; 140: 771-776.
[24] Franceschi C, Bonafe M, Valensin S, *et al*. Inflamm-aging: An evolutionary perspective on immunosenescence. Ann NY Acad Sci 2000; 908: 244-254.
[25] Caruso C, Lio D, Cavallone L, Franceschi C. Aging, longevity, inflammation and cancer. Ann NY Acad Sci 2004; 1028: 1-13.
[26] Bürkle A, Caselli G, Franceschi C, *et al*. Pathophysiology of ageing, longevity and age related diseases. Immunol Aging 2007; 4: 4
[27] Turnbaugh PJ, Gordon JI. The core gut microbiome, energy balance and obesity. J Physiol 2009; 587: 4153-4158.
[28] Greenblum S, Turnbaugh PJ, Borenstein E. Metagenomic systems biology of the human gut microbiome reveals topological shifts associated with obesity and inflammatory bowel disease. Proc Natl Acad Sci USA 2012; 109: 594-599.
[29] Turnbaugh PJ, Ley RE, Hamady M, Fraser-Liggett CM, Knight R, Gordon JI. The human microbiome project. Nature 2007; 449: 804-810.
[30] Bell G. Model metaorganism. A review by Graham Bell. Science 1998; 282: 248
[31] Bosch TCG, McFall-Ngai M. Metaorganisms as the new frontier. Zoology (Jena) 2011; 114: 185-190.
[32] Biagi E, Candela M, Fairweather-Tait S, Franceschi C, Brigidi P. Ageing of the human metaorganism: the microbial counter part. Age (Dordr) 2012; 34: 247-267.
[33] Aller MA, Arias JI, Arias J. pathological axes of wound repair: gastrulation revisited. Theor Biol Med Model 2010; 7: 37.
[34] Aller MA, Blanco-Rivero J, Arias JI, Balfagon G, Arias J The wound healing response and upregulated embryonic mechanisms: brothers-in-arms forever. Exp Dermatol*, in press*
[35] Redd MJ, Cooper L, Wood W, Stramer B, Martin P. Wound healing and inflammation: embryos reveal the way to perfect repair. Phil Trans R Soc Lond B 2004; 359: 777-784.
[36] Poss KD. Advances in understanding tissue regenerative capacity and mechanisms in animals. Nat Rev Genet 2010; 11: 710-722.
[37] Chandramore K, Ghaskadbi S. Evo-devo: Hydra raises its Noggin. J Biosci 2011; 36: 517-529.
[38] Aller MA, Arias N, Fuentes-Julian S, Blazquez-Martinez A, Argudo S, De Miguel MP, Arias JL, Arias J. Coupling inflammation with evo-devo. Med Hypotheses 2012; 78: 721-731.
[39] Gilbert SF. The morphogenesis of evolutionary developmental biology. Int J Dev Biol 2003; 47: 467-477.

Send Orders for Reprints to reprints@benthamscience.net

Surgical Inflammation, 2013, 18-50

CHAPTER 2

Surgical Inflammation: From Molecule to Clinic

Jose-Ignacio Arias[1,*], María-Angeles Aller[2], Gregorio Rodríguez-Boto[3], Manuel Giner[4] and Jaime Arias[2]

[1]General Surgery Unit, Monte Naranco Hospital, Oviedo, Asturias, Spain; [2]Surgery Department, School of Medicine, Complutense University of Madrid, Spain; [3]Neurosurgery Unit, San Carlos University Hospital, Surgery Department, School of Medicine, Complutense University of Madrid, Spain and [4]General and Digestive Surgery Unit, San Carlos University Hospital, Surgery Department, School of Medicine, Complutense University of Madrid, Spain

Abstract: Tetrapyrrole molecules are distributed in virtually all living organisms on Earth. In mammals, tetrapyrrole end products are closely linked to oxygen metabolism. Since increasingly complex trophic functional systems for using oxygen are considered in the post-traumatic inflammatory response, it can be suggested that tetrapyrrole molecules and, particularly their derived pigments, play a key role in modulating inflammation. In this way, the diverse colorfulness that the inflammatory response triggers during its evolution would reflect the major pathophysiological importance of these pigments in each one of its phases. Hence, the need of exploiting this color resource could be considered for both the diagnosis and treatment of the inflammation.

Keywords: Post-traumatic inflammatory response, oxygen metabolism, tetrapyrroles, edema, necrosis, ischemia-reperfusion, hypoxia, cyanosis, ecchymosis, hemoglobin, pus, suppuration, scar.

INTRODUCTION

The inflammatory response related to surgery (elective or anesthetized injury) and to trauma (accidental or un-anesthetized injury) could be considered a surgical inflammation [1]. The surgical inflammation, as an inflammatory process, is composed of a series of overlapping successive phases [2]. That is why it is common that each researcher chooses for his study a specific aspect of this

***Address correspondence to Jaime Arias:** Cátedra de Cirugía, Facultad de Medicina, Universidad Complutense, Pza. de Ramón y Cajal s.n., 28040 MADRID, Spain; Tel: +34 91 394 1389; Fax: +34 91 3947115; E-mail: jariasp@med.ucm.es

complex response. At the same time, the interrelation of the knowledge that is successively obtained allows for better understanding of the pathophysiological mechanisms of the surgical inflammation. It also allows for suggesting new possible meanings of this inflammatory response.

A quality of the surgical inflammation that has always been observed is its color. The color in inflammation is one of the components by which the classical description of inflammation accounts for the visual changes seen.

Based on visual observation, the ancients characterized inflammation by four cardinal signs, namely redness, swelling, heat and pain [3].

It could be considered that the color of the injured tissue is changeable because both the traumatic injury (contusion and/or wound) and the inflammatory response related to this aggression are of an evolutive nature.

Especially the post-traumatic acute inflammatory response has been described as a succession of three functional phases with increasingly complex trophic functional systems for using oxygen [2, 4, 5]. And, interestingly enough, it could be imagined that an array of colors is displayed through this evolution.

TISSUE INJURY

In the mechanical trauma, it is considered that the inflammatory response is induced by the tissue injury [1, 2]. However, its special initial superimposition suggests that a "continuous" pathophysiological mechanism is established.

The tissue injury due to mechanical energy can produce a contusion (bruise), that is, damage without tissue breakage or damage with tissue breakage. In this last case, if the tissue is soft, the lesion is called a wound and if the tissue is hard, the lesion is called a fracture [6].

The contusion, according to its severity, could be classified in three degrees: First degree.- Characterized by the temporary loss of function.

Although it could be associated with edema, the alterations are reversible, and therefore, full recovery is possible; Second degree: would occur with ecchymosis, namely with tissue infiltration by red blood cells. The evolution would be ambivalent since cellular and tissue alterations can be reversed or worsened, causing cell death; Third degree: is an irreversible lesion since the injury causes cell death by necrosis and the tissue suffers from infarction [6] (Fig. **1**).

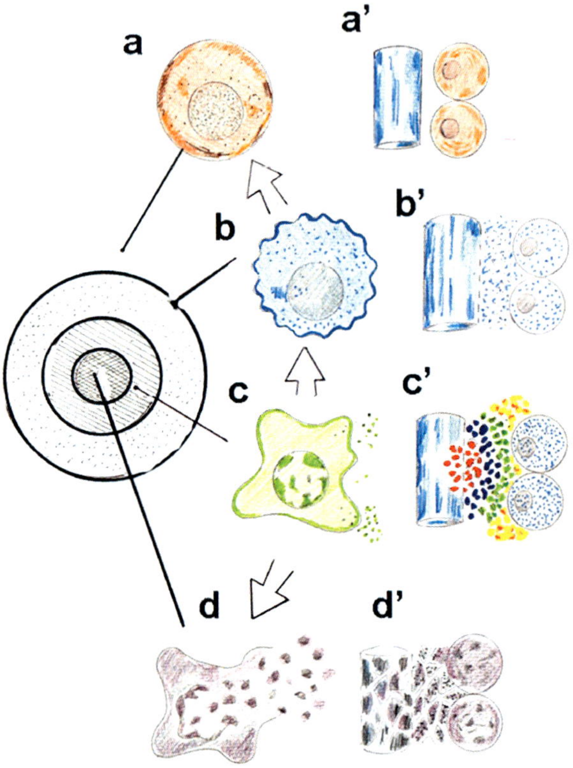

Figure 1: Injury without breakage is produced by blunt etiological agents and is made up of concentric areas of different degrees of severity. From the cellular point of view, the first-degree contusion is a reversible injury. The alteration consists in small plasma bleb formation. In the second-degree contusion, a fusion of the blebs is produced and the plasma membrane permeability increases. In the third-degree contusion, cell death is produced by necrosis. At the same time, contusions can be superficial or deep. From the tissue point of view, edema is produced in the first-degree contusion; ecchymosis would be associated with edema in the second-degree contusion; an infarction would be produced in the third-degree contusion. Ecchymosis means that the red blood cells are the first blood cells to infiltrate the interstitial space in posttraumatic inflammation. Ecchymosis, also called a contusion or a bruise, due to its blue color, from the Latin word *cardinus* (bluish) explains its purple color.

Cellular and tissue lesion is irreversible in the wound and fracture since necrosis is produced [6] (Fig. **2**).

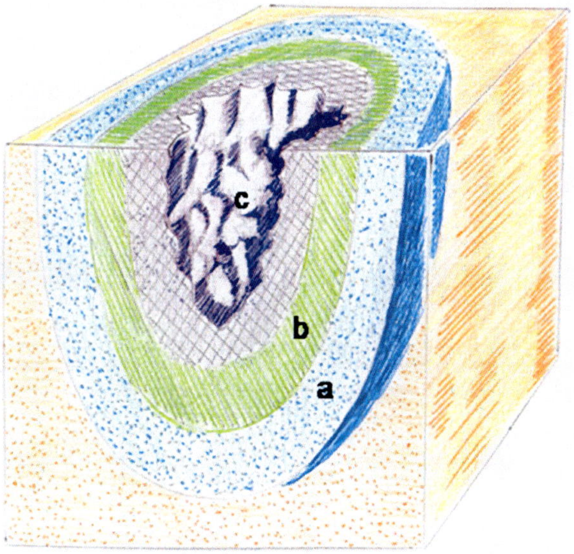

Figure 2: Injury without breakage in the soft tissue can be superficial or deep. The wound enters the tissue suffering from a first, second or third-degree contusion, as the figure shows. The evolution of the second-degree bruised area, whether reversible or irreversible, will determine the evolution of the wound since it can increase the necrosis area. The superficial injury without breakage has external hemorrhaging and the deep injury without breakage has contusions of internal tissue or intraparenchymatous hemorrhage. a: first-degree contusion; b: second-degree contusion; c: third-degree contusion.

Until recently, necrosis has often been viewed as an accidental and uncontrolled cell death process. Nevertheless, growing evidence supports the idea that necrotic cell death may also be programmed [7]. Cellular signaling events have been identified to initiate necrotic destruction that could be blocked by inhibiting discrete cellular processes [8]. The most relevant mechanisms culminating in cell necrosis correspond to: mitochondrial dysfunction and ATP depletion; loss of intracellular ion homeostasis with osmotic swelling and oxidative stress; activation of degradative hydrolases, including proteases, phosphorylases, and endonucleases; and degradation of cytoskeletal proteins with disruption of cytoskeletal integrity [9]. Surprisingly, this list of mechanisms also corresponds to those that occur in the acute inflammatory post-traumatic response [2, 4]. It seems, that in response to injury, the cell can develop a mechanism that would play a defensive role (inflammation) and that could favor reversing the alterations until their inadequate expression would make them harmful (necrotic). Hence, at a specific moment in time, the pathophysiological mechanisms (cellular response to injury) become pathogenic mechanisms (producers of cell death) [4].

THE TISSUE INFLAMMATION

We have proposed that the acute inflammatory response to injury by mechanical energy, regardless of whether it is local or systemic, is based on the successive pathologic functional predominance of the nervous, immune and endocrine systems. This hypothesis implies that the final and prevalent pathologic functions of these systems may represent the consecutive phases of the response to stress developed by the body, all of which may have a trophic meaning for the injured tissue [4, 5, 10].

Perhaps the leading role in this response is played by the relation between the blood and the interstitial space. This assumption is based on the fact that the different blood components escape the intravascular space one by one in order to occupy the interstitial space, where they play the main role in the successive phases of the inflammatory response. Therefore, the endothelium plays a bidirectional mediating role between blood flow and the interstitial space, which is where inflammation mainly takes place [2, 4].

Since the phases of the inflammatory response go from ischemia to the development of an oxidative metabolism, the successive pathophysiological mechanisms that develop in the interstitium of tissues when they undergo inflammation are considered increasingly complex trophic functional systems for using oxygen [2, 4, 5, 10].

PHASES OF THE INFLAMMATORY RESPONSE

It could be considered that the acute post-traumatic inflammatory response is made up of three overlapping phases (Fig. **3**).

The first or immediate phase has been referred to as the nervous phase, because the sensory (pain and analgesia) and motor alterations (contraction and relaxation) respond to the injury [2, 4]. This early pathological activity, in essence, could reflect the predisposition of the body's nervous tissue to suffer inflammation first.

Furthermore, this nervous response coexists almost completely with the tissue injury evolution and, therefore, conditions it.

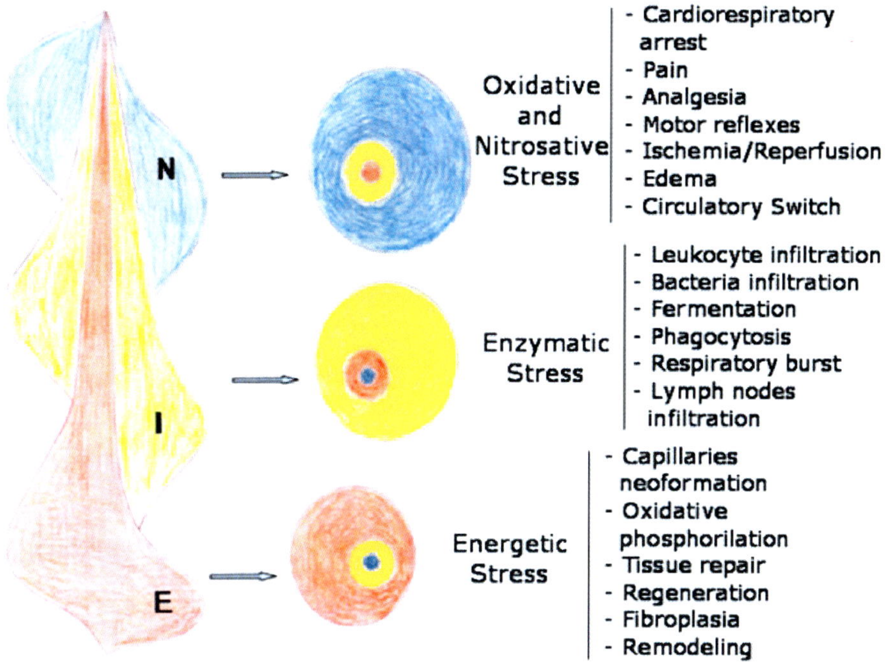

Figure 3: The post-traumatic inflammatory response is considered to be made up of three overlapping phases with increasingly complex trophic functional systems for using oxygen. During the first or nervous phase, oxidative and nitrosative stress are produced. In the second or immune phase, enzymatic stress is produced and in the third or endocrine phase, oxidative phosphorylation is reached and therefore, energetic stress is produced. N: Nervous phase with oxidative stress and edema which progressively subsides. I: Immune phase with enzymatic stress and its subsequent neutralization. E: Endocrine phase with its initial tissue de-structuring and subsequent tissue repair through regeneration and/or fibroplasia.

The nervous or immediate functional system presents ischemiarevascularization and edema, which favor nutrition by diffusion through the injured tissue. This trophic mechanism has a low energy requirement that does not require oxygen (ischemia) or in which the oxygen is not correctly used, with the subsequent development of reactive oxygen and nitrogen species (ROS/RNS) (reperfusion). In this phase, while the progression of the interstitial edema increases in the space between the epithelial cells and the capillaries, the lymphatic circulation is simultaneously activated (circulatory switch). Thus, the injured tissues adopt an ischemic phenotype (hypoxia) [4] (Figs. **3** and **4**).

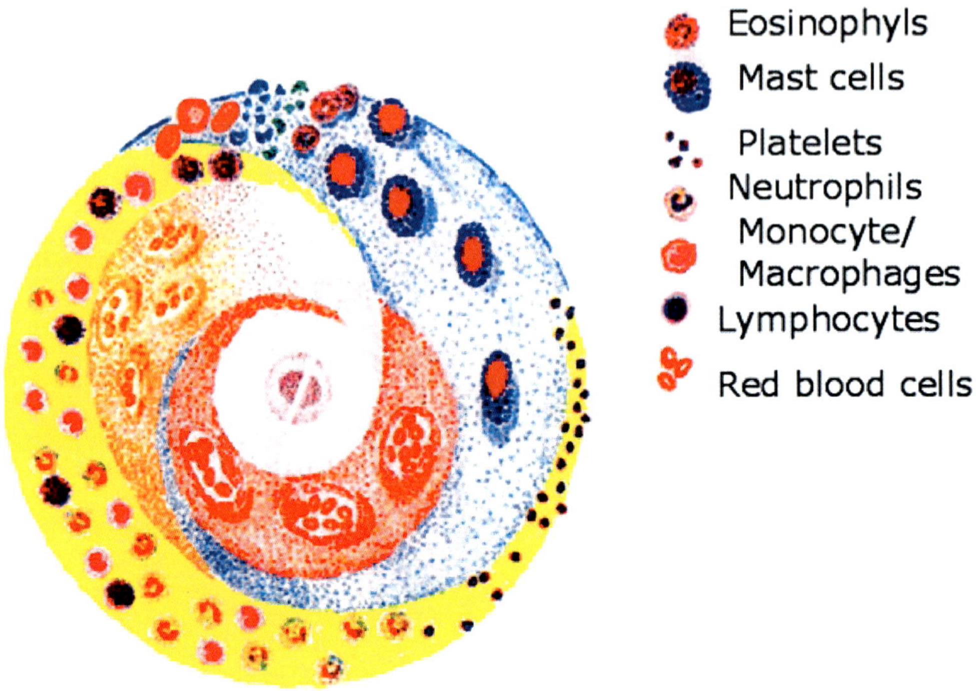

Figure 4: Schematic representation of the inflammatory response phases revolving around stem cells (structural and hematopoietic) and substrates for producing edema (blue), suppuration (yellow), granulation tissue (orangey),with fibrosis (striped area) and tissue regeneration (red). The three function systems (nervous, immune and endocrine) overlap in different evolutive periods (acute, central and chronic, peripheral) can lead to resolution (regeneration) or organization (fibrosis).

In the following immune or intermediate phase of the inflammatory response, the tissues and organs which have suffered ischemia-reperfusion, are infiltrated by inflammatory cells and bacteria. Interstitial inflammation is favored by the concurrent activation of hemostasis and complement cascades. In the tissues and organs which suffer oxidative stress, symbiosis of the inflammatory cells and bacteria for extracellular digestion by enzyme release (fermentation) and by intracellular digestion (phagocytosis) could be associated with a hypothetical trophic capacity. Improper use of oxygen persists in this immune phase and is also associated with enzymatic stress. Furthermore, lymphatic circulation plays a major role and macrophages and dendritic cells migrate to lymph nodes where they activate lymphocytes [2, 4, 11] (Figs. **3** and **4**).

It is considered that angiogenesis characterizes the last or endocrine phase of the inflammatory response, so nutrition mediated by the blood capillaries is established [2, 4, 5]. However, the angiogenic process becomes active earlier and excessive proliferation of endothelial cells occurs which in turn, develops a great density of endothelial sprouts. Through this initial and excessive proliferation, the endothelial cells could successively perform antioxidant and antienzymatic functions. These functions would favor the evolution of the inflammatory response towards tissue repair through specialized capillary development. If so, it would be in this last phase of the inflammatory response when the process of angiogenesis would be responsible for tissue nutrition through capillaries. Oxygen and oxidative metabolisms are an excellent combination through which cells can obtain an abundant energy supply (energetic stress) for tissue repair by epithelial regeneration or wound healing [2, 4, 5, 10, 11] (Fig. **3**).

THE COLOR OF THE INFLAMMATORY PHASES

The colors of inflammation can be represented in three groups:

1. Cold Colors

The tissue color that initially is associated with mechanical injury is white. When mechanical energy acts on the tissue, especially if this occurs through a blunt etiological agent, an abrupt crushing is produced that takes the blood out of the tissue. The bloodless tissue is white, a color that brings together the entire light spectrum, but if it continues it becomes ominous since it can signal sphacelation. Thus, in a third-degree contusion, the tissue suffers a crush injury with vasospasm, endothelial damage and thrombosis [12] (Fig. **1**).

Decreased transcutaneous oxygen tension, reduced arterial hemoglobin saturation and increased transcutaneous carbon dioxide tension revealed reduced blood flow and poor tissue perfusion as the earliest warning signs of shock and death [13]. Again the paleness, in this case generalized, implies a poor prognosis.

Morbidity and mortality from blood loss remains a leading cause of traumatic death [14]. Control of bleeding and correction of intravascular volume are the hallmarks of conventional resuscitation after massive blood loss [14].

After cardiopulmonary resuscitation of trauma patients with cardiac arrest, the survival rates are only 0% to 5% [15, 16]. Only cardiac resuscitation (chest compression without ventilation) by bystanders is the preferable approach to resuscitation [17]. In blunt and/or penetrating trauma patients efforts should be withheld in cases of evidence of a significant time lapse since pulselessness, including lividity, *rigor mortis* and decomposition [18] (Fig. **5**).

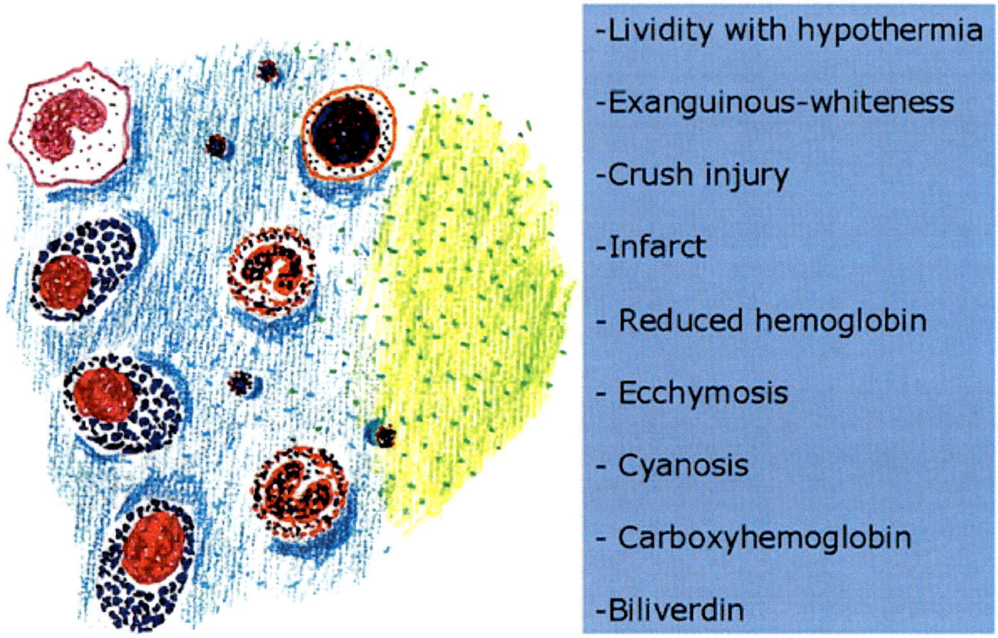

Figure 5: Cold colors of the inflammatory response. Ecchymosis and cyanosis with edema

Early care of the severely injured patient and intervention for hypothermia, coagulopathy and acidosis, components of the trauma triad of death, would improve shock resuscitation [19-21]. Since cardiac arrest is an evolutive injury, it has been suggested that the optimal treatment is phase specific and includes: the electrical phase (0-4 minutes), the circulatory phase (4-10 minutes) and the metabolic phase (beyond 10 minutes after cardiac arrest) [22]. In any case, early initiation of cardiopulmonary resuscitation is the most effective measure [23].

Inflammatory pain is caused by tissue damage [24] and its pathogeny also seems to be phase-specific. Thus, after the initial electrical phase, with upregulation of ionic channels expression in the nociceptive circuits that causes the spontaneous neural firing [24, 25], the following would be an immune phase, with cytokines, chemokines and prostaglandins derived from glial and immune cells, acting as pain mediators and modulators [26, 27]. Lastly, in an endocrine phase, neurotrophic factors, including nerve growth factor (NGF), brain-derived neurotrophic factor (BDNF) and neurotrophins 3 and 4, would be associated with structural neural remodeling [28]. If so, the velocity in which the phases of inflammation are expressed in the neural tissue, would allow it to play a modulating role in the post-mechanical injury inflammatory response in the rest of the tissues and organs of the body.

An immediate component of the stress response to pain is the efferent nervous response mediated by the somatic motor and autonomic nervous systems [29]. The somatic motor response usually consists in the withdrawal of the affected part of the body from the source of irritation. Withdrawal reflexes are the simplest centrally organized responses to painful stimuli [30].

Furthermore, the fight-or-flight response is the behavioral response to a threat, in which the somatic motor response stands out [29]. With respect to the autonomic nervous system, both the sympathetic and parasympathetic nervous systems participate in inflammation. An early pathological motor response, where the smooth muscular fiber is prominent, particularly in the vascular system, is triggered [2, 4,10]. The whey-face is one of the most visible consequences of these vasomotor responses.

The vasomotor response with vasoconstriction, which collaborates in the production of ischemia and vasodilation, cause the redistribution of the local vascular and systemic blood flow. The intensity and duration of this ischemia-reperfusion phenomenon will modify the color of the tissues and organs and will possibly determine their evolution during the subsequent inflammatory response [2, 4].

In this first phase of the inflammation, the tone or group of dominating colors are those called "cold· colors", namely, blue and green, which produce sedative effects.

In particular, the color blue, more or less dark, can be found after a mechanical injury, both local (ecchymosis) and systemic (cyanosis) (Figs. **4** and **5**).

The second-degree contusion initiates its evolution with edema and ecchymosis (Fig. **1**). The initial dark blue color of the ecchymotic lesion comes from the carboxyhemoglobin, which is the result of the bounding of carbon monoxide to hemoglobin. Then, the release of hemoglobin into the interstitial space is a phenomenon associated with hemolysis. Hemoglobin, released from red blood cells, is the major source of heme for bile pigment synthesis [31, 32]. Heme is a prosthetic group of various types of proteins, such as hemoglobin, myoglobin, cytochrome C, cytochrome p450, catalase and peroxidase [33]. Heme is converted by heme-oxygenase (HO) forming biliverdin, with blue-green color, carbon monoxide and iron [32, 34] (Table **1**).

Table 1: Tetrapyrroles and other pigment compounds involved in color production and in the inflammatory response evolution.

• Haem. An alternative spelling for heme
• Heme. Heme a – $C_{49}H_{56}O_6N_4Fe$ – Cytochrome a refers to the heme A in specific combination with membrane protein forming a portion of Cytochrome C oxidase.
Heme b – $C_{34}H_{32}O_4N_4Fe$
Heme c – $C_{34}H_{36}O_4N_4S_2Fe$
• Hemoglobin (Hb). A metalloprotein (globin)
Hemoglobin A ($\alpha_2\beta_2$) is the most common in human adults.
• Carboxyhemoglobin – Complex of carbon monoxide and hemoglobin (COHb)
• Nitrix oxide synthase (NOS) – A eukaryotic enzyme calmodulin-containing cytochrome P450-like hemoprotein.
• Peroxidase – Can contain a heme cofactor in their active site. It is an electron donor. The optimal substrate is hydrogen peroxide (H_2O_2).
• Catalase – Contains four porphyrin heme groups that allow the enzyme to react with the H_2O_2 to form water and oxygen.
• Porphyrin – A natural pigment containing a fundamental skeleton of four pyrrole nuclei united by methine groups.
• Photosynthetic pigments:
- Chlorophylls – A green pigment found in most plants, *algae* and
Cyanobacteria.
Chlorophyll a ($C_{55}H_{72}O_5N_4Mg$)
- Carotenoids – Organic pigments that naturally occur in chromoplasts of plants and

some other photosynthetic organisms like algae, fungus and some bacteria. There are two classes:
. xanthophylls
And
. carotenes – A yellow-orange-red pigments
(tetraterpenoids)
- Phycobilins – Light capturing molecules (chromophores).
- blue (phycocyanobilin)
- orange (phycourobilin) and
- red (phycoerythrobilin)
All of them in *cyanobacteriae.*
• Biliverdin – A green pigment formed as a by-product of heme breakdown ($C_{33}H_{34}N_4O_6$).
• Bilirubin – A yellow breakdown product of normal heme catabolism ($C_{33}H_{34}N_4O_6$).
• Bilirubin glucuronides – Bilirubin glucoronidation reaction is catalyzed by UGT (uridine diphosphate (UDP)-glucuronyl transferase).
- Bilirubin monoglucuronide.
- Bilirubin diglucuronide.
• Bile salts
- Urobilinogen is a colorless product of bilirubin reduction ($C_{33}H_{44}N_4O_6$).
- Urobilin is a yellow linear tetrapyrrole produced when urobilinogen is oxidized by intestinal bacteria. This produces a brown pigment excreted in urine ($C_{33}H_{42}N_4O_6$).
. Cytochromes
- Cytochrome C oxidase. The last enzyme in the respiratory electron transport chain. The complex contains two hemes, a cytochrome a and cytochrome a_3 and two copper centers.
- Cytochrome P450 (CYP450). A large superfamily of hemoproteins found in all domains of life. Acts as terminal oxidase in multicomponent electron-transfer chains, called P450-containing monooxygenase systems.
Myoglobin. A globular protein containing a heme prosthetic group. It is the primary oxygen-carrying pigment of muscle tissues and responsible for making these tissues red.
• Oxyhemoglobin. Heme group contains one iron atom that can bind one oxygen molecule through ion-induced dipole forces (HbO2). It is the oxygen-loaded form of hemoglobin.

Three isoforms, HO-1, HO-2 and HO-3, are expressed in most tissues. HO-1 is an inducible enzyme, also known as heat shock protein 32, activated by oxidative stress and cytokines [34]. HO-1 has antioxidant activity related to the elimination of pro-oxidant heme, and to the antioxidant properties of biliverdin [34, 35]. Interplay between HO-1 and nitric oxide synthase systems has recently been addressed. These systems share many common features and overlap in biological functions. Particularly, HO activity is involved in the inhibitory effect of NO on neutrophil migration to the inflammatory site [36].

HO-2 and HO-3 display a constitutive expression. HO-2 may have an essential role in the execution of self-resolving inflammatory-reparative processes [37]. HO-3 in turn, has a great structural homology with HO-2 and acts as a heme-sensing/binding protein [38]. HO-2 may also regulate the expression of HO-1 by modulating the cellular heme level [39]. Therefore, the pathophysiological mechanisms as a whole that are established in the second degree contusions due to their antioxidant, anti-inflammatory and reparative roles, would prevent the harmful evolution of the lesion towards necrosis. In essence, the effects are sedative where the expression of cold colors predominates.

Cyanosis, a word derived from the Greek term *"kyanos",* is the blue coloration of the skin and mucosas that frequently are associated with the traumatic pathology that has a systemic effect with hypoxia and hypotension [40, 41]. Central cyanosis, with blueness of skin, lips and mucous membranes is always a manifestation of hypoxemia. As a result of hypoxemia an excess amount of hemoglobin is not saturated with oxygen; in currently accepted terminology this unsaturated hemoglobin is said to be reduced [42]. It is the quantity of reduced hemoglobin per deciliter of capillary blood that accounts for the bluish color of cyanosis [43] (Figs. **4** and **5**).

2. Warm Colors

During the immune phase of the inflammatory response, the colors tend to be warmer. Thus, the yellow coloration arises.

The contused tissue becomes yellowish because of the emergence of bilirubin, a bile pigment [31]. Bilirubin is produced *via* reduction of heme-derived biliverdin by biliverdin-reductase [31, 32]. However, biliverdin-reductase also serves in a catabolic pathway because it is an evolutionarily conserved protein found across the spectrum of metazoans. Homologs of the reductase are found in unicellular organisms and plants [44, 45]. Plants use biliverdin produced by ferredoxin-dependent heme-oxygenase for the synthesis of phytochromes, the sensory photoreceptors [44, 45].

Biliverdin-reductase may function as a protein-kinase [44]. Thus the functions are broadened since protein phosphorylation by kinases and dephosphorylation by phosphatases are essential components and mechanisms of signal transduction in the cell [44]. So, biliverdin-reductase plays an important role in mediating cytoprotective effects of HO-1 against hypoxia induced injury [44, 46]. Also the existence of a link between biliverdin-reductase and the cytokine-activated stress signaling, suggest its main role in mediating the inflammatory response [44].

Bilirubin has a number of new and interesting biochemical and biological properties [47]. In addition to having a protective role against oxidative stress [47, 48] bilirubin also has antiapoptotic [47, 49] and antimutagenic properties [49]. Therefore, the increase in the production of bilirubin in the contused tissue may have beneficiary effects as an inflammatory modulator.

In the immune phase of the inflammatory response, the interstitium is infiltrated first by platelets and later by leukocytes [5, 51, 52, 59]. In these injured tissues showing oxidative stress, symbiosis of the inflammatory cells and bacteria, could produce enzymatic stress [11].

Usually pyogenic bacteria, such as *Staphylococcus aureus*, make the inflammatory process yellow [53]. The genus *Staphylococcus* describes a grapelike cluster of bacteria found in pus from surgical abscesses, since *staphylo* means “grape” in Greek. *Aureus* is the species name, and means “golden” in Latin, that is its characteristic surface pigmentation in comparison with less virulent *staphylococci.* Studies of the *staphylococcus aureus* pigment have unraveled a biosynthetic pathway that produces carotenoids, which are also a type of plant coloring with antioxidants [53].

The formation of yellow, milky yellow, greenish yellow or white-yellow pus characterizes suppuration or purulent inflammation [54, 55] (Figs. **4** and **6**). In addition to the enzymes released by granulocytes during the process of phagocytosis and bacterial killing, the bacteria themselves produce a number of exoenzymes that cause tissue destruction as well as localization of infection [56, 57]. In particular, almost all *Staphylococcus aureus* strains have the ability to secrete an array of enzymes including nucleases, proteases, lipases, hyaluronidase, and collagenase [57]. Matrix metalloproteinases would also collaborate in the development of enzymatic stress in the acute inflammatory tissue injury [58, 59]. Pus mainly contains necrotic tissue debris and dead neutrophils and, when the collection of pus is localized, and abscess is established [56, 57].

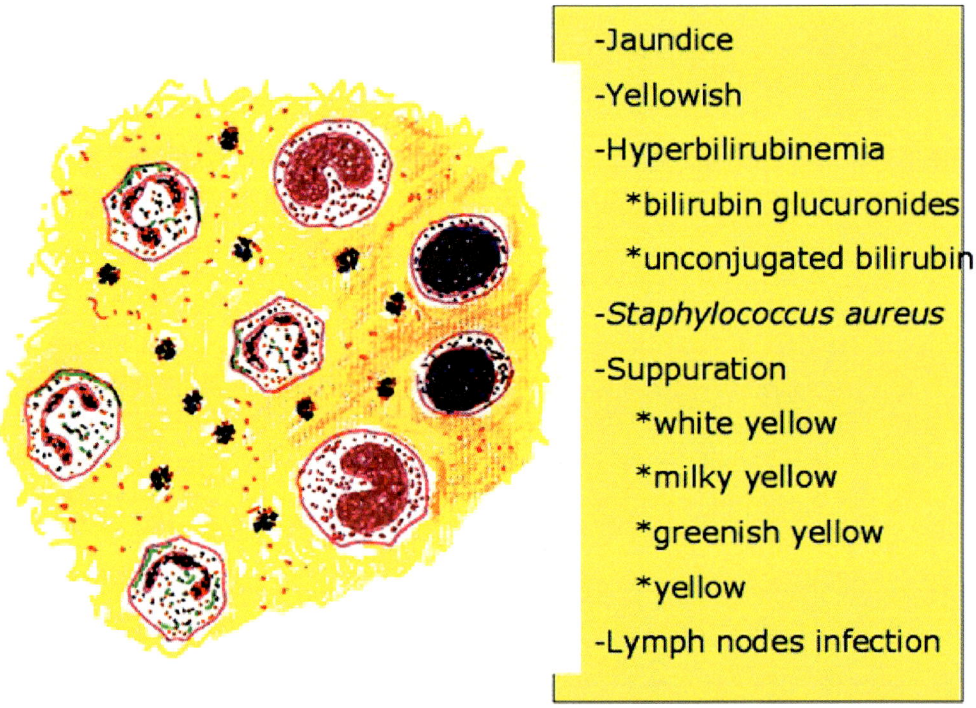

Figure 6: Warm colors of the inflammatory response. Jaundice and suppuration

Compensation of the acute phase response includes the production of positive acute phase proteins, like α2-macroglobulin, that binds proteolytic enzymes, and α1-antitrypsin and α1-antichymotrypsin, which are inhibitors of leukocyte and lysosomal proteolytic enzymes [60]. Likewise, the natural inhibitors of matrix metalloproteinases (TIMPs) could promote antienzymatic stress [58].

Also, unconjugated bilirubin is a potent inhibitor of the digestive proteases trypsin and chymotrypsin [61]. In the gut, bilirubin glucuronides are deconjugated by beta-glucuronidase, which exist in the gut mucosa, and could also be found in some strains of bacteria such as *Escherichia coli* and *Streptococcus pyogenes*. Therefore, it has been accepted that a dramatic decrease of beta-glucuronidase-positive bacteria, which in turn results in impaired inactivation of digestive enzyme from the pancreas in the large intestine, would favor the development of inflammation in this location [61, 62].

The ability of *staphylococcus aureus* to cause infection is absolutely dependent on the acquisition of iron from the host. Particularly, the most abundant iron source is in the form of the porphyrin heme [63, 64]. That is why it has been suggested that the ultimate fate of exogenously acquired heme in *staphylococcus aureus* also depends on the intracellular and extracellular availability of both iron and heme, and plays a significant role in the infectious process [64] (Fig. **4**).

The yellowish coloring of the skin and mucosas is called icterus (or jaundice). This means yellowness, "*ikteros*" in Greek. Postoperative jaundice is associated with elevated serum bilirubin, mainly conjugated, above 3 mg per dl. Although hyperbilirubinemia seems to be multifactorial, perioperative hypotension and/or hypoxia are important pathogenic factors in the development of postoperative jaundice and multiple organ failure [65]. In patients with sepsis and multiple organ failure a serum total bilirubin greater than 2 mg per dl is a significant factor in predicting mortality [66] (Fig. **6**).

Jaundice is an important and transient clinical sign seen in most healthy newborns. They have hyperbilirubinemia but finding the cause is not often possible [67]. Nevertheless, increased concentrations of IL-1 beta in the colostrum from breast-feeding mothers, whose infants had neonatal jaundice, have been demonstrated. Therefore, cytokines could be involved in the pathophysiological events that can lead to neonatal jaundice [68].

However the relation of the biliary pigments with infection is ambivalent since increasing serum levels of biliverdin and bilirubin were shown to be beneficial in the setting of inflammation [69]. Thus in a mouse model of endotoxemia, a single-dose administration of bilirubin in addition to its antioxidant effects also exerts potent anti-inflammatory activity [69] (Table **1**).

The maximum intensity of the immune response may be reached when an associated systemic infection is produced. Failure of the intestinal barrier resulting in bacterial translocation worsens the systemic inflammatory response syndrome in the polytraumatized patient, and it is an important etiological factor of sepsis and multiple organ failure [70-72].

Hypovolemic shock, severe hemorrhage or major surgery, leads to priming the host and the exposure to a posterior bacterial stimulus can produce an excessive response to an otherwise low-grade inflammatory trigger [73, 74]. Most likely a current definition of sepsis is too broad and encompasses heterogeneous groups of patients suffering similar but different immune syndromes that are historically grouped under the general diagnosis of sepsis [75]. Cholestatic jaundice also occurs in the setting of sepsis [76]. Liver abnormalities in sepsis include cholestasis and hyperbilirubinemia. Gram negative infections used to be the cause of cholestasis associated with sepsis [76]. Hyperbilirubinemia develops in sepsis particularly in the setting of bacteremia. Hyperbilirubinemia precedes positive blood cultures in one third of cases [77].

3. Hot Colors

The evidence shows the intensity and duration of the nervous and immune phases of the inflammatory response condition of the evolution of the last or endocrine phase. Thus, oxidative and enzymatic stress which dominates the initial phases of the inflammation, according to their intensity and duration, would regulate the type of response that is produced during the final or endocrine phase [2, 4].

Platelets [78], mast cells [79], neutrophils [80, 81], macrophages [82-84] and T cells [79, 84] are characterized by expert functions in assisting and modulating the inflammatory response. Even today the potential role of leukocyte-derived neuropeptides and hormones in inflammation as a localized hypothalamic-pituitary-like axis has been proposed [85]. As the inflammatory response progresses, certain “stop signals” at appropriate “checkpoints” prevent further edema production and leukocyte traffic into tissues [83, 86]. The proinflammatory mechanisms are counterbalanced by endogenous anti-inflammatory signals, that serve to temper the severity and limit the duration of the early phases, which leads to their resolution [83, 86-88] (Fig. **4**).

However, the interstitium is considered as the "battle field" where inflammation develops [2, 4, 5] and its equivalent in tissues and organs is the stroma. At the same time, the most abundant cell type of tissue stroma comprises the fibroblasts, an active heterogeneous population of cells [89]. Fibroblasts can modify the quality, quantity and length of the inflammatory infiltration during the induction of the inflammatory response [90]. Fibroblasts can also contribute to the resolution of inflammation by withdrawing survival signals and normalizing chemokine gradients, thereby allowing infiltrating leukocytes to undergo apoptosis or to leave the tissues through the draining lymphatics [91]. Lastly, fibroblasts may also provide important positional cues for wound healing and tissue regeneration. In addition to their role of producing an extracellular matrix, they may facilitate angiogenesis by production and release of growth factors [89].

The color red is the first of the solar spectrum and is applied to the color of arterial blood, namely, when the blood contains oxyhemoglobin (HbO_2). The reflectance spectra for human skin have a characteristic signature, due to the absorption spectrum of oxygenated hemoglobin in the blood, and provide leads about the evolution of primate color vision [92, 93] (Fig. **7**).

Oxyhemoglobin reaches the cells through the capillaries as a result of angiogenesis. This process, with neoformation of capillaries, would characterize the last or endocrine phase of the inflammatory response [4, 11]. Hemoglobin is the respiratory protein in the red blood cells of vertebrates. Its physiological functions are transport of oxygen from lungs to tissues and transfer of carbon dioxide from tissues to lungs [94]. The oxygen dissociation curve of hemoglobin has profound clinical importance being applicable in numerous situations of health and disease, such as in the neonatal period, aging, anesthesia, surgery, hemorrhages and septic shock [95].

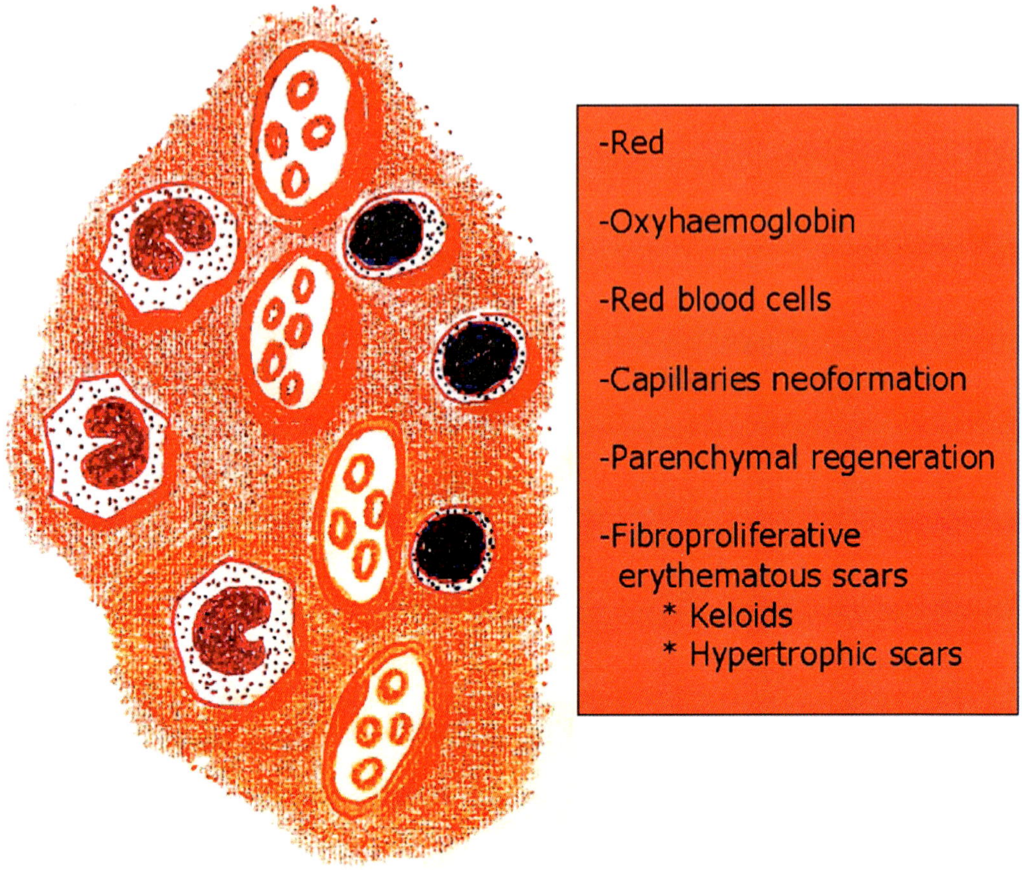

Figure 7: Hot colors of the inflammatory response. Angiogenesis (capillaries) of the granulation tissue (orangey) and tissue regeneration (red)

Flesh color is the common color of the tissues due to its content of oxyhemoglobin. The ability to use the oxygen, when it is disassociated from hemoglobin in the oxidative metabolism, is recovered when patients recover their capillary function and therefore, nutrition is mediated by them in the so called endocrine or late phase. This type of metabolism is characterized by a large production of ATP (coupled reaction), which is used to drive multiple specialized cellular processes (energetic stress) with limited heat generation and it would determine the onset of healing [2, 4, 11].

Therefore, the blood cells that occupy the interstitial space in this latter phase of the inflammatory response are red blood cells [2, 4]. To carry out this interstitial occupation, the red blood cells are transported by the newly formed blood capillaries [96] and, therefore, angiogenesis is considered to play the main role in this inflammatory period [2, 4,10, 11] (Fig. **4**).

The best way to finish the post-traumatic inflammatory response is with regeneration since the tissue and/or organ physiology returns to their normal state [86]. Regeneration is a process well known by the body since it is produced right afterwards and in particular by the epithelial tissues. Regeneration could be considered a good method of fighting against the energetic stress that the oxidative metabolism imposes on the epithelial cells [4, 11]. Epithelial organs par excellence, including the lungs and liver, show dark red grayish-brown color, basically a yellowish red or the result of the mix of the colors red black and some yellow or orange.

Recently, lipoxins, resolvins, protectins [97-99] and vasoinhibins [100] have emerged as signaling molecules that regulate many cell functions and ample evidence emphasizes their role in the resolution of the inflammatory response [86]. Resolution is an active and tightly regulated process controlled by anti-inflammatory and pro-resolving mediators and cellular moieties [86, 98].

Emerging evidence now suggests that this process of resolution initiates in the first few hours after an inflammatory response begins [83]. Therefore, this process could be characterized as being similar to the elaboration of bread.

First, the flour is mixed with water, salt (edema; oxidative stress) and yeast (inflammatory and bacterial cells; enzymatic stress) and it ferments. Then it is baked in the oven to obtain bread, one of the most important foods acquired by humanity.

Like in a cooking recipe, it is possible that the final product of the posttraumatic inflammatory response depends on the amount of the components used, as well as the time employed in each phase of the elaboration.

The ideal result is the resolution with tissue and organ recovery to a normal state. However, there are other alternative solutions. By default, an impairment of wound healing and chronic inflammation is produced. At the same time, by excess, the healing is produced by repair with fibrous scar or by fibroproliferative scars [51, 84, 101, 102]. Chronic non-healing wounds generally are due to ischemia and multiple factors that contribute to their resistance to treatment [88, 102]. The fibrous scar is pearly white, namely, iridescent white, since colors of the rainbow can be produced. The fibrous scar is secondary to excessive traumatic tissue necrosis with formation of rosy granulation tissue [51]. Lastly, prolonged inflammation in wounds contributes to the development of fibroproliferative scars, in other words, keloids and hypertrophic scars, both erythematous [103]. Free heme plays a major role in the expression of chronic inflammation. It activates neutrophil functions and delays neutrophil apoptosis and for these reasons heme is considered as a pro-inflammatory molecule [104].

The fibrotic component of the wound healing response is mediated by myofibroblasts or by cells that gain a myofibroblasts-like phenotype, and their activities include the abundant synthesis of fibrillar collagens [105]. In this way, the remodeling of tissues by fibrosis could be a useful solution to combat the energetic stress associated with the oxidative metabolism since the cellular content diminishes and the metabolic demand increases the extracellular component of reduced vitality (Fig. **4**).

During prolonged critical illness, lean tissue is wasted despite feeding, a problem that often persists even after the underlying disease has resolved. In this chronic phase of the critical illness, the wasting syndrome is associated with a neuroendocrine dysfunction characterized by a hypothalamic rather than pituitary dysfunction [1, 2,106]. During the evolution of the nervous and immune phases of the systemic inflammatory response, the body loses its more specialized functions and structures. In this progressive deconstruction, there is a depletion of the hydrocarbonate, lipid and protein stores, as well as multiple or successive dysfunction and posterior failure or necrosis of the specialized epithelium, *i.e.*, the pulmonary, gastrointestinal, renal and hepatic ones [2, 4,107].

However, consumption of the substrate deposits and the dysfunction or failure of the specialized epithelia of the body could also represent an accelerated process of dedifferentiation [2, 4]. The hypothetical ability of the body to involute or dedifferentiate could represent a return to early stages of development. Therefore, it could form an effective defense mechanism against injury since it could make retracing a well-known route possible, that is, the prenatal specialization phase during the endocrine phase of the systemic inflammatory response. This last phase of the inflammatory response has the disadvantage that it develops in an extrauterine environment without the functional support of the mother with her placenta [2, 4]. The elevated incidence of post-traumatic stress syndromes would thus be explained as a consequence of a frustrated recovery of homeostasis.

LIGHT, PIGMENTS AND LIFE

The importance of color in the surgical pathology could be attributed to the benefits for the diagnosis and treatment of diseases. However, this coloring can also have an added-value related to its possible pathophysiological importance. This possibility has not yet been fully discovered, which would allow us to better understand its meaning in Nature.

Color depends on light, which is a kind of energy that the sun emits in the form of radiation. The spreading of solar light constitutes a spectrum that we perceive as a series of colors (red, orange, yellow, green, blue, indigo and violet) [92, 93]. The use of the sun's light energy by photosynthetic organisms provides the foundation for virtually all life on Earth [108].

Photosynthesis efficiently converts light energy to electrochemical energy for oxidation-reduction ("redox") reactions. The excitation of light harvesting pigments by a photon of light causes an electron to be transferred along biochemical pathways that lead to the reduction of CO_2. When the reductant is water, then oxygen is produced. But photosynthesis may use reductants other than water, such as H_2S, H_2 and Fe^{2+}. The direct products of oxygenic photosynthesis are carbohydrates and oxygen [108].

Photosynthetic pigments are categorized into three chemical groups: chlorophylls, carotenoids and phycobilins. Chlorophylls are essential molecules of green algae and land plants. They are responsible for harvesting solar energy in photosynthetic systems but also influence processes such as photosynthetic gene expression, growth rates and cell-death [109, 110] (Fig. **8**).

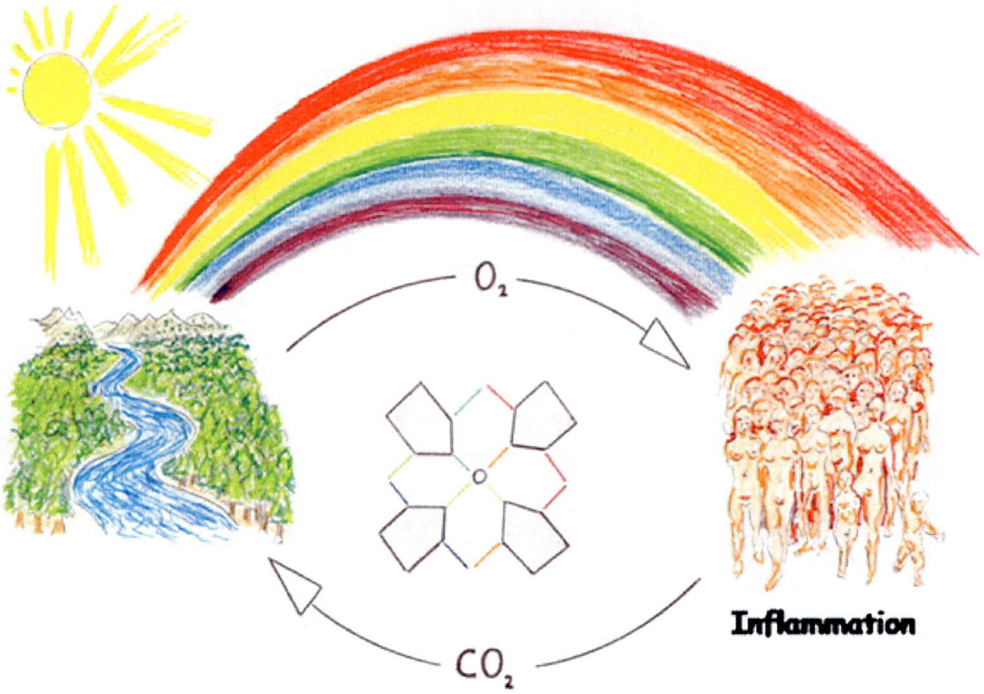

Figure 8: Tetrapyrrole products allow plants to use CO_2 and mammals to use O_2. These molecules in their color version take advantage of the solar spectrum, produced by the dispersion of sunlight and so they would play the main role in the origin of plant and animal life, and therefore, in inflammation.

The appearance of chlorophyll in land plants during springtime and its disappearance in autumn demonstrate the season-dependent nature of processes that can even be seen from outer space. Thus the chlorophyll biosynthetic and degradation reactions belong to the most important biochemical pathways known [109]. But in addition to chlorophylls, other tetrapyrrole end products are synthesized through the same pathway including heme, hemoglobin, myoglobin, cytochromes, nitric oxide synthase, peroxidase and catalases [33, 109].

Tetrapyrrole molecules, such as heme, are employed in a number of biochemical processes in algae plants [108, 109], bacteria [108, 111] and mammals [112] and therefore allow for establishing links between their metabolism and functions. Proteins containing heme continue to be one of the most studied classes of biomolecules due to their diverse range of biological functions [113] (Table **1**).

This large functional capacity of the tetrapyrrole molecules, explains why plants, through their mediation, can use the sunlight energy selectively for life, through the reduction of CO_2 [108, 109, 114]. In a similar way, mammals can use oxygen produced by plants to obtain, through its reduction, biochemical energy for life [115]. In summary, photosynthesis and respiration are complemented in the creation of increasingly more complex forms of life. Therefore, photosynthetic pigments and oxygen on extra solar planets are considered strong biomarkers for detecting life [116].

PIGMENTS, OXYGEN AND INFLAMMATION

Due to the major importance of the tetrapyrrole molecules in the evolution of life on Earth [108] we could also presuppose that these molecules play a leading role in inflammation, both in its production and in its evolution since this is a vital process for the body.

Inflammation has been linked to the nutritional alteration in affected tissues from ancient times. In 1877 Santiago Ramón y Cajal, to obtain his doctor's degree, presented a manuscript titled "*Pahtogeny of the Inflammation*", (the original version can be read at the Complutense University Medical School Library, although it has also been published in a facsimile edition) [117]. The future Spanish Nobel Prize winner cited the existence of disorders or perturbations of the nutritional activity in the organic territory subject to irritation, seconding Virchow. These authors considered that the essential phenomenon of the inflammatory process was irritation of the cell, which would be expressed by feeding the cell itself most actively, while exaggerating its function and by cell genesis [117].

Thus, we have proposed that the sequence in the expression of progressively more elaborated and complex nutritional systems could hypothetically be considered the essence of the inflammation, regardless of what its etiology or localization may be [2, 4, 5, 10]. The successive pathophysiological mechanisms that develop in the interstitium of tissues when they undergo acute post-traumatic inflammation are considered increasingly complex trophic functional systems for using oxygen. The expression of the nervous (oxidative and nitrosative stress), immune (enzymatic stress) and endocrine (energetic stress) functional systems during the inflammatory response makes it possible to differentiate three successive phases, which progress from ischemia, through a metabolism that is characterized by defective oxygen use (reperfusion, oxidative burst and heat hyperproduction), up to an oxidative metabolism (oxidative phosphorylation) with the correct use of oxygen that produces usable energy. Hence, the incidence of harmful influences during their evolution could involve regressing to the most primitive trophic stages, in which nutrition by diffusion (nervous phase) takes place. This is simpler, but also less costly and facilitates temporary survival until a more favorable environment makes it possible to initiate more complex nutritional methods (immune and endocrine phases) [2, 4, 10, 11].

Thus, it is also tempting to speculate on whether the body reproduces the successive stages from which life passes from its origin without oxygen [118] until it develops an effective, although costly, system for the use of oxygen every time we suffer acute inflammation [4, 10, 11].

Oxygen availability is coupled with an increase in network complexity beyond what is reachable by any anoxic network, and they highlight enzymes and metabolic pathways that might have been important in the adaptation to the oxic atmosphere produced only by a single biological reaction: oxygenic photosynthesis. Therefore, a correlation between the increased organism complexity and the development of the use of the atmospheric oxygen could be established [118-120]. This correlation also seems to exist in the evolutive phases of the inflammatory response since progressive cellular and tissue complexity occur parallel to a gradual oxygenation process (Fig. **8**).

Tetrapyrrole end products also accompany the evolution of the inflammatory response since its beginning with ischemia to its end with oxidative phosphorylation. Thus traumatic injury with cell damage and hemolysis can lead to high tissue concentrations of free heme, causing oxidative stress [121, 122] and chemotactic call for leukocytes [121]. Catalase and peroxidase have an antioxidative effect [33]. Biliverdin and bilirubin downregulate proinflammation [36, 47-49, 69]. Hemoglobin transports oxygen in the erythrocytes and cytochrome-C-oxidase is the terminal enzyme in the respiratory chain which allows for the synthesis of ATP, where the energy of food consumption and respiration is stored [123]. Therefore, it could be considered that the continuous interaction of tetrapyrrole molecules and oxygen, dominates the inflammatory response and perhaps reflects the thorough control that animal life should carry out with regards to this toxic cell potential, which is oxygen. Perhaps this is why once oxygen reaches the capillaries of the new formed tissues, whether by regeneration or by fibroplasia, the cells have to pay a very high price for obtaining energy, since they overly increase their turnover (regeneration) or reduce energy to the maximum, until acquiring a tissue with the least amount of cells, and therefore, one with very little vitality (fibrosis).

We could conclude that the close relationship that the tetrapyrrole end products establish with oxygen to acquire forms of life on Earth is based on the oxidative metabolism. This would also explain the tetrapyrrole end products location in the successive phases of the inflammatory response and so, phylogeny could be recapitulated [5] (Fig. **8**). Furthermore, the profusion with which nature uses tetrapyrrole derivates, including pigments in virtually all living organisms on Earth [116, 124], perhaps makes necessary their incorporation into our diagnostic and therapeutic arsenal. Then, the final aim of their use in the clinical area would be to achieve a similar efficiency in maintaining our life, when threatening factors arise [125].

ACKNOWLEDGEMENTS

We would like to thank Maria Elena Vicente for preparing the manuscript, Elizabeth Mascola for translating it into English and librarians of Complutense University Medical School, particularly the Director, Francisco Javier Jorge García-Reyes, and Manuela Crego and María José Valdemoro and B. Braun Surgical S.A. for their technical assistance.

This study was carried out in part with grants from Mutua Madrileña Research Foundation (Ref. nº PA 3077/2008 and AP5966/2009), MICINN PSI2010-19348 and with the special collaboration of the INEUROPA (Instituto de Neurociencias del Principado de Asturias).

CONFLICT OF INTEREST

The author(s) confirm that this chapter content has no conflict of interest.

ABBREVIATIONS

ATP = Adenosin triphosphate

BDNF = Brain-derived neurotrophic factor

CO_2 = Carbon dioxide

HbO_2 = Oxyhemoglobin

HO = Heme-oxygenase

H_2S = Hydrogen sulfide

IL-1β = Interleukin 1-beta

NGF = Nerve growth factor

RNS = Reactive nitrogen species

ROS = Reactive oxygen species

TIMPs = Tissue inhibitors metalloproteinases

REFERENCES

[1] Kohl BA, Deutschman CS. The inflammatory response to surgery and trauma. Curr Opin Crit Care 2006; 12:325-332.
[2] Aller MA, Arias JL, Nava MP, Arias J. Post-traumatic inflammation is a complex response based on the pathological expression of the nervous, immune and endocrine functional systems. Exp Biol Med (Maywood) 2004; 229:170-181.
[3] Punchard NA, Whelan CJ, Adcock I. The journal of inflammation. J Inflamm (Lond) 2004; 1: 1.
[4] Aller MA, Arias JL, Sanchez-Patan F, Arias J. The inflammatory response: An efficient way of life. Med Sci Monit 2006; 12:RA225-234.
[5] Aller MA, Arias JL, Arias JI, Sanchez-Patan F, Arias J. The inflammatory response recapitulates phylogeny through trophic mechanisms to the injured tissue. Med Hypotheses 2007; 68:202-209.

[6] Arias J, Aller MA, Arias JI, Lorente L. Traumatismos mecánicos: Contusión. Herida. Fractura. In *Fisiopatología Quirúrgica. Chapter 2*. Edited by Arias J, Aller MA, Arias JI, Lorente L. Madrid: Ed. Tébar; 1999; 35-49.

[7] Vande Velde C, Cizeau J, Dubik D, Alimonti J, Brown T, Israels S, Hakem R, Greenberg AH. BNIP3 and genetic control of necrosis-like cell death through the mitochondrial permeability transition pore. Mol Cell Biol 2000; 20:5454-5468.

[8] Jin Z, El-Deiry WS. Overview of cell death signaling pathways. Cancer Biol & Ther 2005; 4:139-163.

[9] Rosser BG, Gores GJ. Liver cell necrosis: Cellular mechanisms and clinical implications. Gastroenterology 1995; 108:252-275.

[10] Aller MA, Arias JL, Nava MP, Arias J. Evolutive trophic phases of the systemic acute inflammatory response, oxygen use mechanisms and metamorphosis. Psicothema 2004; 16:369-372.

[11] Aller MA, Arias JL, Arias J. The mast cell integrates the splanchnic and systemic inflammatory response in portal hypertension. J Transl Med 2007; 5:44.

[12] Yang JG, Rowe DJ, Dzwierzynski W, Yan YH, Zhang LL,Sanger J, Matloub HS. Pathophy-siological process of traumatic vascular spasm in multiple crush injury. J Reconstr Microsurg 2007; 23:237-242.

[13] Chien LC, Lu KJ, Wo CC, Shoemaker WC. Hemodynamic patterns preceding circulatory deterioration and death after trauma. J Trauma 2007; 62:928-932.

[14] Garrison RN, Zakaria ER: Peritoneal resuscitation. Am J Surg 2005; 190:181-185.

[15] Alanezi K, Alanzi F, Faidi S, Sprague S, Cadeddu M, Baillie F, Bowser D, McCallum A, Bhandari M. Survival rates for adult trauma patients who require cardiopulmonary resuscitation. Can J Emerg Med 2004; 6:263-265.

[16] Willis CD, Cameron PA, Bernard SA, Fitzgerald M. Cardiopulmonary resuscitation after traumatic cardiac arrest is not always futile. Injury 2006; 37:448-454.

[17] SOS-KANTO study group: Cardiopulmonary resuscitation by bysbystanders with chest compression only (SOS-KANTO): an observational study. Lancet 2007; 369:920-926.

[18] Hopson LR, Hirsh E, Delgado J, Domeier RM, McSwain NE, Krohmer J. Guidelines for withholding or termination of resuscitation in prehospital traumatic cardiopulmonary arrest: joint position statement of the national association of EMS physicians and the american college of surgeons committee on trauma. J Am Coll Surg 2003; 196:106-112.

[19] Gentilello LM, Pierson DJ. Trauma critical care. Am J Respir Crit Care Med 2001; 163:604-607.

[20] Moore FA, McKinley BA, Moore EE. The next generation in shock resuscitation. Lancet 2004; 363:1988-1996.

[21] Ho AMH, Karmakar MK, Dion PW. Are we giving enough coagulation factors during major trauma resuscitation? Am J Surg 2005; 190:479-484.

[22] Weisfeldt ML, Becker LB. Resuscitation after cardiac arrest: A 3-phase time-sensitive model. JAMA 2002; 288:3035-3038.

[23] Ali BA, Zafari AM. Cardiopulmonary resuscitation and emergency cardiovascular care: Review of the current guidelines. Ann Intern Med 2007; 147:171-179.

[24] Pace MC, Mazzariello L, Passavanti MB, Sansone P, Barbarisi M, Aurillo C. Neurobiology of pain. J Cell Physiol 2006; 209:8-12.

[25] Waxman SG, Dib-Hajj S, Cummins TR, Black JA. Sodium channels and pain. Proc Natl Acad Sci USA 1999; 96:7635-7639.

[26] McMahon SB, Cafferty WBJ, Marchand F. Immune and glial cell factors as pain mediators and modulators. Exp Neurol 2005; 192:444-462.
[27] Rittner HL, Brack A. Chemokines and pain. Curr Opin Investig Drugs 2006; 7:643-646.
[28] Pezet S, McMahon SB. Neurotrophins: Mediators and modulators of pain. Ann Rev Neurosci 2006; 29:507-538.
[29] McEwen BS. Physiology and neurobiology of stress and adaptation: Central role of the brain. Physiol Rev 2007; 87:873-904.
[30] Clarke RW, Harris J. The organization of motor responses to noxious stimuli. Brain Res Rev 2004; 46:163-172.
[31] Schmidt R, McDonagh AF. The enzymatic formation of bilirubin. Ann NY Acad Sci 1975; 244:533-552.
[32] Maines MD, Cohn J. Bile pigment formation by skin heme oxygenase: Studies on the response of the enzyme to heme compounds and tissue injury. J Exp Med 1977; 145:1054-1059.
[33] Furuyama K, Kaneko K, Vargas PD. 5th: Heme as a magnificient molecule with multiple missions: Heme determines its own fate and governs cellular homeostasis. Tohoku J Exp Med 2007; 213:1-16.
[34] Otterbein LE, Soares MP, Yamashita K, Bach FH. Heme oxygenase-1: unleashing the protective properties of heme. TRENDS in Immunol 2003; 24:449-455.
[35] Tang LM, Wang YP, Wang K, Pu LY, Zhang F, Li XC, Kong LB, Sun BC, Li GQ, Wang XH. Exogenous biliverdin ameoliorates ischemia-reperfusion injury in small-for-size rat liver grafts. Transplant Proc 2007; 39:1338-1344.
[36] Freitas A, Alves-Filho JC, Secco DD, Neto AF, Ferrerira SH, Barja-Fidalgo C, Cunha FQ. Heme oxygenase/carbon monoxide-biliverdin pathway down regulates neutrophil rolling, adhesion and migration in acute inflammation. Br J Pharmacol 2006; 149:345-354.
[37] Seta F, Bellner L, Rezzani R, Regan RF, Dunn MW, Abraham NG, Gronert K, Laniado-Schwartzman M. Heme oxygenase-2 is a critical determinant for execution of an acute inflammatory and reparative response. Am J Pathol 2006; 169:1612-1623.
[38] McCoubrey WKJr, Huang TJ, Maines MD. Isolation and characterization of a cDNA from the rat brain that encodes hemeprotein heme oxygenase-3. Eur J Biochem 1997; 247:725-732.
[39] Ding Y, Zhang Y-Z, Furuyama K, Ogawa K, Igarashi K, Shibahara S. Downregulation of heme oxygenase-2 is associated with the increased expression of heme oxygenase-1 in human cell lines. FEBS J 2006; 273:5333-5346.
[40] Orlinsky M, Shoemaker W, Reis ED, Kerstein MD. Current controversies in shock and resuscitation. Surg Clin North Am 2001; 81:1217-1262.
[41] Keel M, Trentz O. Pathophysiology of polytrauma. Injury 2005; 36:691-709.
[42] Martin L, Khalil H. How much reduced hemoglobin is necessary to generate central yanosis? Chest 1990; 97:182-185.
[43] Lundsgaard C, Van Sylke DD. The Quantitative Influences of Certain Factors Involved in the Production of Cyanosis. Proc Natl Acad Sci USA 1922: 8: 280-282.
[44] Maines MD: Biliverdin reductase. PKC interaction at the cross-talk of MAPK and PI3K signaling pathways. Antioxid Redox Signal 2007; 9:1-9.
[45] Kohchi T, Mukougawa K, Frankenberg N, Masuda M, Yokota A, Lagarias JC. The arabidopsis HYE gene encodes phytochromobilin synthase, a ferredoxin-dependent biliverdin reductase. Plant Cell 2001; 13:425-436.

[46] Pachori AS, Smith A, McDonald P, Zhang L, Dzau VJ, Melo LG. Hemeoxygenase-1induced protection against hypoxia/reoxygenation is dependent on biliverdin reductase and its interaction with Pi3k/AKT pathway. J Mol Cell Cardiol 2007; 43: 580-592.
[47] Vitek L, Schwertner HA. The heme catabolic pathway and its protective effects on oxidative stress-mediated diseases. Adv Clin Chem 2007; 43:1-57.
[48] Ollinger R, Wang H, Yamashita K, Wegiel B, Thomas M, Margreiter R, Bach FH. Therapeutic applications of bilirubin and biliverdin in transplantation. Antioxid Redox Signal 2007; 9: 2175-2185.
[49] Bulmer AC, Ried K, Blanchfield JT, Wagner KH. The anti-mutagenic properties of bile pigments. Mutat Res 2008; 658: 28-41.
[50] Cone JB. Inflammation. Am J Surg 2001; 182:558-562.
[51] Monaco JL, Lawrence WT: Acute wound healing. An overview. Clin Plastic Surg 2003; 30:1-12.
[52] Sherwood ER, Toliver-Kinsky T: Mechanisms of inflammatory response. Dest Pract Res Clin Anesth 2004; 18:385-405.
[53] Liu GY, Essex A, Buchanan JT, Datta V, Hoffman HM, Bastia NJF, Fierer J, Nizet V. *Staphylococcus aureus* golden pigment impairs neutrophil killing and promotes virulence through its antioxidant activity. JEM 2005; 202:209-215.
[54] Deitch EA. Infection in the compromised host. In *Surgical Infections*. Volume 68. Edited by Howard RJ. *Surg Clin North Am* 1988; 68: 181-197.
[55] Ohkusu K. Cost-effective and rapid presumptive identification of gramnegative bacilli in routine urine, pus and stool cultures: evaluation of the use of CHRO Magar orientation medium in conjuntion with simple biochemical tests. J Clin Microbiol 2000; 38:4586-4592.
[56] Hau T, Haaga JR, Aeder MI. Pathophysiooogy, diagnosis and treatment of abdominal abscesses. Curr Probl Surg 1984; 21:1-82.
[57] Iwatsuki K, Yamasaki O, Morizane S, Oono T. Staphylococcus cutaneous infections: Invasión, evasión and aggresion. J Dermatol Sci 2006; 42:203-214.
[58] Loo WTY, Sasano H, Chow LWC. Pro-inflammatory cytokine, matrix metallopro- teinases and TIMP-1 are involved in wound healing after mastectomy in invasive breast cancer patients. Biomed Pharmacother 2007; 61:548-552.
[59] Nerusu KC, Warner RL, Bhagavathula N, McClintock SD, Johnson KJ, Varani J. Matrix metalloproteinase-3 (stromelysin-1) in acute inflammatory tissue injury. Exp Mol Pathol 2007; 83:169-176.
[60] Gruys E, Toussaint MJM, Niewold TA, Koopmans SJ. Acute phase reaction and acute phase proteins. J Zhejiang Univ Sci 2005; 6B:1045-1056.
[61] Qin X. Inactivation of digestive proteases by deconjugated bilirubin: the possible evolutionary driving force for bilirubin or biliverdin predominance in animals. Gut 2007; 56:1641-1642.
[62] Qin XF. Impaired inactivation of digestive proteases by deconjugated bilirubin: the possible mechanism for inflammatory bowel disease. Med Hypotheses 2002; 59:159-163.
[63] Ascenzi P, Bocedi A, Visca P, Altruda F, Tolosano E, Beringhelli T, Fasano M. Hemoglobin and heme scavenging. IUBMB Life 2005; 57:749-759.
[64] Reniere ML, Torres VJ, Skaar EP. Intracellular metalloporphyrin metabolism in *staphylococcus aureus*. Biometals 2007; 20:333-345.
[65] Mastoraki A, Karatzis E, Mastoraki S, Kriaras I, Sfirakis P, Geroulands S. Postoperative jaundice after cardiac surgery. Hepatobiliary Pancreat Dis Int 2007; 6:383-387.

[66] Chou FF, Sheen-Chen SM, Chen YS, Chen MC, Chen FC, Tai DI. Prognostic factor for pyogenic abscess of the liver. J Am Coll Surg 1994; 179:727-732.

[67] Maisels MJ. What's in a name? Physiologic and pathologic jaundice: The conundrum of defining normal bilirubin levels in the newborn. Pediatrics 2006; 118:805-807.

[68] Zanardo V, Golin R, Amato M, Trevisanuto D, Favaro F, Faggian D, Plebani M. Cytokines in human colostrum and neonatal jaundice. Pediatric Res 2007; 62:191-194.

[69] Kadl A, Pontiller J, Exner M, Leitinger N. Single bolus injection of bilirubin improves the clinical outcome in a mouse model of endotoxemia. Shock 2007; 28: 582-588.

[70] Carrico CJ, Meakins JL, Marshall JC, Fry D, Maier RV. Multiple-organfailure syndrome. Arch Surg 1986; 121:196-208.

[71] Marshall JC, Christou NV, Meakins JL. The gastrointestinal tract. The "undrained abscess" of multiple organ failure. Ann Surg 1993; 218:111-119.

[72] Gatt M, Reddy BS, MacFie J. Bacterial translocation in the critical ill. Evidence and methods of prevention. Aliment Pharmacol Ther 2007, 25:741-757.

[73] Cheadle WG, Turina M. Infection and organ failure in the surgical patient: a tribute to seminal contributions by Hiram C. Pok, Jr, MD. Am J Surg 2005, 190:173-177.

[74] Luyer MD, Buurman WA, Hadfoune M, Wolfs T, Van't Veer C, Jacobs JA, Dejong CH, Greve JWM. Exposure to bacterial DNA before hemorrhagic shock strongly aggravates systemic inflammation and gut barrier loss *via* an IFN-γ-dependent route. Ann Surg 2007; 245:795-802.

[75] Ulloa L, Tracey KJ. The "cytokine profile": a code for sepsis. Trends Mol Med 2005; 11:56-63.

[76] Moseley RH. Sepsis and cholestasis. Clin Liver Dis 1999; 3:465-475.

[77] Marrero J, Martinez FJ, Hyzy R. Advances in critical care hepatology. Am J Respir Crit Care Med 2003; 168:1421-1426.

[78] Von Hundelshausen P, Weber C. Platelets as immune cells. Bridging inflammation and cardiovascular disease. Circ Res 2007; 100:27-40.

[79] Oberyszyn TM. Inflammation and wound healing. Front Biosci 2007; 12:2993-2999.

[80] Borregaard N, Sørensen OE; Theilgaard-Mönch K. Neutrophil granules: a library of innate immunity proteins. Trends Immunol 2007; 28:340-345.

[81] Heideman SM, Glibetic M. Comparison of the systemic and pulmonary inflammatory response to endotoxin of neutropenic and non-neutropenic rats. J Inflammation 2007; 4:7.

[82] Duffield JS. The inflammatory macrophage: a story of Jekyll and Hyde. Clin Sci 2003; 104:27-38.

[83] Serhan CN, Savill J. Resolution of inflammaton: the beginning programs the end. Nature Immunol 1005; 6:1191-1197.

[84] Meneghin A, Hogaboam GM. Infections disease, the innate immune response, and fibrosis. J Clin Invest 2007; 117:530-538.

[85] Smith EM. Neuropeptides as signal molecules in common with leukocytes and the hypothalamic-pituitary-adrenal axis. Brain Behav Immun 2007; 22: 3-14.

[86] Serhan CN, Brain SD, Buckley CD, Gilroy DW, Haslett C, O'Neill LAJ, Peretti M, Rossi AG, Wallace JL. Resolution of inflammation: state of the art, definitions and terms. FASEB J 2007; 21:325-332.

[87] Rajakariar R, Yaqoob MM, Gilroy DW. Cox-2 in inflammation and resolution. Mol Interv 2006; 6:199-207.

[88] Lawrence T, Gilroy DW. Chronic inflammation: a failure of resolution? Int J Exp Path 2007; 88:85-94.

[89] Flavell SJ, Hou TZ, Lax S, Filer AD, Salmon M, Buckley CD. Fibroblasts as novel therapeutic targets in chronic inflammation. Br J Pharmacol 2008; 153 Suppl 1: S241-246.

[90] Parsonage G, Filer AD, Haworth O, Nash GB, Rainger GE, Salmon M, Buckley CD. A stromal address code defined by fibroblasts. Trends Immunol 2005; 26:150-156.

[91] Buckley CD, Pilling D, Lord JM, Akbar AN, Scheel-Toellner D, Salmon M. Fibroblasts regulate the switch from acute resolving to chronic persistent inflammation. Trends Immunol 2001; 22:199-204.

[92] Jacobs GH. Primate photopigments and primate color vision. Proc Natl Acad Sci USA 1996; 93:577-581.

[93] Changizi MA, Zhang Q, Shimojo S. Bare skin, blood and the evolution of primate colour vision. Biol Lett 2006; 2:217-221.

[94] Madjdpour C, Heindl V,Spahn DR. Risks, benefits, alternatives and indications of allogenic blood transfusions. *Minerva Anestesiol* 2006, 72:283-298.

[95] Leow MKS. Configuration of the hemoglobin oxygen dissociation curve desmystified: a basic mathematical proof for medical and biological sciences undergraduates. Adv Physiol Educ 2007; 31:198-201.

[96] Ribatti D, Conconi MT, Nussdorfer GG. Nonclassic endogenous novel [corrected] regulators of angiogenesis. Pharmacol Rev 2007; 59:185-205.

[97] El Alwani M, Wu BX, Obeid LM, Hannun YA. Bioactive sphingolipids in the modulation of the inflammatory response. Pharmacol Ther 2006; 112:171-183.

[98] Ariel A, Serhan CN. Resolvins and protectins in the termination program of acute inflammation. Trends Immunol 2007; 28:176-183.

[99] Yacoubian S, Serhan CN. New endogenous anti-inflammatory and proresolving lipid mediators: implications for rheumatic diseases. Nat Clin Pract Rheumatol 2007; 3:570-579.

[100] Clapp C, Aranda J, Gonzalez C, Jeziorski MC, Martinez de la Escalera G. Vasoinhibins: endogenous regulators of angiogenesis and vascular function. Trends Endocrinol Metabol 2006; 17:301-307.

[101] Meier K, Nanney LB. Emerging new drugs for wound repair. ExpertOpin Emerging Drugs 2006; 11:23-37.

[102] Burns JL, Mancoll JS, Phillips LG. Impairments to wound healing. Clin Plastic Surg 2003; 30:47-56.

[103] Rahban SR, Garner WL. Fibroproliferative scars. Clin Plastic Surg 2003; 30:77-89.

[104] Arruda MA, Graça-Souza AV, Barja-Fidalgo C. Heme and innate immunity: a new insights for an old molecule. Mem Inst Oswaldo Cruz 2005; 100:799-803.

[105] Iredale JP. Models of liver fibrosis: exploring the dynamic nature of inflammation and repair in a solid organ. J Clin Invest 2007; 117:539-548.

[106] Van Den Berghe G. Neuroendocrine axis in critical illness. Curr Opin Endocrinol Diabetes 2001; 8:47-54.

[107] Yasuhara S, Asai A, Sahani ND, Martín JA. Mitochondria, endoplasmic reticulum, and alternative pathways of cell death in critical illness. Crit Care Med 2007; 35:S488-S495.

[108] Kiang NY, Siefert J, Govindjee, Blankenship RE. Spectral signatures of photosynthesis. I. Review of earth organisms. Astrobiology 2007; 7:222-251.

[109] Eckhardt U, Grimm B, Hörtensteiner S. Recent advances in chlorophyll biosynthesis and breakdown in higher plants. Plant Mol Biol 2004; 56:1-14.

[110] Tanaka A, Tanaka R. Chlorophyl metabolism. Curr Opin Plant Biol 2006; 9:248-255.
[111] Sasaki K, Watanabe M, Suda Y, Ishizuka A, Noparatnaraporn N. Applications of photosynthetic bacteria for medical fields. J Biosci Bioeng 2005; 100:481-488.
[112] Latunde-Dada GO, Simpson RJ, McKie AT. Recent advances in mammalian haem transport. Trends Biochem Sci 2006; 31:182-188.
[113] Reedy CJ, Elvekrog MM, Gibney BR. Development of a heme protein structure-electrochemical function database. Nucleic Acids Res 2007, *in press*.
[114] Tanaka R, Tanaka A. Tetrapyrrole biosynthesis in higher plants. Ann Rev Plant Biol 2007; 58:321-346.
[115] Hosler JP, Ferguson-Miller S, Mills DA. Energy transduction: Proton transfer through the respiratory complexes. Ann Rev Biochem 2006; 75:165-187.
[116] Kiang NY, Segura A, Tinetti G, Govindjee, Blankenship RE, Cohen M, Sieffert J, Crisp D, Meadows VS. Spectral signatures of photosynthesis. II. Coevolution with other stars and the atmosphere on extrasolar worlds. Astrobiology 2007; 7:252-274.
[117] Ramon y Cajal S. Patogenia de la inflamación. *Discurso de Doctorado.* Edición facsímil. Universidad de Zaragoza y Gobierno de Aragón. INO Reproducciones S.A. Zaragoza 2007; 1-109.
[118] Raymond J, Segre D. The effect of oxygen on biochemical networks and the evolution of complex life. Science 2006; 311:1764-1767.
[119] Falkowski PG. Tracing oxygen's imprint on Earth's metabolic evolution. Science 2006; 311:1724-1725.
[120] Acquisti C, Kleffe J, Collins S. Oxygen content of transmembrane proteins over macroevolutionary time scales. Nature 2007; 445:47-52.
[121] Porto BN, Alves LS, Fernandez PL, Dutra TP, Figueiredo RT, Graça-Souza AV, Bozza MT. Heme induces neutrophil migration and reactive oxygen species generation through signaling pathways characteristics of chemotactic receptors. J Biol Chem 2007; 282:24430-24436.
[122] Takahashi T, Shimizu H, Morimatsu H, Inoue K, Akagi R, Morita K, Sassa S. Heme oxygenase-1: a fundamental guardian against oxidative tissue injuries in acute inflammation. Mini Rev Med Chem 2007; 7:745-753.
[123] Siegbahn PEM, Blomberg MRA. Energy diagrams and mechanism for proton pumping in cytochrome C oxidase. Biochem Biophys Acta 2007; 1767:1143-1156.
[124] Suo Z, Avci R, Schweitzer MH, Deliorman M. Porphyrin as an ideal biomarker in the search for extraterrestrial life. Astrobiology 2007, 7:605-615.
[125] Arias JI, Aller MA, Arias J.Surgical inflammation: a pathophysiological rainbow. J Transl Med. 2009; 7:19.

Send Orders for Reprints to reprints@benthamscience.net
Surgical Inflammation, 2013, 51-98

CHAPTER 3

The Embryological Bases of Surgical Inflammation

Maria-Angeles Aller[1], Jose-Ignacio Arias[2], Carlos Gilsanz[3], Vicente Martínez[4], Patri Vergara[4] and Jaime Arias[1,*]

[1]Surgery Department, School of Medicine, Complutense University of Madrid, Madrid, Spain; [2]General and Digestive Surgery Unit, Monte Naranco Hospital, Asturias, Oviedo, Spain; [3]General and Digestive Surgery Unit, Sudeste Hospital, Arganda del Rey, Madrid, Spain and [4]Department of Cell Biology, Physiology and Immunology, Veterinary School, Autonoma University of Barcelona, Barcelona, Spain

Abstract: Post-traumatic inflammation is formed by molecular and cellular complex mechanisms whose final goal seems to be injured tissue regeneration. In the skin, an exterior organ of the body, mechanical or thermal injury induces the expression of different inflammatory phenotypes that resemble similar phenotypes expressed during embryo development. Particularly, molecular and cellular mechanisms are involved in gastrulation return. This is a developmental phase that delineates the three embryonic germ layers: ectoderm, endoderm and mesoderm. Consequently, in the post-natal wounded skin primitive functions related with the embryonic mesoderm, *i.e.* amniotic and yolk sac-derived, are expressed. Among the primitive function mechanisms involved, neurogenesis and hematogenesis stand out as the prominent ones.

Interestingly, in these phases of the inflammatory response, whose molecular and cellular mechanisms are considered as traces of the early phases of the embryonic development, the mast cell, a cell that is supposedly inflammatory, plays a key role. The correlation that can be established between the embryonic and the inflammatory events suggests that the results obtained from the research regarding both great fields of knowledge must be interchangeable to obtain the maximum advantage.

Keywords: Mesoderm, endoderm, ectoderm, amniotic, yolk sac, mesenchyma, granulation tissue, gastrulation, wound repair, angiogenesis, inflammatory pain, fetal, embryonic, remodeling.

INTRODUCTION

Inflammation is considered the fundamental scientific principle underlying the

***Address correspondence to Jaime Arias:** Cátedra de Cirugía, Facultad de Medicina, Universidad Complutense, Pza. de Ramón y Cajal s.n., 28040 MADRID, Spain; Tel: +34 91 394 1389; Fax: +34 91 3947115; E-mail: jariasp@med.ucm.es

practice of surgery [1]. Although nowadays the main role of the inflammatory response is due to its close relationship with illness and therefore is pathological, the origin of these mechanisms may have a different meaning, even physiological. In this way, we have previously proposed that the evolutive phases of the post-traumatic inflammatory response may have a trophic meaning for the injured tissue [2]. Under this supposition it would not be unreasonable to consider most of the inflammatory mechanisms as remnants of ancestral times when life depended on their trophic activity [3]. Fortunately, these mechanisms do not only represent the remnants from the past in the case of injury, but also they assume their ancient phenotypes to favor survival [2, 3].

When acute tissue damage is produced by a mechanical or thermal harmful stimulus, both types of energy are etiologically involved, either in tissue injury production, usually a wound [4], or in triggering an inflammatory response [5]. Cellular lesions are irreversible in the wounds produced by mechanical and thermal energy since necrosis is produced [5]. Until recently, necrosis has often been viewed as an accidental and uncontrolled cell death process. Nevertheless, growing evidence supports the idea that necrotic cell death may also be programmed [6]. Cellular signaling events have been identified to initiate necrotic destruction that could be blocked by inhibiting discrete cellular processes [7].

The most relevant mechanisms culminating in cell necrosis correspond to mitochondrial dysfunction and ATP depletion; loss of intracellular ion homeostasis, with osmotic swelling and oxidative stress; activation of degradative hydrolyses, and degradation of cytoskeletal proteins with disruption of cytoskeletal integrity [8]. Surprisingly enough, this list of mechanisms also corresponds to those that occur in the acute inflammatory post-injury response [2, 3]. It seems that, in response to injury, cells can develop mechanisms that would play a defensive role, *i.e.* inflammation, and that could favor reversing the alterations until their inadequate expression would make them harmful, *i.e.* cell death [9]. Hence, at a specific moment in time, the pathophysiological mechanisms, *i.e.* cellular response to injury, become a pathogenic mechanism, *i.e.* producers of cell death [3]. Thus, it could be considered that the cells can "escape" death in attacked tissues. Taken all together these mechanisms would in turn constitute the post-injury inflammatory response [2, 3, 10].

WOUNDS AND INFLAMMATION

The skin protects the organism against physical, chemical and microbial impacts of the environment [11, 12]. It represents the second largest organ in adult humans, only surpassed by the vascular system [12]. The skin consists of an outer squamous epithelium, the epidermis and its appendages (sweat glands, pilosebaceous follicles and nails) and two inner layers of connective tissues, the dermis and the hypodermis [11, 13]. Therefore, a wound that includes the three layers of this organ may damage its parenchyma, or epidermis, and its stroma, made up in turn, by dermis and hypodermis (Fig. **1**).

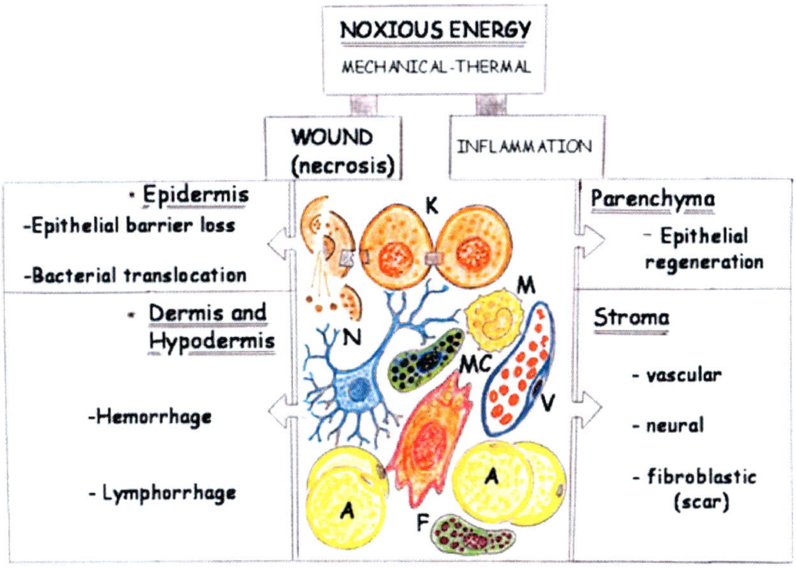

Figure 1: Consequences of noxious -mechanical and thermal energy- over the skin organ that is formed by epidermis (parenchyma), and dermis and hypodermis (stroma). A: adipocyte; F: fibroblast; K: keratinocyte;; L: lymphatic capillary; M: macrophage; MC: mast cell; N: neuron; V: post-capillary venule.

The inflammatory response is expressed by this organ after a wound can have exogenous and endogenous inducers [9]. Noxious mechanical or thermal stimuli as exogenous signals and cellular necrosis, as endogenous signals, can initiate the inflammatory response [14, 15]. Thus mechanical or thermal energy, as an exogenous damage/alarm signal [14, 15], has the ability to produce a wound, *i.e.* damage, as well as initiate an inflammatory response, *i.e.* alarm.

Today, the role that inflammation *"per se"* plays in cutaneous wound repair is quite rare and limited. Thus, it is accepted that inflammation is only another component of the repair process. Thus, the common description of wound repair evolution includes three classic types: inflammation, new tissue formation and remodeling [16-19]. However, some authors describe four healing phases: Hemostasis, inflammation, repair and remodeling [20] and even five phases: Hemostasis, inflammation, cellular migration and proliferation, protein synthesis and wound contraction and remodeling [21].

Nowadays, we need integrative pathophysiology to integrate all the new knowledge into an understanding of the inflammatory response because the distance between new molecular knowledge and every day patient care is increasing. Now we need to understand cell biology and genetics of inflammation to better identify gene and metabolic targets in order of modulating aspects of the inflammatory response [22]. We have therefore proposed that the inflammatory wound response recapitulates ontogeny and phylogeny through trophic mechanisms of increasing complexity to the injured tissue [2, 10].

PHASES AND PHENOTYPES DURING WOUND REPAIR

The inflammatory response that is induced in the injured tissue could be described as a succession of three overlapped phases, during which the phenotypes of metabolic progressive complexity related with the use of oxygen are expressed. Each one of these phases emphasizes the trophic role of the mechanisms developed in the damaged tissue. Hence, the first phase is predominated by nutrition by diffusion; in the second phase, trophism is mediated by inflammatory cells and finally, in the third phase, the blood circulation and oxidative metabolism play the most significant nutritive role [10].

Since these trophic mechanisms are of increasing complexity, progressing from anoxia to total specialization in the use of oxygen to obtain usable energy, it could be speculated that they represent the successive reappearance of the stages that took place during the evolution of life without oxygen on Earth from ancient times. In this sense, the inflammatory response not only could recapitulate phylogeny, but also ontogeny, through the successive expression of phenotypes that have a trophic meaning to the injured tissue [2, 3, 10] (Fig. **2**).

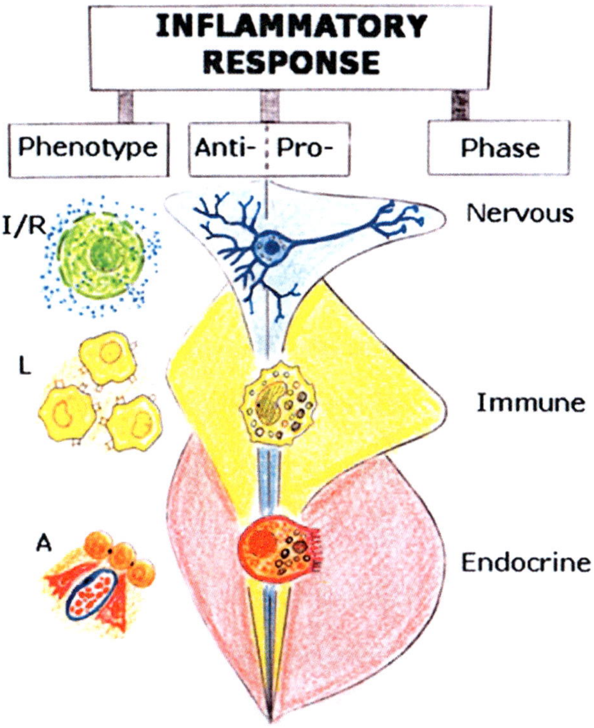

Figure 2: The Inflammatory response which is developed after skin injury is divided into evolutive vascular phenotypes and phases. Ischemia-reperfusion (I/R), leukocytic (L) and angiogenic (A) phenotypes are successively expressed during the vascular inflammation. The injured tissue losses its normal structure and acquires functional autonomy during ischemia-reperfusion and leukocytic phenotype expression. Then, when the angiogenic phenotype is progressively expressed, the tissue is re-structured and specialized. In the immediate nervous phase, depolarization and repolarization of cell membranes would be the key pathophysiological mechanism. During the immune phase, the transient synthesis of adhesion molecules favors cellular and bacterial translocation. Lastly, in the endocrine phase the skin tries to recover its parenchymatous structure, or epithelium (regeneration), as well as its stroma or connective tissue (scarring).

The successive inflammatory phenotypes are expressed mainly in the interstitial space. Therefore, the interstitial space always seems to be the battlefield for inflammation, whether it is due to trauma [2, 3], infection [3] or tumors [23-25].

In the first or immediate phase of the inflammatory response, interstitial hydroelectrolytic alterations stand out. This phase has been referred to as the nervous phase, because the sensory (pain and analgesia) and motor alterations (contraction and relaxation of smooth and skeletal muscle fibers) respond to the injury. Particularly, the vasomotor response with vasoconstriction and vasodilatation is responsible for the ischemia-reperfusion phenomenon, with the subsequent excessive production of reactive oxygen and nitrogen species (ROS/RNS) that causes oxidative and nitrosative stress in the injured tissue. In this phase, during the progression of the interstitial edema, the space between the epithelial cells and the capillaries increases, and the lymphatic circulation is simultaneously activated (circulatory switch) [2, 10].

In the following intermediate or immune phase of the inflammatory response, the tissues which have suffered ischemia-reperfusion suffer an immunological activation. In addition, they are infiltrated by inflammatory blood-born cells, particularly leukocytes. The chemotactic call, that activates and induces the recruitment of blood cells, is also taken as an advantage of bacteria to infiltrate the interstitial space. In the tissue which suffers oxidative and nitrosative stress, symbiosis of the leukocytes and bacteria for extracellular digestion by enzyme release, *i.e.* fermentation, and by intracellular digestion, *i.e.* phagocytosis, produces enzymatic stress. Furthermore, macrophages and dendritic cells take advantage of activation of the lymphatic circulation, and migrate through them until reaching the lymph nodes, where they activate lymphocytes [2, 3].

During the third phase of the inflammatory response, angiogenesis permits numerous substances, including hormones, to be transported by the blood circulation. For this reason, it has been considered that the predominance of angiogenesis during the last phase of the inflammatory response would allow for calling it the endocrine phase. Although the final objective of the angiogenic phenotype is to form new mature vessels for oxygen, substrates and blood cells, other functions could be carried out before the new mature vessels are formed. Thus, angiogenesis could have antioxidant and antienzymatic properties, favoring the resolution of the inflammation as well as wound repair by epithelial regeneration and scarring. Therefore, in this phase the new formed tissue is structured, specialized and matured by remodeling [2, 3,10] (Fig. **2**).

The three overlapped trophic phases of the post-traumatic inflammatory response could also be named, by their corresponding length, as acute, sub-acute and chronic, respectively. The acute phase is characterized by the quick molecular infiltration of the interstitial space that would in turn favor the establishment of a trophic axis based in the interstitial fluid flow. In the following or sub-acute phase, the cellular infiltration of the interstitial space predominates. In this phase, the invasion of the interstitium by blood cells would create another trophic axis based on a hypothetical enzymatic digestive ability that is assumed by the leukocytes in the injured tissue. Finally, it could be interpreted that through the confluence in the interstitial space of both trophic axes, molecular and cellular, the appropriate metabolic conditions would be generated so that tissue repair takes place during the last so-called chronic phase of the inflammatory response.

EMBRYONIC BASES OF INFLAMMATION: THE AMNION AND THE YOLK SAC

The inflammatory response could recapitulate ontogeny through the expression of the two hypothetical trophic axes, molecular and cellular, in the interstitial space of the injured tissue.

We have previously proposed the hypothesis that inflammation would represent the debut during the post-natal life of ancestral biochemical mechanisms that were used for normal embryonic development. The re-expression of these old mechanisms, with a prenatal solvent path, is perhaps inappropriate and hard to recognize since they are anachronistic during post-natal life and because they are established in a different environmental medium [3, 26].

The early mammalian embryon already has the ability to manage fluids in the interstitial space. In the human blastocyst, the inner cell mass or embryoblast differentiates into two layers, the hypoblast and epiblast. The epiblast is the source of all three germ layers and develops within a small cavity named amniotic cavity [27]. At the early stages of pregnancy, amniotic fluid consists of a filtrate of maternal blood. That is why in this period drugs taken by the mother can enter the amniotic fluid by diffusion across the placenta [28]. Amniotic fluid is an essential component for fetal development and maturation during pregnancy [29]. During these stages, amniotic fluid is a bioactive medium actively secreted by the cells lining the amniotic cavity and as gestation progresses it includes significant volume of fetal urine [30] (Fig. **3**).

AMNIOTIC AXIS

* Interstitial hidroelectrolitic management
* Neurogenic phenotype
* Biogenic monoamines
* Cytokines/Growth factors

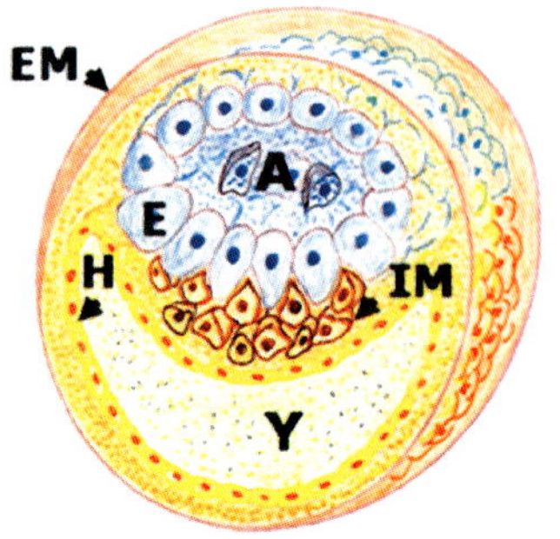

YOLK SAC AXIS

* Hematopoietic and angiogenic phenotype
* Glycolipoprotein store
* Cholesterol/Steroids
* Enzymatic phenotype

Figure 3: Schematic representation of the early mammalian embryo during gastrulation. The extraembryonic mesoderm (EM) is represented surrounding the amniotic cavity (A) and the yolk sac cavity (Y). Between the epiblast (E) and the hypoblast (H) the mesoderm interiorizes (IM) by epithelial-mesenchymal transition. In the figure top some of the characteristics of the amniotic axis are summarized. On the other hand, in the bottom some of the characteristics of the yolk sac axis are exposed.

Body fluid is distributed among three major fluid spaces: Intracellular fluid, interstitial fluid and plasma. Nevertheless, the fluid distribution in each of these compartments is dramatically different in the fetus compared to the adult. Particularly, the amniotic fluid that surrounds the fetus may be considered an extension of the extracellular space of the fetus [31]. Thus, the lymphatic system plays an essential role in the regulation of fluid distribution between the plasma and the interstitial fluid and, probably with the amniotic fluid [31]. It could also be hypothesized that similar functions, *i.e.* development and maturation, that the amniotic-lympathic-interstitial fluid axis has in the embryo, could have interstitial edema and activated lymphatic circulation (circulatory switch) in the traumatized tissue.

The yolk sac is the final destination of migrating visceral endoderm cells that in turn are derivatives of the hypoblast (Fig. **3**). The yolk sac begins to form during gastrulation [32]. The visceral yolk sac expands and blood islands, structures consisting of hematopoietic progenitors surrounded by a loose network of endothelial cells, appear [32]. Endothelial cell precursors associated with blood islands differentiate and coalesce to form a primitive circulation bed, which later becomes connected with the embryo *via* the vitelline vessels [32, 33].

Mammalian development requires the rapid *de novo* formation of embryonic blood cells to support embryonic and fetal growth prior to the establishment of the adult hematopoietic system. The very first blood cells to appear in the embryonic circulation arise in the extra-embryonic yolk sac [34]. Particularly, primitive macrophages first develop in the yolk sac [35]. As the embryo develops, newly formed hematopoietic stem cells are found in the aorta-gonad-mesonephros region, then in the fetal liver, thymus and spleen and ultimately, for adult hematopoiesis, in the bone marrow [36]. The yolk sac suffers a rapid involution following completion of their hemopoietic and angiogenic functions (Fig. **4**).

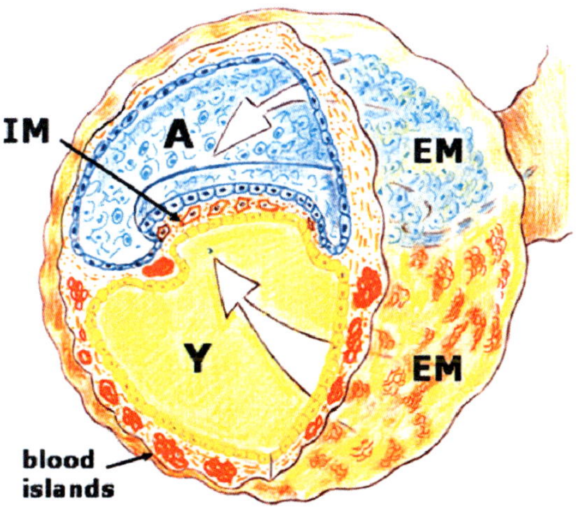

Figure 4: Schematic representation of the gastrulating embryo under the hypothetical influence of an amniotic-interstitial fluid-neurogenic axis (A) and yolk sac-hematopoietic-angiogenic axis (Y). EM: Extraembryonic mesoderm; IM: intraembryonic mesoderm.

Thus, the yolk sac-hematopoietic-angiogenic axis coordinates blood cell differentiation and vessel formation and plays an essential role supporting embryonic and fetal growth [32]. It could also be hypothesized that a similar trophic cellular axis is developed by the traumatized patient [37].

The confluence during mammalian development of the amniotic-interstitial fluid axis and the yolk sac-hematopoietic-angiogenic axis could be one essential factor to drive gastrulation (Fig. **5**). Although the details of gastrulation differ among different species, the cellular mechanisms involved in gastrulation are common to all animals. After induction of the germ layers, the blastula, composed by pluripotent stem cells, is transformed by gastrulation movements into a multilayered embryo, including ectoderm, endoderm and mesoderm with head, trunk and tail rudiments [38]. During the internalization process, cells of the mesoderm move through the blastopore under the ectoderm. Mesoderm, the middle or interstitial germ layer, gives rise to hematopoietic, endothelial, heart, skeletal muscle and connective tissues [38].

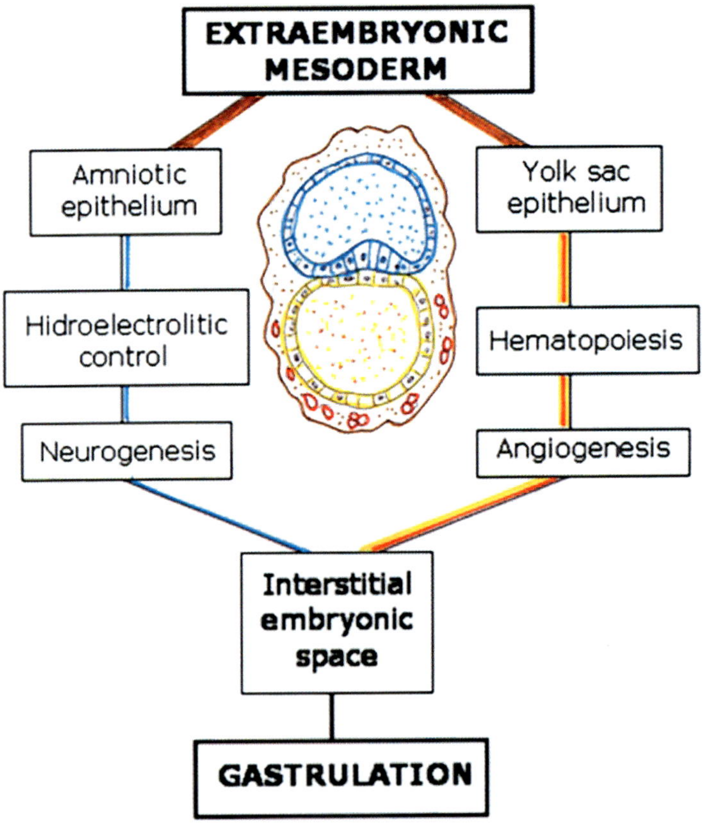

Figure 5: Hypothetical embryonary interstitial confluence of amniotic and yolk sac trophic axis to induce gastrulation.

In the current review we suggest that in the traumatized tissue both rudimentary and hypothetical trophic axes could be re-expressed with a similar aim, that is, the creation of a specialized tissue once again. If so, probably during damaged tissue repair, a similar set of morphogenetic cell behaviors are used as during gastrulation, including a series of changes in cell motility, cell shape and cell adhesion. This post-traumatic recreation of embryonic processes in the adult tissues is a hypothesis that would be supported by the recent findings about pluripotent stem resident cells in specialized tissues [36, 39]. Stem cells with pluripotent/multipotent capacity were thought to be restricted to the early embryonic stages. However, recent evidence challenged this idea by confirming the presence of pluripotent/multipotent stem cells in adult tissues and organs. These cells may participate in cellular turnover and the rebuilding pool of the tissue circumstances such as tissue injury [39]. However, their expression in the post-natal body under the influence of multiple anomalous environmental factors could induce pathological actions associated to tissue reparation.

It has been accepted that the impairments or pathologies associated with the wounded tissue repair during post-natal life have an interstitial origin because they are supposedly in this space, which is successively occupied by the mesoderm and then, by the connective tissue, where the hypothetical embryonic trophic axes are re-expressed after trauma [37]. Maybe, this is the reason behind the commonness of the alterations of those structures that ocupan in the tissues the space equivalent to the interstitium, that is the stroma. Particularly, the vascular, blood and lymphatic and nervous inflammatory alterations appear. These inflammatory changes have been grouped for their study in pathological axes that are predominantly expressed in the interstitial space (Fig. **6**).

Given the confluence of the two rudimentary trophic axes in the injured tissue, we have supposed that the underlying intention is to carry out a similar phenomenon to gastrulation. Therefore, it is possible that the resulting vasculo-nervous inflammatory alterations represent morphogenetic processes related to this crucial step in early embryogenesis.

PATHOLOGICAL AXES OF INFLAMMATION

The inappropriate expression of the inflammatory phenotypes induces evolutive post-traumatic complications. Normally, the abnormal post-traumatic inflammatory phenotypes are predominantly expressed in the vasculo-nervous structures and, for this reason their pathophysiological mechanisms play the main role in the study of wound repair complications.

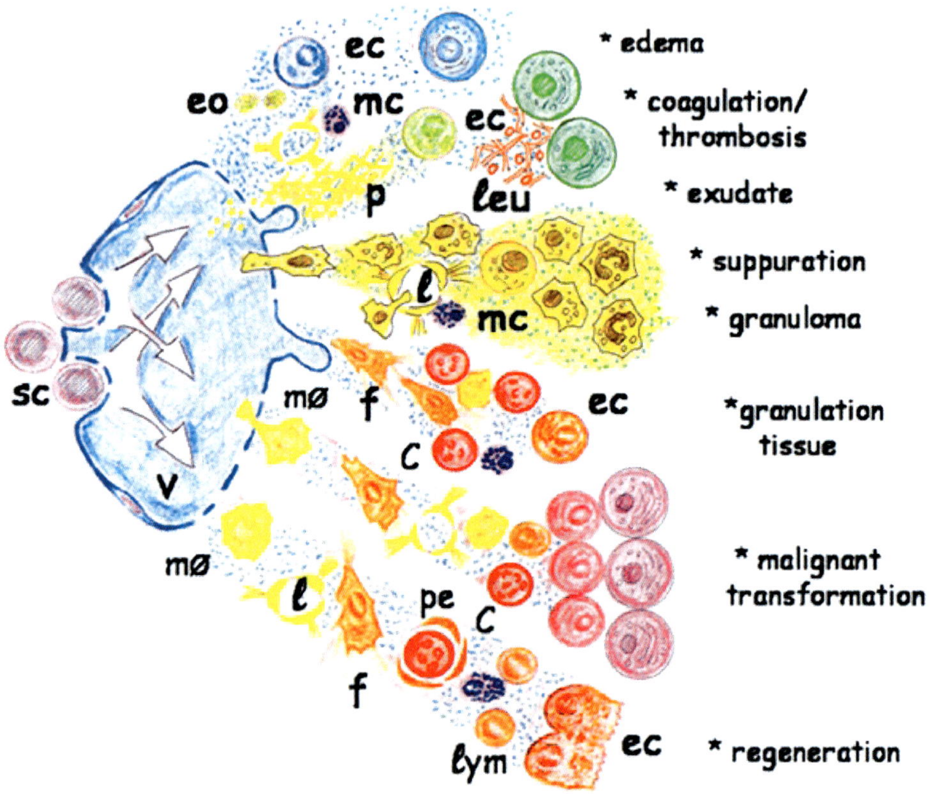

Figure 6: Schematic representation of the pathological axes expression during vascular inflammation, which is developed in the interstitial space of the injured tissue. c: capillary; ec: epithelial cell; eo: eosinophils; f: fibroblast; l: lymphatic vessel; leu: leucocytes; lym:lymphocyte; mc: mast cell; mØ: macrophage; p: platelets and fibrin; pe: pericyte; sc: stem cell; v: post-capillary venule.

1. Pathological Axis of Vascular Inflammation

The concept of the inflammatory response as distributed in the successive phases of ischemia-reperfusion, leukocytic infiltration and angiogenesis [40] is based on the normal microcirculatory, lymphatic and blood changes suffered by the injured tissue. Consequently, the inappropriate expression of these vascular inflammatory phenotypes, either by excess or by defect, is an obligatory reference (Fig. **6**).

- *Edema*

The abnormal expression of the ischemia-reperfusion phenotype during repair can produce disturbances in ion transport associated with cellular dysfunction.

There is increasing evidence that conditions characterized by an intense local inflammatory response are associated with abnormal ion transport [41]. Inflammatory mediators which influence ion transport are bradykinin, leukotriens, cytokines, thrombin, and transforming growth factor (TGF). They trigger the release of specific messengers, like prostaglandins, nitric oxide and histamine which alter the ion transport function through specific receptors, intracellular second messengers and protein kinases [41]. It has been stated that small fluctuations in cell hydration or cell volume act as a potent signal for cellular metabolism and gene expression [42]. Also, the exposure of cells to higher osmolarity results in the secretion of pro-inflammatory cytokines and extends normal macrophage half-life [43].

Interstitial edema causes a steady separation of the cells from the capillaries and widens the diffusion distance for oxygen and nutrients, favors the insufficiency of the lymphatic circulation and reduces tissue defense mechanism leading to a susceptibility to infections [3]. Also interstitial flow is important for lymphangiogenesis [44]. The interstitial fluid flow associated with edema, even though it can be extremely slow, can have important effects on tissue morphogenesis and function, cell migration and differentiation and matrix remodeling, among other processes [45, 46]. Insights into the mechanisms linking mechanical forces to cell and tissue differentiation pathways are important for understanding many diseases, including inflammation [46]. Abnormally increased interstitial flow rates can occur during inflammation and can also trigger fibroblasts to differentiate or remodel the extracellular matrix, contributing to the development of tissue fibrosis [44, 45].

The impaired function or formation of lymphatic vessels after trauma, could be associated with lymphedema, which is characterized by interstitial fluid accumulation. Lymphedema can lead to increased susceptibility to infections, impaired wound healing and chronic swelling [47].

Limiting swelling is extremely important because the injured area cannot return to normal until swelling is gone. In musculoskeletal injuries this is best accomplished with the "RICE" technique, which involves Rest, Ice, Compression and Elevation [48].

- *Coagulation*

When post-capillary venular membranes become permeable to complex molecules, including coagulation factors, the extravasation of fluids leads to interstitial coagulation. Cellular interstitial infiltration of the injured tissue is favored by the action of intrinsic and extrinsic components of the coagulation cascades. This results in the production of thrombin and catalyzes the conversion of fibrinogen of intravascular origin to fibrin [21, 49]. In most pathophysiological situations, it seems that the activation of both coagulation and complement cascades occurs simultaneously [50]. The complement and coagulation systems are organized into proteolytic cascades composed of serine proteases belonging to the chymotrypsin family. An explanation for the structural and functional similarities between the clotting and complement system is that they originate from a common ancestral developmental-immune cascade [51]. Thus the functional linkages between development, hemostasis and immunity in vertebrates would be explained [50, 51].

Mechanical and thermal injuries are conditions predisposed to thrombosis [21]. The mechanisms underlying this increased tendency for thrombus formation are, in part, related to the pro-coagulant properties of the inflammatory mediators produced and released as a response to injury [50]. Complement contributes significantly to thrombosis by directly enhancing blood clotting properties, by augmenting the inflammatory response, which in turn potentiates inflammation [52].

Inadequate fibrin formation is associated with impaired wound healing. Any process that removes fibrin from the wound will disrupt the formation of the extracellular matrix and consequently will also delay wound healing [53]. Mast cells strategically located in the vicinity of blood and lymph vessels as well as nerve fibers are among the first responders to the stimuli that initiate inflammation [50, 54]. While initially mast cells were identified as only participating in allergic responses, it is now clear that they participate in other phenomena such as wound healing and fibrosis [54, 55]. Particularly, they contribute to hemostasis through the expression of tissue plasminogen activator and heparin production, thereby preventing uncontrolled local activation of the coagulation system [50].

- *Exudation*

Chronic wound fluid is biochemically different from acute wound fluid. Chronic wounds may produce large amounts of exudate as a by-product of inflammation that contains elevated levels of enzymes. Exudate from chronic wounds has been shown to impede or block the proliferation of key cells in the wound healing process, such as keratinocytes, fibroblasts and endothelial cells [56].

- *Suppuration*

The formation of yellow, milky-yellow, greenish yellow or white-yellow pus characterizes suppuration or purulent wound inflammation [5]. In addition to the enzymes released by granulocytes during the process of phagocytosis and bacterial killing, the bacteria themselves produce a number of exoenzymes that cause tissue destruction as well as localization of infection. Particularly, almost all *Staphylococcus aureus* strains have the ability to secrete an array of enzymes including nucleases, proteases, lipases, hyaluronidase and collagenase [57]. Matrix metalloproteases would also collaborate in the development of enzymatic stress in the acute inflammatory tissue injury [58]. Pus mainly contains necrotic tissue debris and dead neutrophils and, when the collection of pus is localized, an abscess is established [57].

Phagocytosis of bacteria typically accelerates neutrophil apoptosis, which ultimately promotes the resolution of infection [59]. Although neutrophil apoptosis is critical for granulocyte homeostasis and the resolution of inflammation, many pro-inflammatory molecules extend the survival of polymorphonuclear leukocytes during the initial stages of the inflammatory response. However some bacterial pathogens alter neutrophil apoptosis to survive and thereby cause disease [60].

Colonization is defined as the presence of replicating bacteria and adherent microorganism without tissue damage. However, critical colonization is a novel concept that states that the bacterial burden in the chronic wound does not elicit the typical symptoms of an infection, but delays healing [61, 62].

Acute lymphangitis is often the consequence of a purulent wound inflammation. It is mostly caused by *Staphylococcus pyogenes* or *Streptococci.* Acute lymphangitis is recognizable as linear erythematous streak extending from the primary lesion, *i.e.* wound, towards the regional lymph nodes [63, 64].

Lymph nodes are essential for the initiation of immune responses by creating an environment in which lymphocytes and antigen-presenting cells can optimally interact [65]. Antigen-presenting cells as dendritic cells, macrophages and mast cells, first reach the subcapsular sinus and then, move into the paracortex where they aggregate around high-endothelial venules [65, 66]. These venules allow the active immigration of T and B lymphocytes from the blood into the paracortex compartment of the lymph node [65, 67]. However, wound infection by pyogenic bacteria frequently causes nodular lymphangitis with nodular subcutaneous swelling along the involved lymph nodes [63].

- *Granuloma*

Within hours of wounding, neutrophils are attracted to the wound site, followed by monocytes which mature into macrophages as they invade tissues [68]. In some invertebrates, mesenchymal cells, endothelial cells or fibroblast-like cells can transform into macrophages [35]. In vertebrates macrophages are involved in modulating the inflammatory process during the pathogenesis and resolution of tissue injury and inflammation [59, 69, 70].

Macrophages have remarkable plasticity that allows them to efficiently respond to environmental signals and change their phenotype [35, 70, 71]. Three macrophages populations based on three different homeostatic activities have been proposed: Host defense, wound healing and immune regulation [71]. Foreign bodies are indigestible particles and the macrophages form a granuloma around it. In some cases macrophages can fuse with each other to form "giant cells" that encapsulate the foreign body [9].

- *Granulation Tissue and Remodeling*

Angiogenesis is closely associated with granulation tissue formation and remodeling as the newly forming cellular complex must be supplied with oxygen and nutrients [72]. Excessive angiogenesis participates in the formation of granulation tissue, starting about three or four days after injury. The main cell types driving the excessive generation of the new tissue are macrophages, endothelial cells, fibroblasts and keratinocytes [17]. Mast cells also play a role in coordinating neovascularization in the wound [54].

Angiogenesis is regulated by numerous "classic" factors among which are vascular endothelial growth factor (VEGF), fibroblast growth factor-2 (FGF-2), transforming growth factors (TGFs), angiopoietins, platelet-derived growth factor (PDGF), thrombospondin-1 and angiostatin. "Non classic" endogenous stimulators of angiogenesis include erythropoietin, angiotensin II, endothelins, adrenomedullin, adipokines (leptin, adiponectin), neuropeptide-Y, vasoactive intestinal peptide (VIP) and substance P [73, 74]. They act in synergy to stimulate endothelial cell function during angiogenesis in tissue repair [74].

As granulation tissue forms in the healing wound, the vascular cells intermingle with the provisional matrix, which is composed mainly of fibrin, fibronectin and vibronectin [74]. Then, the new blood vessels associated with fibroblast and macrophages replace the fibrin matrix with granulation tissue, which forms a new substrate for keratinocyte migration [17, 21].

Remodeling begins two to three weeks after injury and lasts for a year or more. A framework of collagen and elastin fibers replaces the granulation tissue and produces progressive tissue sclerosis [75, 76]. Finally, most of the endothelial cells, with macrophages and fibroblasts undergo apoptosis, leaving a mass that contains few cells and consists mostly of collagen and other extracellular-matrix proteins [21].

2. Pathological Axis of Neuronal Inflammation

The inflammatory mechanisms also develop a fundamental role in the production of post-traumatic pain.

- *Inflammatory Pain*

Inflammatory pain is associated with sensitization of the nociceptive system. Central sensitization represents an enhancement in the function of neurons and circuits in nociceptive pathways caused by increases in membrane excitability and synaptic efficacy. It also reduces inhibition and is a manifestation of the remarkable plasticity of the somatosensory nervous system in response to inflammation [77]. To induce central sensitization, the noxious stimulus must be intense, repeated and sustained. Peripheral tissue injury is not necessary, although the degree of noxious stimulation that produces frank tissue injury almost always induces central sensitization [77, 78].

Peripheral inflammation induces a phenotypic switch in primary sensory neurons that comprises a change in their neurochemical character and properties due to alterations in transcription and translation [77]. However, it could be considered that the inflammatory pain pathogeny is phase-specific. Thus, after the initial electrical phase, with upregulation of ionic channel expression in the nociceptive circuits that causes, in turn, the spontaneous neural firing [78, 79], the following would be an immune phase with the leading role of cytokines and immune cells acting as pain mediators and modulators [80, 81]. Lastly, in an endocrine phase, neurotrophic factors, including nerve growth factor (NGF), brain-derived neurotrophic factor (BDNF) and neurotrophins 3 and 4, would be associated with structural neural remodeling [77, 82].

An immediate component of the stress response to pain is the efferent nervous response, which is mediated by the somatic motor and autonomic nervous system [83]. The somatic motor response usually consists in the withdrawal of the affected part of the body from the source of irritation. Withdrawal reflexes are the simplest centrally organized response to painful stimuli [77, 84]. Furthermore, the fight-or-flight response is the behavioral response to a threat, in which the somatic motor response stands out [83].

With respect to the autonomic nervous system, both the sympathetic and parasympathetic nervous systems, participate in the acute inflammatory response [83]. Catecholamines are found in adrenergic neurons, but their highest concentration is found in the peripheral pre-synaptic nerve terminals. After depolarizing the stimulation of these nerves, rapid secretory release of stored catecholamines occurs. Besides the adrenomedullary chromaffin cell and neuron derived catecholamines, lymphocytes and phagocytes represent a third category of catecholamine-producing cells [85].

In addition, the inflammatory reflex of Tracery is a pathway in which the autonomic system detects the presence of inflammatory stimuli and modulates inflammation. Particularly, afferent signals are transmitted to the brain, *via* the vagus nerve, which activates a reflex response that culminates in efferent vagus nerve signaling termed the "cholinergic anti-inflammatory pathway" [86].

Also, by anterograde inflammatory signals, neural cells contribute to local tissue responses. Noxious stimuli cause nerves to release neuropeptides in the injured tissue, *i.e.* substance P and Calcitonin gen related peptide (CGRP). When released into injured tissues, neuropeptides contribute to the pro-inflammatory responses against injury. The evidence that neuropeptides contribute to inflammation includes changes in endothelial cell shape, leading to capillary leak, smooth muscle cell relaxation leading to vasodilatation, mast cell degranulation leading to histamine, serotonine, and proteolytic enzymes and growth factor release, induction of inflammatory cell chemotaxis, increased expression of adhesion molecule and increased cytokine and growth factor production [87-90]. Experimental and clinical research has shown that excessive neuropeptide activity induces exuberant inflammation in hypertrophic scars [89]. Moreover, the functional impotence of the somatic motor system, which controls voluntary movements, *i.e. functio laesa*, favors vascular blood and lymphatic stasis and interstitial edema [48].

- *Complex Regional Pain Syndrome Type I*

Complex Regional Pain Syndrome type I is formerly identified as "reflex sympathetic dystrophy". This syndrome is the new term for "causalgia" that always coexists with documented nerve injury [91]. Complex Regional Pain Syndrome type I cause chronic pain, skin hypersensitivity, vasomotor instability with hyperemia, swelling and trophic alterations. It develops in the extremities mostly after minimal injury and it has been proposed that most of their features are explicable by small-fiber dysfunction [92]. Ectopically generated ongoing activity in afferent fibers conducted antidromically could generate neurogenic inflammation in the peripheral tissues, consisting of arteriolar vasodilation by release of CGRP and substance P, and postcapillary venular plasma extravasation by release of substance P [93, 94]. Nonetheless, these peripheral inflammatory changes cannot be seen independently of the changes in the central nervous system, including the spinal cord. Both, the central and peripheral nervous systems interact with each other *via* afferent and efferent signals, some of which may not be electrical but hormonal signals or by changes of axoplasmic transport [94].

THE INFLAMMATORY MESENCHYMA: A ROUND-TRIP TICKET

Fetal wounds heal by regenerating normal epidermis and dermis with restoration of the extracellular matrix architecture, strength and function [22, 95]. Also adult partial-thickness wounds are repaired by regeneration, *i.e.* replication of similar cells. In contrast, however, adult full-thickness wounds repair by connective scar tissue [56]. Therefore, the prognosis of extensive and deep wounds is not entirely satisfactory because of scar formation and the loss of normal function and skin appendages [96]. As a result, reducing the formation of scars and re-establishing the normal anatomy and function of the skin and its appendages have become the aim of regenerative medicine research [95, 96] (Fig. 7).

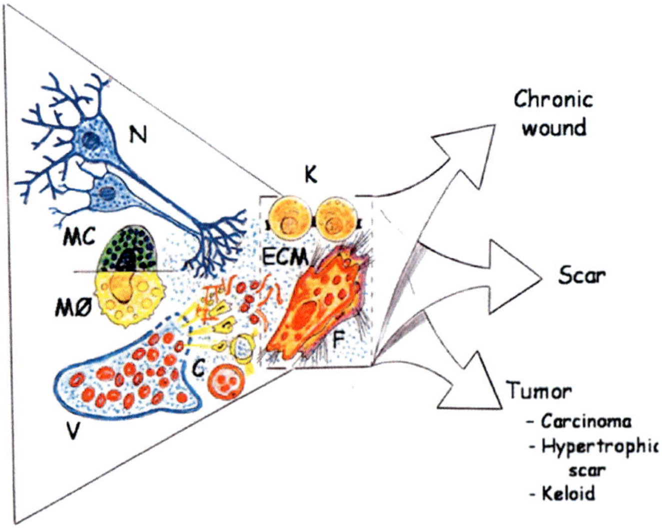

Figure 7: Influence of the pathological axis of neuronal and vascular inflammation in the skin parenchyma (keratinocytes) and stroma (fibroblast). C: arterial capillary; ECM: extracellular matrix; F: fibroblast; K: keratinocyte; MC: mast cell; MØ:macrophage; N: neuron; V: vein.

The spectrum of scarring includes normal scars, hypertrophic scars and keloids [97]. Hypertrophic scars are often red, inflamed, itchy and even painful. They generally regress spontaneously within one month to years after the initial injury [97-99]. Keloid scars are also raised, erythematous and often pruritic, however, they extend beyond the original wound boundaries and rarely regress over time [97-100].

Recently, the role of mast cells in wound repair and the remodeling process has been attracting attention. Mast cell proteases may provoke matrix degradation; histamine stimulates fibroblast migration and thus may contribute to regulation of wound healing [101]. Particularly, keloids and hypertrophic scars have a fourfold increase in the number of mast cells compared with normal skin. In addition, hypertrophic scar mast cells release more histamine than normal skin mast cells after stimulation by substance P [102].

Although after the traumatism, vascular and neuronal inflammations are the main clinical manifestations, it must not be forgotten that the principal cells that constitute the skin organ, or parenchyma, are the keratinocytes, and the fibroblasts, whose primary function is to establish, maintain and modify the connective skin stroma [103] (Fig. **7**).

In the human body the fibroblasts form a heterogeneous collection of mesenchymal cells [103-105] and they are the principal cellular constituents of connective tissues [103]. Skin fibroblasts constitute a heterogeneous population of contractile (myofibroblasts, pericytes and smooth muscle cells), pro-inflammatory, highly proliferative, proangiogenic and profibrogenic cells [103, 106]. Also in the hypodermis the connective tissue has the ability to accumulate lipids, *i.e.* adipose cells [103].

Fibroblasts are mesodermal-derived cells and perhaps this embryonic origin could justify their great postnatal plasticity. The mesodermal cells of the embryo participate in the extraembryonic structures, including the corion, the amnios and the yolk sac [36]. Also, in the embryonic mesoderm "blood islands", consisting in erythroid cells and surrounding endothelial cells, which are formed in the vascular plexus of the yolk sac, develop [36, 107]. The differentiation of amnion from the epiblast occurs before gastrulation and the specification of the three germ layers and cells from the amniotic fluid shows stem cell characteristics although most of the properties reported suggest that these cells are more similar to mesenchymal stem cells than to amnion epithelial cells [27]. The major role of the mesodermal cells and their ability to differentiate from the first stages of embryonic development allow for considering them as the cell protype that should be resorted to when the repair of any tissue in the body is needed [36]. And for this reason, perhaps the post-traumatic inflammatory response has the same intentions, namely, to use the embryonic mesodermal phenotype with a therapeutic objective.

If the post-traumatic tissue repair is based on the re-expression of metabolic, histologic and functional conditions that make the first stages of embryo development possible, then the fibroblast would have a fundamental role in this repair process. In fact, this cell is recognized as a mesoderm or embryonic trace and perhaps the most qualified cell for re-expressing this original phenotype [108] (Fig. **8**).

Local fibroblasts residing in the skin are considered the most prominent source of myofibroblasts [106, 109]. However, a variety of other precursor cells contribute to the myofibroblast population, depending on the nature of the injured tissue and the particular microenvironment [106]. Activated myofibroblasts are generated from a variety of sources including resident mesenchymal cells, epithelial and endothelial cells *via* epithelial/endothelial mesenchymal transition as well as from circulating fibroblast-like cells called fibrocytes, derived from bone-marrow stem cells [103-112]. In addition circulating monocytes have the capacity to differentiate into non-phagocyte *i.e.* mesenchymal cells and endothelial cells [113].

The reason why the myofibroblast is attractive to a broad scientific and clinical audience is due to the large panel of cells that can develop this phenotype upon activation. It appears that myofibroblast can be recruited from any of the local cell type and it is suitable to rapidly repair injured tissue [106]. Fibroblast can be induced to acquire the myofibroblast phenotype during wound repair. Then, the myofibroblast, by virtue of its ability to express high levels of α-smooth muscle actin, cytokines and extracellular matrix, is expected to have key roles in the post-traumatic inflammatory skin response [104].

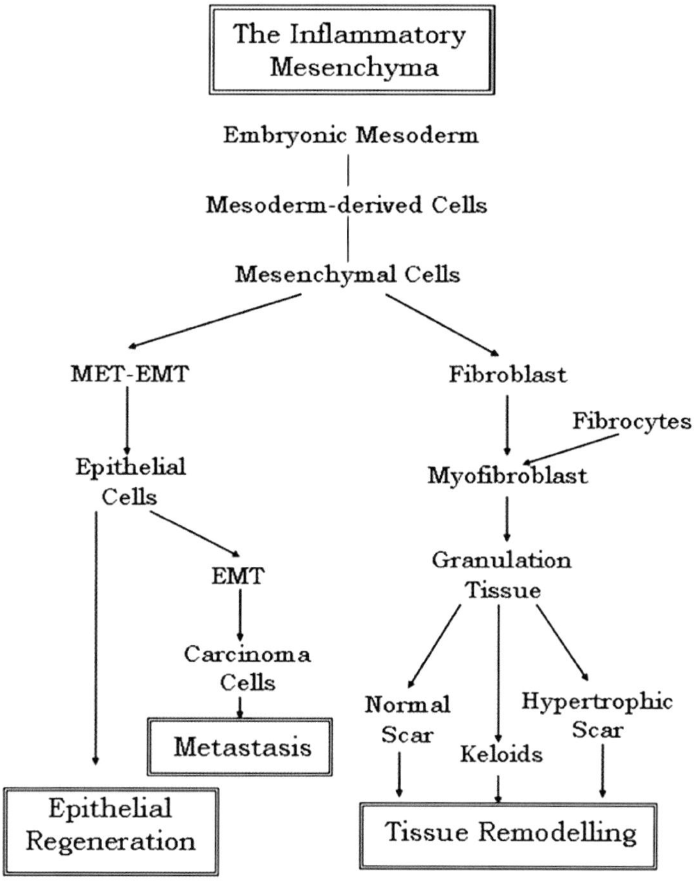

Figure 8: Protagonism of the mesenchymal cells in the inflammatory interstitium.

Several days after injury a subset of wound fibroblast can differentiate into myofibroblasts which are responsible for repopulating the wounded area in parallel to angiogenesis, thus forming the granulation tissue [2, 21, 99]. Also myofibroblasts are responsible for wound contraction. However to highlight the fact that contractile cytoskeleton is not a feature of normal tissue fibroblast, Boris Hinz introduced the term "proto-myofibroblast" for stress fiber-containing but α-smooth muscle actin-negative fibroblast that would consist of the early granulation tissue and preorganize the provisional extracellular matrix [106].

Gastrulation is the first major shape change of the developing embryo and cell-directed mechanical forces have a critical role [114]. Contraction of the actin cytoskeleton, driven by nonmuscle myosins and regulated by the Rho family GTPases, is a recurring mechanism for controlling morphogenesis throughout development, from gastrulation to cardiogenesis [115-117]. Visualizing the location of nonmuscle myosin by immunostaining strongly suggests the role of myosin in regulating tension and compression during gastrulation [116]. The presumed mechanical effect is that myosin causes the outer or apical surface to contract. Individual mesoderm cells constrict apically and leave the epithelium in a process known as ingression. Simultaneously, a loss of tension around the inner surface is produced. This causes the cell layer to buckle in wards leading to invagination [115, 116].

Granulation tissue is then repopulated with fibroblasts to produce a more densely collagenous extracellular matrix which is more akin to the matrix found in interstitial stroma [118]. Recently it has been demonstrated that subcutaneous granulation tissue induced by a large foreign body is a source of adult stem cells. This granulation tissue is derived from a local resting stem cell pool particularly from dedifferentiate pericytes [119].

Tissue remodeling requires the removal of granulation tissue and maturation of collagen is oxygen dependent. Indeed increasing wound oxygenation results in increased collagen deposition and tensile strength [102]. However, hypoxia benefits the expansion, differentiation, adhesion, growth factor secretion and regenerative potential of mesenchymal stem cells derived from subcutaneous adipose tissue [121].

The synthesis and deposition of extracellular matrix largely occur in response to mechanical signals mediated *via* cell receptors [115, 116], cytokines and growth factors [118]. Particularly, the extracellular matrix can bind to and release certain growth factors, *i.e.* FGF-2, VEGF and PDGF, thereby exerting direct control over their activity [118].

The notochord is an embryonic structure that could be a candidate for comparison with this phase of tissue remodeling. This anatomical structure of the embryo dominates early morphogenesis as a source of molecular signals *i.e.* growth factors, and later as a mechanical structure [122].

Degradation and remodeling of the extracellular matrix by proteases, particularly matrix metalloproteases (MMPS) are key features of re-epithelization and tissue remodeling [17]. Interestingly, the differentiation of an antifibrotic myofibroblast phenotype in response to tissue injury could inhibit collagen production as well as fibroblast proliferation. The fact that fibrosis may be due to loss of antifibrotic properties rather than activation of a fibrotic process suggests that, in normal tissues, active mechanisms to suppress fibrosis may be constitutively important in maintaining tissue homeostasis [104].

The phenotypic changes caused by the keratinocytes during re-epithelialization suggest a partial epithelial-mesenchymal transition (Fig. 7). Following the completion of wound-repair, keratinocytes revert their mesenchymal-like phenotype to epithelial phenotype [18, 123]. During the immediate keratinocyte response to the injury, one of the principal transducer signals can be electrical, by depolarization and hyperpolarization of the plasma membranes. Free ion movement occurs suddenly through membrane pores that can either be opened or closed in response to a great variety of gating mechanisms including voltage gating [124].

A cut in the skin produces a current that can be detected. This "injury" potential represented the short circuiting of a transepithelial potential that generated electrical field vectors as current flowed from areas of high resistivity, namely, with intact tight junctions, to the cut, where resistivity is low. Thus the short circuiting of transepithelial potentials can be sensed over 1-2 mm from the wound and it will persist until repair and re-epithelization are complete [124, 125].

One to two days after injury, the migration of keratinocytes from the epidermis at the wound edge and from injured appendages is produced [18, 21]. Epithelial cell migration requires the disassembly of desmosomes and hemidesmosomes which provide anchorage of the basal keratinocytes with neighboring epithelial cells and the underlying basement membrane respectively [126]. This disassembly and keratinocytes migration require cross-talk between growth factors, MMPs, integrins and structural proteins. In addition to lamellipodia extension, basal keratinocytes leapfrog over the basal cell near the wound [126].

The keratinocytes that are behind the leading edge in larger wounds proliferate and mature and finally restore the barrier function of the epithelium [18, 21, 49]. This could involve the proliferation of epidermal stem cells [18]. The proteins involved in re-epithelization include various extracellular matrix proteins and their receptors, proteases and cytoskeletal proteins. Growth factors that are known to stimulate wound re-epithelialization include hepatocyte growth factor (HGF), FGF, TGF-α and heparin-binding epidermal growth factor (HB-EGF). The signaling pathways initiated by these growth factors activate the transcription factors signal transducer and activator of transcription 3 (STAT 3) and activator protein (AP)-1, which help to regulate wound re-epithelialization [18].

It has long been known that chronic wounds are at risk for neoplastic progression. Chronic inflammation is a major risk for various types of cancer [127]. The risk of squamous cell carcinoma is markedly increased, suggesting that keratinocytes are especially vulnerable to malignant transformation [17]. The main difference between the migration of wound keratinocytes and cancer cells is the complete epithelial-mesenchymal transition that is frequently seen in cancer cells [128]. The epithelial-mesenchymal transition that is associated with cancer progression is considered a type 3 epithelial-mesenchymal transition [123]. Carcinoma cells undergoing a type 3 epithelial-mesenchymal transition lose all cell-cell contacts, acquire a fibroblast-like morphology and express mesenchymal marker proteins. These processes resemble those that are activated during early embryogenesis (type 1) [123], and following injury of skin (type 2) [123, 128].

There is now ample evidence that tumor cells depend on metabolic alterations for their continued growth and survival, and that these changes make cancer cells peculiarly addicted to the rapacious uptake of glucose and glutamine [129, 130]. This means that glucose and glutamine supply most of the carbon, nitrogen, free energy and reducing equivalents needed to support cell growth and division [124, 131]. Proliferating cells during tumor progression, immune response or wound repair, have a similar metabolic regulation that allows for maximizing their rate of anabolic growth and proliferation [131]. This type of cell metabolism directed at growth and proliferation, is also efficiently used during mammals embryogenesis [129]. This is why it has been proposed that the alterations in metabolic control during wound repair and tumorigenesis may result from reverting to an embryonic program [131]. If so, inflammation, a common process to wound repair, tumorigenesis and embryogenesis could have a trophic purpose for the cells [2, 10, 24, 40, 132, 133].

WHEN EMULATE GASTRULATION IS NOT ENOUGH TO HEAL WOUNDS BY REGENERATION

In the current review, we have proposed that the inflammatory response employed by the adult for wound repair could resemble the early phases of embryogenic development. This hypothesis is based on the comparison of the successive phases of the inflammatory response, particularly in the mechanisms that regulate the earliest steps in amniote gastrulation (Figs. **3** and **4**).

Gastrulation is a developmental phase that delineates the three embryogenic germ layers: Ectoderm, endoderm and mesoderm. Haeckel coined the term gastrulation derived from the Greek word "*gaste*", meaning stomach or gut, that transforms the rather un-structural early embryo into a gastrula with several specific characteristics: The three primary germ layers are formed; the basic body plan is established, including the construction of the rudimentary body axes; and the cells assume new positions, allowing them to interact with cells that were initially not close to them [134].

In essence, gastrulation could be represented as the creation of an interstitial space that is successively infiltrated by molecules and cells, in a similar fashion as the inflammatory interstitium of the traumatized tissue. In this way, during gastrulation the extraembryonic mesoderm interiorizes and occupies the space located between the amnion and the yolk sac. The primitive streak is a subpopulation of the epiblast in the organizing center for amniote gastrulation [135]. Once the initial primitive streak is established, germ layer formation begins. At the primitive streak the epiblast, cells undergo epithelial-mesenchymal transition to form the primary mesenchyma between the amnion and the yolk sac [136]. Afterwards, this is followed by mesenchymal-epithelial transitions to create secondary epithelium as part of somito genesis and further commitment and diversification of cells forming mesoendodermal structures [136, 137]. The concept that fibroblasts are simple residual embryonic mesenchymal cells explains the incorrect and often interchangeable substitution of the term "fibroblast" for "mesenchymal cell" [137].

The vast arrangement of the mesenchyma around and between the developing amniotic and yolk sac cavities suggests an important role of the mesenchyma in orchestrating embryo development. Mesenchymal stem cells are a versatile group of cells derived from mesodermal progenitors and can be found in several fetal and adult tissues [138]. The amnion is comprised of two layers, an epithelial monolayer and a stromal layer. From the human amnion it is possible to isolate two cell types, amniotic epithelial cells, derived from the embryonic ectoderm, and amniotic mesenchymal stromal cells, originating from the extraembryonic mesoderm [139, 140]. Mesenchymal stem cells isolated specifically from the amniotic membrane could differentiate into neuronal-like cells which are identified to secrete dopamine [141]. Cells derived of amniotic fluid also have a neuronal, dopaminergic phenotype [142]. These results allow for considering the amnion as an embrionary functional axis with strong neural potential [141, 142]. In addition, mesenchymal stem cells derived from the amnion are a transplantable cell population with therapeutic potential for multiple central nervous system disorders, especially stroke [140]. Experimental and clinical studies have demonstrated that amniotic membrane transplantation has important biological properties including anti-inflammatory, anti-microbial, anti-fibrosis and anti-scarring, as well as low immunogenicity. It also favors re-epithelization [139, 140]. Amnion-derived multipotent progenitor cells secrete a unique combination of cytokines and growth factors, known as amnion-derived cellular cytokine solution, that establish a communication network between mesenchymal and epithelial cells during embryo development. That is why using the amnion to accelerate wound healing through its functions has been proposed, which regulates migration, proliferation and differentiation of fibroblast and keratinocytes [143].

The extraembryonic visceral yolk sac in mammals is composed of two layers and the visceral endoderm, which is active in endocytosis/digestion and has large lysosomes and the underlying mesoderm layer [144]. In the embryonic mesoderm layer "blood islands" develop, supporting hematopoiesis and angiogenesis [36]. Also a major function of the yolk sac is associated with the accumulation of carbohydrates, proteins and lipids for embryo nutrition (*vitellum*) [145]. Particularly, the yolk sac plays a vital role in providing lipids and lipid-soluble nutrients to embryos during the early phases of development [145, 146]. The yolk sac uses high-density lipoproteins (HDL) and very low-density lipoproteins (VLDL) as carriers to incorporate cholesterol from the material circulation and to transfer it to the embryonic side [145]. Interstitial lipid accumulation of cholesterol, a precursor molecule of many hormones, like aldosterone, corticoides, androgens, strogens and progesterone, may favor fluid infiltration and cell migration, proliferation and differentiation during embryo development [147].

The molecular and cellular contribution that makes both embryo structures amnion and yolk sac to the interstitial space located between them, that is, the mesoderm, is essential for organogenesis. However, both in the amnion as in the yolk sac structures the extraembryonic mesenchyma plays an important role (Fig. **4**). It could be assumed that both cavities, which are surrounded by epithelium, are controlled by an array of inductive and inhibitory signals originating from the adjacent extraembryonic mesenchyma. If so, the amnion wall, represented by the amniotic-mesenchymal-epithelial unit, plays the leading role in primitive interstitial hidroelectrolitico changes [28, 31] and favors the development of a rudimentary neurogenesis [141, 142]. In regards to the yolk sac wall, represented by the vitelline-mesenchymal-epithelial unit, it could exert functions fundamentally associated with hematopoiesis and angiogenesis [32, 37] (Fig. **9**).

It could be accepted that these primitive functions are all together interiorized during the gastrulation to create the mesoderm. In this way, this germ layer would integrate the amnion- and yolk sac-related functions and thus would strengthen its functional ability compared to the extraembryonic mesenchyma (Fig. **9**). Thus, the epithelial cells located near the dorsal midline of the neural tube undergo primary epithelial-mesenchymal transition and differentiate into many diverse derivates including neurons of the peripheral nervous system, glial cells and pigment cells, *i.e.* melanocytes [136, 148]. In turn, the mesoderm and the endoderm contribute cells to other tissues of the developing animal. Thus, the yolk sac is an early source of hemangioblast, a common precursor of endothelial and hematopoietic cell lineages, and the cells of the visceral endoderm constitute a subpopulation of cells within the developing gut tube and therefore, have functions involved in digestion [149-151] (Fig. **10**).

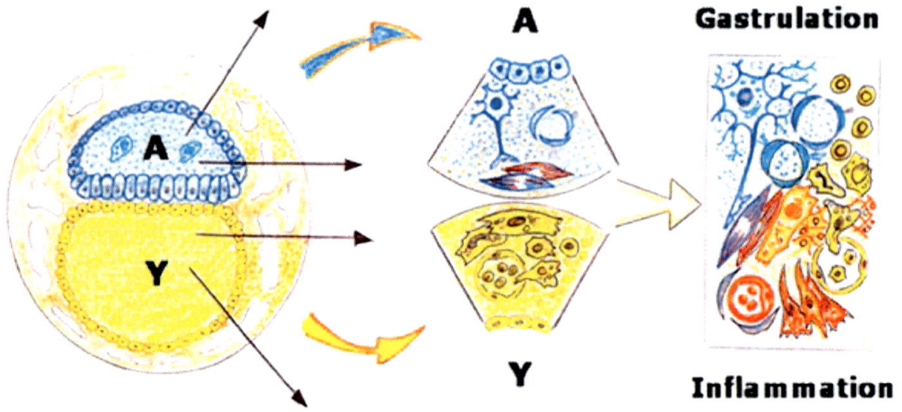

Figure 9: The amniotic embryo. The extraembryonic mesenchyma constitutes the walls of the amnion (A) and the yolk sac (Y). During gastrulation it could be considered that the extraembryonic mesenchyma interiorizes with its functions: hydroelectrolytic control and neurogenesis in the amniotic side and angiogenesis and hematopoiesis in the yolk sac side. The interiorization of the extraembryonic mesenchymal functions could integrate the amnion and the yolk sac original functions into the intraembryonic mesenchyma. Nonetheless, during the inflammatory response, the dedifferentiation process suffered by the tissues could re-express with clarity the primitive axes of the amnion and yolk sac.

In the adult organism many pathways that play an essential role during embryological development are inactivated later in life although some of them may be transiently expressed during adult repair [152]. This hypothetical ability of the tissues to involute or dedifferentiate could be an effective defense mechanism against injury since it could make retracing a well-known route using the appropriate mechanisms for their repair. However, it is possible that the great dedifferentiation reached by the traumatized tissues has been underestimated. That is why in the current review we have considered that wound repair would require the upregulation of signaling pathways characteristic of the extraembryonic mesenchymal function, as well as of its posterior interiorization during gastrulation. If so, emulation by the wounded tissue of the extraembryonic mesenchymal functions perhaps requires retracing the mechanisms that produce and distribute the extracellular fluid, including the amniotic fluid [37]. These extraembryonic mesenchymal functions induce and regulate the neurogenic amniotic phenotype and activate the yolk sac-lipid metabolism associated with hemangioblast differentiation. It could be proposed that traces of these functions, based on stem cell lineages, are developed in the early phases of the post-traumatic inflammatory response (Fig. **2**) and they would be expressed mainly in the interstitial space of the tissues [37] (Figs. **6** and **7**).

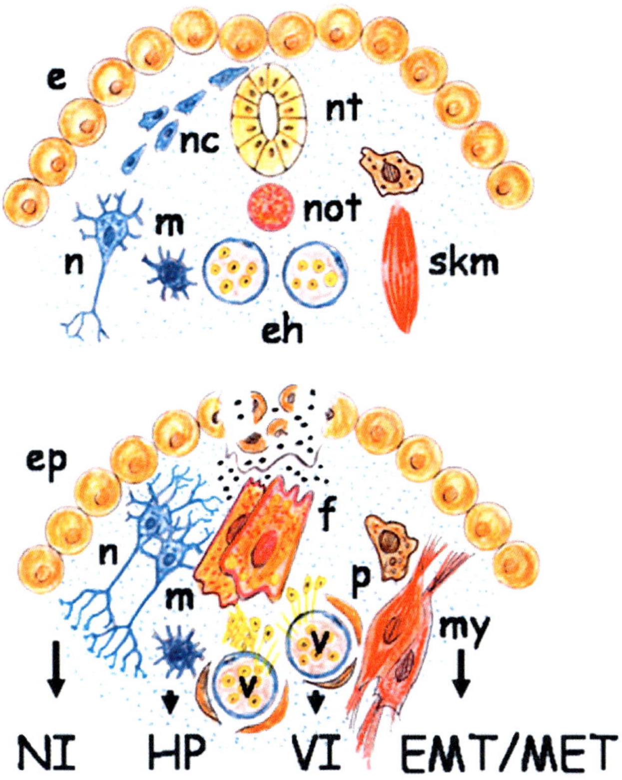

Figure 10: Schematic representation of the gastrulation process (top) and of a skin wound (bottom). The hypothetical functional reactivation of embryonic development axes after a tissue injury would reproduce the embryonic biochemical pathways in the mature organism. e: epiblast; eh: endothelial-hematopoietic cell lineages; ep: epithelium; EMT/MET: epithelial mesenchymal transition/mesenchymal epithelial transition; f: fibroblast; HP: hyperpigmentation; m: melanocyte; my: myofibroblast; n:neuron; nc: neural crest cell; NI: neuronal inflammation; nt: neural tube; not: notochord; p: pericyte; skm: skeletal muscle; v:blood vessels; VI: vascular inflammation.

As in the gastrulation process, it is possible that the primitive functions of the extra-embryonic mesenchyma, whose re-expression is induced by the wound, would be interiorized by the adult body. But, this mechanism would produce a serious loss of its health. So, if embryonic developmental pathways, representative of its primitive life, would re-emerge in the adult organism, they would take the place of post-natal specialized functions, impeding or hindering their actual life.

Nonetheless, according to the proposed hypothesis, the failure of adult skin regeneration after a wound suggests the need of researching about those factors and mechanisms that must be upregulated and those that must be reduced or even avoided to efficiently reproduce the early embryonic conditions for the development. Understanding the process that gives rise to early embryonic development may lead to advances in wound therapies. Perhaps, the mechanisms of scarless wound healing in the fetus are related to this supposed ability to maintain the memory of their origin while undergoing reprogramming events that could allow them to re-enter the embryonic programs of tissue formation to obtain the regeneration after injury [153, 154].

MAST CELLS AS EXECUTORS OF THE PATHOLOGICAL AXIS OF INFLAMMATION: GUARDIANS WHEN NOT TERRORIST

Mast cells are ubiquitous in the interstitial spaces of the body and normally reside in the connective tissue close to blood vessel nerves and epithelia [155]. Current evidence suggests that mast cells exert their role, in all the inflammatory response phases, and that is why they are an ideal candidate for playing a role in wound healing [156] (Fig. **10**).

Particularly, mast cells could orchestrate the inflammatory response inducing the expression of embryonic programs of tissue formation. Mast cells are derivatives of hematopoietic progenitor cells that migrate into virtually all vascularized tissues, where they complete their maturation. Upon activation their "plasticity" renders them greater flexibility and diversity of responsiveness to meet the requirements of the inflammatory response in which these cells are involved [155]. In this sense, activated mast cells can induce the expression of the proposed neurovascular axes of the inflammation. Thus, mast cells secrete numerous biogenic monoamines, *i.e.* histamine, serotonin, and nociceptive molecules that can sensitize sensory neurons which further activate mast cells by releasing neurotransmitter or neuropeptides, *i.e.* acetylcholine, neurotensin, substance P and somatostatin [157, 158]. Mast cells are also the source of many biologically active mediators involved in the process of neovascularization [155, 159]. Mast cells are topographically associated with microvessels and their number rises in angiogenesis-dependent events such as inflammation [159, 160]. The role of mast cells in angiogenesis is mediated by the release of their stored substances to a variety of stimuli [155, 160, 161]. Mast cell mediators include histamine, chymases, cytokine and growth factors like PDGF and VEGF, all of which exhibit pro-angiogenic properties [159-162]. In addition post-traumatic inflammation is a strong pro-hematopoietic stimulus. Mast cells are one of the cells that produce pro-inflammatory pleiotropic mediators that induce hematopoiesis [163]. Hematopoietic stem cells, in turn, give rise to a hierarchically organized set of progenitors for erythroid, myeloid, lymphoid and megakaryocyte lineages [36]. Particularly, neutrophils, monocyte/macrophages and T cells from the bone marrow are always present in the interstitial connective tissue during inflammatory response progression [17, 21]. Mast cells infiltrating injured tissues, through the release of granulocyte-macrophage colony stimulating factor (GM-CSF), can act on the bone marrow requesting the inflammatory cells that are needed for repair. A polarized hematopoietic axis from the bone marrow up to the mesenchymal interstitial space of the injured tissue would be established (Fig. **10**).

Mesenchymal post-traumatic dedifferentiation induced by activated mast cells could favor the expression of extraembryonic mesenchymal associated functions. In this way, embrionary mesenchymal functional axes are again expressed in the injured tissue, favoring in turn neurogenesis, hematopoiesis and angiogenesis. But mast cells also could simultaneously activate the mechanisms associated with gastrulation and this would mean the interiorization of the above mentioned mesenchymal functional axes. In this developmental process, generation of the mesoderm from the ectoderm, that is the epiblast, by epithelial to mesenchymal transition [164], is associated with mesoderm cell constriction, leading to invagination [115, 116]. Therefore, it is not surprising that during wound healing the excessive mesenchymal cell production and matrix deposition predominate, as well as the coexistence of wound contraction, which requires the presence of both, mast cells and contractile fibroblasts [156]. It is possible that in the inflammatory responses in which mast cells predominate, *i.e.* allergic and autoimmunes [165, 166] this primitive embryonic mesenchymal response predominates. This hypothetical comparison could help to better understand the pathophysiological mechanisms and the histological characteristics that these type of chronic inflammatory responses develops, particularly, the type of bidirectional interactions established between epithelial and mesenchymal phenotypes [165, 167].

Mast cells could also participate in the worsening of the inflammatory response when a noxious factor is associated [168]. Mast cells are components of the innate immune system that act as sentinels stationed around blood vessels, including swelling, redness and leukocyte recruitment [169]. Histamine, serotonin, proteases and VEGF stand out among the mediators released by mast cells, which cause vasodilation, edema and exudation due to increased vascular permeability [155]. The persistence of edema induced by mast cell mediators could maintain hypoxia in the wounded tissue and consequently inflammation [120, 169]. However, chronic interstitial edema could also induce mesenchymal dedifferentiation. If so, mesenchymal fibroblasts embedded in the interstitial fluid could migrate and preserve their proliferation potential.

Under conditions of long-lasting inflammation, wound healing is associated with excessive interposition of fibrotic tissue. Prolonged inflammation in wounds contributes to the development of fibro-proliferative scars, in other words, keloids and hypertrophic scars, both with erithematous and increased mast cell density [101, 102]. Interactions between mast cells and fibroblasts are paramount in the genesis of fibrosis [168]. Fibrosis is characterized by excessive matrix deposition and reduced remodeling. Often fibrotic lesions are associated with increased densities of mast cells [170]. It has been shown that mast-cell secreted factors, specifically PDGF, could contribute to inflammation-associated fibrosis, inducing the expression of osteopontin by wound granulation tissue fibroblasts [171]. The fibro-proliferative scars constitute solid cords along the wound axis which are related to wound remodeling. This excessive stiffness of the repair tissue resembles the notochord in the early embryo and, if so, it could be an ancestral trace of the mesenchyme also related to gastrulation. Particularly, mesoderm creation includes the development of a solid structure with great stiffness essential for correct morphogenesis, that is the notochord, and which is precisely what dominates the chordates.

Growth factors pivotal for repair in mammalians are PDGF/VEGF. In general, fibroblasts could respond in a pathological fashion to PDGF/VEGF promoting fibrotic tissue scarring [17]. Inflammatory cells, such as activated macrophages and mast cells, can produce inflammatory mediators that promote up-regulation of PDGF receptors on mesenchymal cells. As a result, PDGF-mediated proliferation of mesenchymal cells may be a hallmark of all chronic inflammation [172]. However, important developmental roles for PDGF and their receptor-like proteins have also been demonstrated in mammalian and non-mammalian vertebrates. Several observations suggest that PDGF has early developmental functions, particularly during gastrulation. PDGF receptors expression occurs in the developing mesoderm, mediating mesoderm cell migration, and upon PDGF receptor inhibition, the mesodermal cell detaches from the ectoderm and undergoes apoptosis [172, 173]. PDGF signaling has an evolutionary conserved role during gastrulation and it has been implicated in neural development and function as well as in the early differentiation of hematopoietic/endothelial precursor [172].

If we hypothesize that during the wound healing a process similar to the embryonic gastrulation with interiorization of the primitive extra-embryonic functions is developed, we could deliberate on about the original nature of these functions and their corresponding mediators. Therefore, it could turn to the mast cell functions and mediators because of its ubiquity during all the phases of the inflammatory response [156]. Mast cells are able to take up, store and release a variety of biogenic amines through which it is hypothesized that they participate in inflammatory reactions, mainly monoamines like histamine and serotonin [157]. These monoaminergic systems play a variety of roles in animals as neurotransmitters, autocrine and paracrine factors and hormones. However, also the venoms of many different animals, *i.e.* coelenterates, octopus, scorpions, centipedes, insects, amphibians and snakes contain histamine, in addition to other monoamines [174]. Also, the most ubiquitous effect of venoms on monoaminergic systems is venom-induced release of histamine from mast cells [174, 175].

Likewise, the venoms of some species of coelenterates, octopus, spiders, scorpion, cone snails, centipedes, insects, amphibians and snakes contain serotonin [174]. For both histamine and serotonin it is thought that their most common function in venom is to produce pain and paralysis in the prey. Therefore, for histamine and serotonin, characteristics mast cells mediators, are venoms developed for both offensive and defensive purposes [174, 175].

Examination of the effects of venoms on monoaminergic systems points out the great diversity of venom effects and also the cases of evolutionary convergence.

For example, the venoms of scorpions, spiders and jellyfish cause catecholamine storm in the victim [174, 176-178].

A common feature of the *Phylum Cnidaria, i.e.* hydroids, anemones, corals and jellyfish, is tentacles with stinging cells, *i.e.* nematocytes or cnidocytes, which contain un-discharged nematocyst. The nematocyst neurotoxins can paralyze and often kill the small prey, which are their food [178, 179]. Both mechanical and chemical stimuli cause nematocysts to be discharged suggesting the involvement of both chemoreceptors and mechanoreceptors in the discharge process [179].

It is possible that during the evolution these invertebrate armaments -defensive and offensive- were interiorized into in the mesenchyma. If so, an evolutive advantage was associated with the risk of self-poisoning when the body suffered an injury that caused the cells to be stuffed with toxic products, *i.e.* the mast cells. Even psychological stress [180] because of the mutual association between mast cells and nerves [157] is a potential cause of mast cell inflammatory activation [155]. Interactions between the nervous system and the immune system, *i.e.* mast cells, are increasingly recognized as important in the pathophysiology of inflammation, including itch [181].

Mast cells exhibit phenotypical and functional heterogeneity in different anatomical sites [155]. Two types of mast cells have been identified in rodents, connective tissue-type mast cells (CTMC) and mucosal mast cells (MMC) [155, 182]. Particularly fetal skin-derived mast cells have many characteristic features of CTMC [182]. Mast cells are being preferentially localized at host-environment interface [155], although it is also accepted that they occupy strategic locations with respect to the basic structural division of the tissues and organs in parenchyma, *i.e.* MMC and stroma, *i.e.* CTMC. This distribution suggests the involvement of the mast cell subtypes in the differentiation of the tissue structure. Perhaps thanks to these privileged locations in organs and tissues, mast cells may participate in the pathogenesis of a wide array of diseases, including allergic, inflammatory, angiogenic and fibrotic diseases [163, 168, 182]. In these anatomical locations mast cells, as interstitials cells, could exert a key role in modulating the epithelial-mesenchyma interaction, both in the physiological as in the pathological status (Fig. **11**).

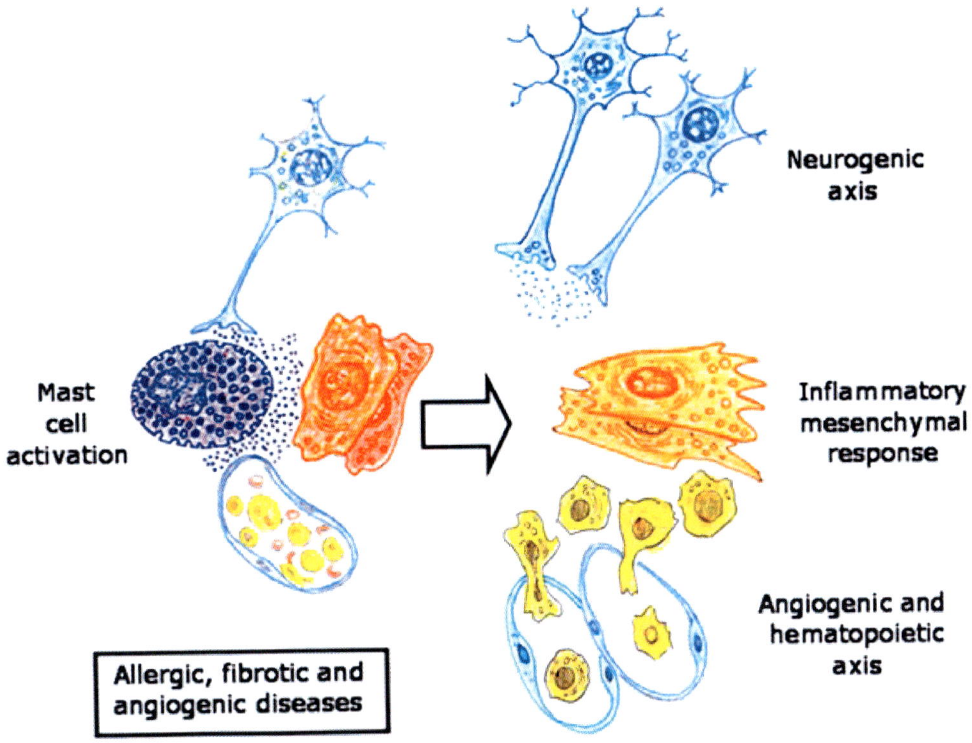

Figure 11: Mast cell key role in orchestrating the inflammatory axis. Upon activation, mast cells could induce the expression of both the inflammatory axes, the neurovascular axis and the mesenchymal axis.

Taken all together the above-mentioned considerations and results, we can conclude that the ability of the tissues to involute or dedifferentiate could represent a return to early stages of development. Therefore, it could form an effective defense mechanism to escape death after injury since it could make retracing a well-known route possible, *i.e.* the initial phases of embryonic development during the evolution of the inflammatory response. Particularly, the up-regulation of signaling pathways during gastrulation, in which the interiorization of extraembryonic functions would be made, could help explain the meaning of the diverse and complex mechanisms expressed by the mature organism in response to skin injury [37].

If so, even the embryonic mechanisms to generate pigment cells could be responsible of the post-inflammatory hyperpigmentation with higher concentrations of melanocytes [187, 188]. Nowadays, the underlying mechanisms and the individual variability showed for developing post-inflammatory hyperpigmentation are not well understood [184, 185].

This amazing property of the cells to keep a memory of their origin undergoing reprogramming events could allow them post-injury to re-enter the embryonic programs of tissue formation and obtain regeneration [186]. Generally, while the monopotent and tissue-committed stem cells were described in the adult tissue, stem cells with a pluripotent/multipotent capacity were thought to be restricted to the early embryonic stages. However, recent evidence challenged this idea by confirming the presence of pluripotent/multipotent stem cells in adult tissues and organs [39]. Particularly, adult human mesenchymal cell populations, such as skin fibroblasts, contain distinctly multipotent stem cells. These stem cells have the ability to generate the multiple cell types of the three germ layers, like ectodermal (*e.g.* neural marker-positive cells), endodermal and mesodermal lineage cells [187].

Interestingly enough, quiescent and active adult stem cells coexist in several tissues that have the ability to renew and regenerate, like bone marrow, intestinal epithelium and hair follicles, all of them placed in the vicinity of a mesenchymal cell [188]. This stem cell-mesenchymal cell relation takes us back to the initial epiblast mesoderm relationship during gastrulation [36]. Thus, during vertebrate gastrulation, the cell behavior is strictly coordinated in time and space by various signaling pathways. In vertebrates, the non-canonical Wnt/planar cell polarity (Wnt/PCP) pathway is a key regulator of convergence and extension movements, also involved in the internalization of mesodermal cells and their migration [189]. The name Wnt is derived from a combination of two homologous genes; Wg (the Drosophila wingless gene) and Int (the murine homolog mouse mammary tumor virus integration site 1 gene) [190]. Wnt represents a large morphogenic family of secreted lipid-modified glycolproteins that during embryogenesis controls multiple developmental processes [189, 190] and during adult life regulates tissue maintenance and remodeling [188, 190]. At the cellular level, Wnt signals coordinate changes in cellular metabolism favoring either a "quiescent metabolism" or a "proliferating metabolism" [188, 190]. This is why it is tempting to speculate that common alterations in metabolic programming may accompany embryonic and/or stem cell differentiation and these may also be involved in adult tissue development and/or remodeling [190].

In summary, the post-traumatic inflammatory response could be considered a reaction of the body in which the mesenchymal cell plays a leading role during which the early events of embryonic development and particularly gastrulation are recreated. The mesenchymal cell due to its strategic and privileged location in the interstitial space is able to induce the successive phases of inflammation. Therefore, the mesenchymal cell uses the mast cell, to induce the expression of neurovascular inflammatory axes that have an extensive corporal projection and whose activity converges in the wounded skin. The correlation that can be established between the embryonic and inflammatory post-traumatic events suggests that the results obtained from the research about both great fields of knowledge must be interchangeable to obtain the maximum advantage in the daily care of patients' wounds [37].

ACKNOWLEDGEMENTS

We would like to thank Maria Elena Vicente for preparing the manuscript, Elizabeth Mascola for translating it into English and librarians of Complutense University Medical School, particularly the Director, Francisco Javier Jorge García-Reyes, and Manuela Crego and María José Valdemoro and B. Braun Surgical S.A. for their technical assistance.

This study was carried out in part with grants from Mutua Madrileña Research Foundation (Ref. nº PA 3077/2008 and AP5966/2009), MICINN PSI2010-19348 and with the special collaboration of the INEUROPA (Instituto de Neurociencias del Principado de Asturias).

CONFLICT OF INTEREST

The author(s) confirm that this chapter content has no conflict of interest.

REFERENCES

[1] Cone JB. Inflammation. Am J Surg 2001; 182: 558-562.

[2] Aller MA, Arias JL, Nava MP, Arias J. Post-traumatic inflammation is a complex response based on the pathological expression of the nervous, immune and endocrine functional systems. Exp Biol Med (Maywood) 2004; 229: 170-181.

[3] Aller MA, Arias JL, Sanchez-Patan F, Arias J. The inflammatory response: An efficient way of life. Med Sci Monit 2006 12: RA225-RA234.
[4] Singer AJ, Dagun AB. Current management of acute cutaneous wounds. N Engl J Med 2008; 359: 1037-1046.
[5] Arias JI, Aller MA, Arias J. Surgical inflammation: a pathophysiological rainbow. J Transl Med 2009; 7: 19.
[6] Vande Velde C, Cizeau J, Dubik D, Alimonti J, Brown T, Israels S, Hakem R, Greenberg AH. BNIP3 and genetic control of necrosis-like cell death through the mitochondrial permeability transition pore. Mol Cell Biol 2000; 20: 5454-5468.
[7] Jin Z, El-Deiry WS. Overview of cell death signaling pathways. Cancer Biol & Ther 2005; 4: 139-163.
[8] Rosser BG, Gores GJ. Liver cell necrosis: Cellular mechanisms and clinical implications. Gastroenterology 1995; 108: 252-275.
[9] Medzhitov R. Origin and physiological roles of inflammation. Nature 2008; 454: 428-435.
[10] Aller MA, Arias JL, Arias JI, Sanchez-Patan F, Arias J. The inflammatory response recapitulates physiology through trophic mechanisms to the injured tissue. Med Hypotheses 2007; 68: 202-209.
[11] Kanitakis J: Anatomy, histology and immunohistochemistry of normal human skin. Eur J Dermatol 2002; 12: 390-399.
[12] Breitkreutz D, Mirancea N, Nischt R. Basement membranes in skin: unique matrix structures with diverse functions? Histochem Cell Biol 2009; 132: 1-10.
[13] Prost-Squarcioni C. Histology of skin and hair follicle. Med Sci (Paris) 2006; 22: 131-137.
[14] Gallucci S, Matzinger P. Danger signals: SOS to the immune system. Curr Opin Immunol 2001; 13: 114-119.
[15] Matzinger P. The danger model: A renewed sense of self. Science 2002; 296: 301-305.
[16] Yamaguchi Y, Yoshikawa K. Cutaneous wound healing: an update. J Dermatol 2001; 28: 521-534.
[17] Eming SA, Krieg T, Davidson JM. Inflammation in wound repair: Molecular and cellular mechanisms. J Invest Dermatol 2007; 127: 514-525.
[18] Gurtner GC, Werner S, Barrandon Y, Longaker MT. Wound repair and regeneration. Nature 2008; 453: 314-321.
[19] Eming SA, Hammerschmidt M, Krieg T, Roers A. Interrelation of immunity and tissue repair or regeneration. Semin Cell Dev Biol 2009; 20:517-527.
[20] Stojadinovic A, Carlson JW, Schultz GS, Davis TA, Elster EA. Topical advances in wound care. Gynecol Oncol 2008; 111: S70-S80.
[21] Monaco JL, Lawrence T. Acute wound healing. An overview. Clin Plastic Surg 2003; 30: 1-12.
[22] Redd MJ, Cooper L, Wood W, Stramer B, Martin P. Wound healing and inflammation: embryos reveal the way to perfect repair. Philos Trans R Soc Lond B Biol Sci 2004; 359: 777-784.
[23] Freitas I, Baronzio GF, Bono B, Grifini P, Bertone V, Sonzini N, Magrassi GR, Bonandrini L, Gerzeli G. Tumor interstitial fluid: Misconsidered component of the internal milieu of a solid tumor. Anticancer Res 1997; 17: 165-172.
[24] Arias JI, Aller MA, Arias J. The use of inflammation by tumor cells. Cancer 2005; 104: 223-228.
[25] Schäffer M, Werner S. Cancer as an overhealing wound: an old hypothesis revisited. Nat Rev Mol Cell Biol 2008; 9: 628-638.

[26] Aller MA, Arias JL, Nava MP, Arias J. Evolutive trophic phases of the systemic acute inflammatory response, oxygen use mechanisms and metamorphosis. Psicothema 2004; 16: 369-372.
[27] Miki T, Strom SC. Amnion-derived pluripotent/multipotent stem cells. Stem Cell Reviews 2006; 2: 133-142.
[28] Gay T, Huestis M. Bioanalytical procedures for monitoring in utero drug exposure. Anal Bioanal Chem 2007; 388: 1455-1465.
[29] Tong X-L, Wang L, Gao TB, Qin Y-G, Qi Y-Q, Xu Y-P. Potential function of amniotic fluid in fetal development. Novel insights by comparing the composition of human amniotic fluid with umbilical cord and maternal serum at mid and late gestation. J Clin Med Assoc 2009; 72: 368-373.
[30] Wagner CL, Taylor SN, Johnson D. Host factors in amniotic fluid and breast milk that contribute to gut maturation. Clin Rev Allerg Immunol 2008; 34: 191-204.
[31] Bellini C, Boccardo F, Bonioli E, Campisi C. Lymphodynamics in the fetus and newborn. Lymphology 2006; 39: 110-117.
[32] Bielinska M, Narita N, Wilson DB. Distinct roles for visceral endoderm during embryonic mouse development. Int J Dev Biol 1999; 43: 183-205.
[33] Collardeau-Frachon S, Scoazec J-Y: Vascular development and differentiation during human liver organogenesis. Anat Rec 2008; 291: 614-627.
[34] Isern J, Fraser ST, He Z, Baron MH. Development niches for embryonic erithroid cells. Blood Cells Mol Diseases 2010; 44:207-208.
[35] Naito M. Macrophage differentiation and function in health and disease. Pathol Int 2008; 58: 143-155.
[36] De Miguel MP, Arnalich-Montiel F, Lopez-Iglesias P, Blazquez-Martinez A, Nistal M. Epiblast-derived stem cells in embryonic and adult tissues. Int J Dev Biol 2009; 53: 1529-1540.
[37] Aller MA, Arias JI, Arias J. Pathological axes of wound repair: Gastrulation revisited. Theor Biol Med Model 2010; 7: 37.
[38] Wang Y, Steinbeisser H. Molecular basis of morphogenesis during vertebrate gastrulation. Cell Mol Life Sci 2009; 66: 2263-2273.
[39] Zuba-Surma EK, Kucia M, Ratajczak J, Ratajczak MZ. "Small Stem Cells" in adult tissues; very small embryonic-like stem cells (VSELs) stand up! Cytometry 2010; 75:4-13.
[40] Aller MA, Arias JL, Cruz A, Arias J. Inflammation: A way to understanding the evolution of portal hypertension. Theor Biol Med Model 2007; 4: 44.
[41] Eisenhut M. Changes in ion transport in inflammatory disease. J Inflamm 2006; 3: 5.
[42] Häussinger D. The role of cellular hydration in the regulation of cell function. Biochem J 1996; 313: 697-710.
[43] Schwartz L, Guais A, Pooya M, Abolhassani M. Is inflammation a consequence of extracellular hyperosmolarity? J Inflamm (Lond) 2009; 6: 21.
[44] Ng ChP, Helm C-LE, Swartz HA. Interstitial flow differentially stimulates blood and lymphatic endothelial cell morphogenesis *in vitro*. Microvasc Res 2004; 68: 258-264.
[45] Rutwski JM, Swartz HA. A driving force for change: interstitial flow as a morphoregulator. Trends Cell Biol 2006; 17: 44-50.
[46] Patwari P, Lee RT. Mechanical control of tissue morphogenesis. Circ Res 2008; 103: 234-243.

[47] Liersch R, Detmar M. Lymphangiogenesis in development and disease. Thromb Haemost 2007; 98: 304-310.

[48] Baumert PW. Acute inflammation after injury. Quick control speeds rehabilitation. Postgrad Med 1995; 97: 35-49.

[49] Sherwood ER, Toliver-Kinsky T. Mechanisms of the inflammatory response. Best Pract Res Clin Anesth 2004; 18: 385-405.

[50] Markiewski MM, Nilsson B, Ekdahl KN, Mollnes TE, Lambris JD. Complement and coagulation: Strangers or partners in crime? Trends Immunol 2007; 28: 184-192.

[51] Krem MM, Di Cera E. Evolution of enzyme cascades from embryonic development to blood coagulation. Trends Biochem Sci 2002; 27: 67-74.

[52] Esmon CT. The impact of the inflammatory response on coagulation. Thromb Res 2004; 114: 321-327.

[53] Wysocki AB, Grinell F. Fibronectin profiles in normal and chronic wound fluid. Lab Invest 1990; 63: 825-831.

[54] Oberyszyn TM. Inflammation and wound healing. Front Biosci 2007; 12: 2993-2999.

[55] Aller MA, Garcia-Dominguez J, Vergara P, Arias J. Mast cells in wound-healing cholestatic liver response. Burns 2010; 36: 292-294.

[56] Gokoo C. A primer on wound bed preparation. J Am Col Certif Wound Spec 2009; 1: 35-39.

[57] Iwatsuki K, Yamasaki O, Morizane S, Oono T. Staphylococcus cuatenous infections: invasion, evasion and aggresion. J Dermatol Sci 2006; 42: 203-214.

[58] Nerusu RC, Warner RL, Bhagavathula N, McClintock SD, Johnson KJ, Varani J. Matrix metalloproteinase-3 (stromelysin-I) in acute inflammatory tissue injury. Exp Mol Pathol 2007; 83: 169-176.

[59] Nathan C, Ding A. Non resolving inflammation. Cell 2010; 140: 871-882.

[60] Kennedy AD, De Leo FR. Neutrophil apoptosis and the resolution of infection. Immunol Res 2009; 43: 25-61.

[61] Panuncialman J, Falanga V. The science of wound bed preparation. Surg Clin N Am 2009; 89: 611-626.

[62] Guo S, Di Pietro LA. Factors affecting wound healing. J Dent Res 2010; 89: 219-229.

[63] Kostman JR, Dinubile MJ. Nodular lymphangitis: A distinctive but often unrecognized syndrome. Ann Intern Med 1993; 118: 883-888.

[64] Wilting J, Becker J, Buttler K, Weich HA. Lymphatics and inflammation. Curr Med Chem 2009; 16: 4581-4592.

[65] Roozendaal R, Mebius RE, Kraal G. The conduit system of the lymph node. Int Immunol 2008; 20: 1483-1487.

[66] Tammela T, Alitalo K: Lymphangiogenesis. Molecular mechanisms and future promise. Cell 2010; 140: 460-476.

[67] Chaplin DD. Overview of the immune response. J Allergy Clin Immunol 2010; 125: S3-S23.

[68] Stramer BM, Mori R, Martin P. The inflammation-fibrosis link? A Jekyll and Hyde role for blood cells during wound repair. J Invest Dermatol 2007; 127: 1009-1017.

[69] Glaros T, Larsen M, Li L. Macrophages and fibroblasts during inflammation, tissue damage and organ injury. Front Biosci 2009; 14: 3988-3993.

[70] Geissmann F, Manz MG, Jung S, Sieweke MH, Merad M, Ley K. Development of monocytes, macrophages and dendritic cells. Science 2010; 327: 656-661.

[71] Mosser DM, Edwards JP. Exploring the full spectrum of macrophage activation. Nat Rev Immunol 2008; 8: 958-969.

[72] Isenberg JS, Ridnour LA, Espey MG, Wink DA, Roberts DD. Nitric oxide in wound healing. Microsurgery 2005; 25: 442-451.

[73] Ribatti D, Conconi M-T, Nussdorfer GG. Non classic endogenous regulators of angiogenesis. Pharmacol Rev 2007; 59: 185-205.

[74] Chan LKW. Current thoughts on angiogenesis. J Wound Care 2009; 18: 12-16.

[75] Buckley CD, Pilling D, Lord JM, Akbar AN, Scheel-Toellner D, Salmon M. Fibroblasts regulate the switch from acute resolving to chronic persistent inflammation. Trends Immunol 2001; 22, 199-204.

[76] Barrientos S, Stojadinovic O, Golinko MS, Brem H, Tomic-Canic M. Growth factors and cytokines in wound healing. Wound Rep Reg 2008; 16: 585-601.

[77] Latremoliere A, Woolf CJ. Central sensitization: A generator of pain hypersensitivity by central neural plasticity. J Pain 2009; 10: 895-926.

[78] Pace MC, Mazzariello L, Passavanti MB, Sansone P, Barbarisi M, Aurillo C. Neurobiology of pain. J Cell Physiol 2006; 209: 8-12.

[79] Waxman SG, Dib-Jaji S, Cummins TR, Black JA. Sodium channels and pain. Proc Natl Acad Sci USA 1999; 96: 7635-7639.

[80] McMahon SB, Cafferty WBJ, Marchand F. Immune and glial cell factors as pain mediators and modulators. Exp Neurol 2005; 192: 444-462.

[81] Rittner HL, Brack A. Chemokines and pain. Curr Opin Invest Drugs 2006; 7: 643-646.

[82] Pezet S, McMahon SB. Neurotrophins: Mediators and modulators of pain. Ann Rev Neurosci 2006; 29: 507-538.

[83] McEwen BS. Physiology and neurobiology of stress and adaptation: Central role of the brain. Physiol Rev 2007; 87: 873-904.

[84] Clarke RW, Harris J. The organization of motor responses to noxious stimuli. Brain Res Rev 2004; 46: 163-172.

[85] Flierl MA, Rittirsch D, Huber-Lang M, Sarma JV, Ward PA. Catecholamines-crafty weapons in the inflammatory arsenal of immune/inflammatory cells or opening Pandora's box? Mol Med 2008; 14: 195-204.

[86] Czura CJ, Tracey KJ. Autonomic neural regulation of immunity. J Int Med 2005; 257: 156-166.

[87] Holzer P. Neurogenic vasodilatation and plasma leakage in the skin. Gen Pharmacol 1998; 30: 5-11.

[88] Muangman P, Muffley LA, Anthony JP, Spenny ML, Underwood RA, Olerud JE, Gibran NS. Nerve growth factor accelerates wound healing in diabetic mice. Wound Repair Regen 2004; 12: 44-52.

[89] Scott JR, Muangman P, Gibran NS. Making sense of hypertrophic scar: a role for nerves. Wound Repair Regen 2007; 15: S27-S31.

[90] Helle KB. Regulatory peptides from chromogranin A and secretogranin II: Putative modulators of cells and tissues involved in inflammatory conditions. Regul Pept 2009; *in press.*

[91] Hsu ES. Practical management of complex regional pain syndrome. Am J Ther 2009; 16: 147-154.

[92] Oaklander AL, Fields HL. Is reflex sympathetic dystrophy/complex regional pain syndrome type I a small-fiber neuropathy? Ann Neurol 2009; 65: 629-638.

[93] Bove GM. Focal nerve inflammation induces neuronal signs consistent with symptoms of early complex regional pain syndromes. Exp Neurol 2009; 219: 223-227.
[94] Jänig W. The fascination of complex regional pain syndrome. Exp Neurol 2010; 221:1-4.
[95] Buchanan EP, Longaker MT, Lorenz HP. Fetal skin wound healing. Adv Clin Chem 2009; 48: 137-161.
[96] Fu X, Li H. Mesenchymal stem cells and skin wound repair and regeneration: possibilities and questions. Cell Tissue Res 2009; 335: 317-321.
[97] Seifert O, Mrowietz U. Keloid scarring: bench and bedside. Arch Dermatol Res 2009; 301: 259-272.
[98] Rahban SR, Garner WL. Fibroproliferative scars. Clin Plastic Surg 2003; 30: 77-89.
[99] Bloemen MCT, Van Der Veer WM, Ulrich MMW, Van Zuijlen PPM, Niessen FB, Middelkoop E. Prevention and curative management of hypertrophic scar formation. Burns 2009; 35: 463-475.
[100] Butler PD, Longaker MT, Yang GP. Current progress in keloid research and treatment. J Am Coll Surg 2008; 206: 731-741.
[101] Kohyama T, Yamauchi Y, Takizawa H, Kamitani S, Kawasaki S, Nagase T. Histamine stimulates human lung fibroblast migration. Mol Cell Biochem 2009; 337:77-81.
[102] Van der Veer W, Bloemen MCT, Ulrich MMW, Molema G, Van Zuijlen PP, Middelkoop E, Niessen FB. Potential cellular and molecular causes of hypertrophic scar formation. Burn 2009; 35: 15-29.
[103] Sorrel JM, Caplan AI. Fibroblast – A diverse population at the center of it all. Int Rev Cell Mol Biol 2009; 276: 161-214.
[104] Phan SH. Biology of fibroblasts and myofibroblasts. Proc Am Thorac Soc 2008; 5: 334-337.
[105] Vaheri A, Enzerink A, Räsänen K, Salmenperä P. Nemosis, a novel way of fibroblast activation, in inflammation and cancer. Exp Cell Res 2009; 315:1633-1638.
[106] Hinz B. The myofibroblast: Paradigm for a mechanically active cell. J Biomechanics 2010; 43:146-155.
[107] Pera MF, Trounson AO. Human embryonic stem cells: prospects for development. Development 2004; 131: 5515-5525.
[108] Chaffer CL, Thompson EW, Williams ED. Mesenchymal to epithelial transition in development and disease. Cells Tissues Organs 2007; 185: 7-19.
[109] Nakanuma Y, Stao Y, Kiktao A. Pathology and pathogenesis of portal venopathy idiopathic portal hypertension: Hints from systemic sclerosis. Hepatol Res 2009; 39: 1023-1031.
[110] Hinz B. Formation and function of the myofibroblast during tissue repair. J Invest Dermatol 2007; 127: 526-537.
[111] Burchfield JS, Dimmeler S. Role of paracrine factors in stem and progenitor cell mediated cardiac repair and tissue fibrosis. Fibrogenesis Tissue Repair 2008; 1: 4.
[112] Pilling D, Fan T, Huang D, Kaul B, Gomer RH. Identification of markers that distinguish monocyte-derived fibrocytes from monocytes, macrophages, and fibroblasts. PLoS One 2009; 4: e7475.
[113] Seta N, Kuwana M. Human circulating monocytes as multipotential progenitors. Keio J Med 2007; 56: 41-47.
[114] Davidson LA, Joshi SD, Kim HY, Von Dassow M, Zhang L, Zhou J. Emergent morphogenesis: Elastic mechanics of a self-deforming tissue. J Biochem 2010; 43: 63-70.

[115] Maekawa M, Ishizaki T, Boku S, Watanabe N, Fujita A, Iwamatsu A, Obinata T, Ohashi K, Mizuno K, Narumiya S. Signaling from Rho to the actin cytoskeleton through protein kinases ROCK and LIM-Kinase. Science 1999; 285: 895-898.
[116] Patwari P, Lee RT: Mechanical control of tissue morphogenesis. Circ Res 2008; 103: 234-243.
[117] Von Dassow M, Davidson LA. Natural variation in embryo mechanics: gastrulation in xeopus laevis is highly robust to variation in tissue stiffnes. Dev Dyn 2009; 238: 2-18.
[118] Eckes B, Nischt R, Krieg T. Cell-matrix interactions in dermal repair and scarring. Fibrogenesis Tissue Repair 2010; 3: 4.
[119] Patel J, Gudehithlu KP, Dunea G, Arruda JA, Singh AK. Foreign body-induced granulation tissue is a source of adult stem cells. Transl Res 2010; 155:191-199.
[120] Sen CK. Wound healing essentials: let there be oxygen. Wound Rep Reg 2009; 17: 1-18.
[121] Chung HM, Won CH, Sung JH. Responses of adipose-derived stem cells during hypoxia: enhanced skin-regenerative potential. Expert Opin Biol Ther 2009; 9: 1499-1508.
[122] Zhou J, Kim HY, Davidson LA. Actomyosin stiffens the vertebrate embryo during crucial stages of elongation and neural tube closure. Development 2009; 136: 677-688.
[123] Kalluri R, Weinberg RA. The basics of epithelial-mesenchymal transition. J Clin Invest 2009; 119: 1420-1428.
[124] Brown SB, Dransfield I. Electric fields and inflammation: May the force be with you. Scientific World Journal 2008; 8: 1280-1294.
[125] McCaig CD, Rajnicek AM, Song B, Zhao M. Controlling cell behavior electrically: current views and future potential. Physiol Rev 2005; 85: 943-978.
[126] Falanga V. Wound healing and its impairment in the diabetic foot. Lancet 2005; 366: 1736-1743.
[127] Balkwill F, Mantovani A. Cancer and inflammation: Implications for pharmacology and therapeutics. Clin Pharmacol Ther 2010; 87: 401-406.
[128] Kalluri R. EMT: when epithelial cells decide to become mesenchymal-like cells. J Clin Invest 2009; 119:1417-1419.
[129] De Perardinis RJ, Lum JJ, Hatzivassillou G, Thompson CB. The biology of cancer: Metabolic reprogramming fuels cell growth and proliferation. Cell Metab 2008; 7: 11-20.
[130] Vousden KH, Ryan KM. p53 and metabolism. Nat Rev Cancer 2009; 9: 691-699.
[131] Vander Heiden MG, Cantley LC, Thompson CB. Understanding the Warburg effect: The metabolic requirements of cell proliferation. Science 2009; 324: 1029-1033.
[132] Arias JI, Aller MA, Sanchez-Patan F, Arias J. Inflammation and cancer: Is trophism the link? Surg Oncol 2006; 15: 235-242.
[133] Arias JI, Aller MA, Arias J. Cancer cell: using inflammation to invade the host. Mol Cancer 2007; 6: 29.
[134] Wang Y, Steinbeisser H. Molecular basis of morphogenesis during vertebrates gastrulation. Cell Mol Life Sci 2009; 66: 2263-2273.
[135] Mikawa T, Poh AM, Kelly KA, Ishii Y, Reese DE. Induction and patterning of the primltive streak, an organizing center of gastrulation in the amniote. Develop Dynamics 2004; 229: 422-432.
[136] Acloque H, Adams MS, Fishwick K, Bronner-Fraser M, Nieto MA. Epithelial-mesenchymal transitions: the importance of changing cell state in development and disease. J Clin Invest 2009; 119: 1438-1449.

[137] Kalluri R, Neilson EG. Epithelial-mesenchymal transition and its implications for fibrosis. J Clin Invest 2003; 112: 1776-1782.

[138] Feng B, Chen L. Review of mesenchymal stem cells and tumors: Executioner or conspirator? Cancer Biother Radiopharm 2009; 24: 717-721.

[139] Niknejad H, Peirovi H, Jorjani M, Ahmadiani A, Ghanavi J, Seifalian M. Properties of the amniotic membrane for potential use in tissue engineering. Eur Cell Mater 2008; 15: 88-99.

[140] Yu SJ, Soncini M, Kaneko Y, Hess DC, Parolini O, Borlongan CV. Amnion: A potent graft source for cell therapy in stroke. Cell Transplant 2009; 18: 111-118.

[141] Chang YJ, Hwang SM, Tseng CP, Cheng FC, Huang SH, Hsu LW, Tsai MS. Isolation of mesenchymal stem cells with neurogenic potentials from the mesoderm of the amniotic membrane. Cells Tissues Organs 2010; [Epub ahead of print].

[142] McLaughlin PS. *In vitro* differentiation of human amniotic fluid derived cells; augmentation towards a neuronal, dopaminergic phenotype. Cell Biol 2010; [Epub ahead of print].

[143] Uberti MG, Pierpont YN, Ko F, Wright TE, Smith CA, Cruse CW, Robson M, PayWG. Amnion-derived cellular cytokine solution (ACCS) promotes migration of keratinocytes and fibroblasts. Ann Plast Surg 2010; 64:632-635.

[144] Koike S, Keino-Masu K, Ohto T, Sugiyama E, Takahashi S, Masu M. Autotaxin/lysophospholipase D-mediated lysophosphatidic acid signaling is required to form distinctive large lysosomes in the visceral endoderm cells of the mouse yolk sac. J Biol Chem 2009; 284: 33561-33570.

[145] Yoshid S, Wada Y. Transfer of maternal cholesterol to embryo and fetus in pregnant mice. J Lipid Res 2005; 46: 2168-2174.

[146] Terasawa Y, Cases SJ, Wong JS, Jamil H, Jothi S, Traber MG, Packer L, Gordon DA, Hamilton RL, Farese RV. A poliprotein B-releted gene expression and ultrastructural characteristic of lipoprotein secretion in mouse yolk sac during embryonic development. J Lipid Res 1999; 40: 1967-1977.

[147] Rantakari P, Lagerbohm H, Kaimairen M, Suomela J-P, Strauss L, Sainio K, Pakarinen P, Poutanen M. Hydroxysteroid (17β) dehydrogenase 12 is essential for mouse organogenesis and embryonic survival. Endocrinology 2010; 151:1893-1901.

[148] Conti L, Cattaneo E. Neural stem cell systems: physiological players or *in vitro* entities? Nat Rev Neurosci 2010; 11: 176-187.

[149] Dazzi F, Ramasamy R, Glennie S, Jones SP, Roberts I. The role of mesenchymal stem cells in haemopoiesis. Blood Rev 2006; 20: 161-171.

[150] Phinney DG, Prockop DJ. Mesenchymal stem/Multipotent stromal cells: The state of transdifferentiation and modes of tissue repair – current views. Stem Cells 2007; 25: 2896-2902.

[151] Fraser ST, Baron MH. Embryonic fates for extraembryonic lineages: New perspectives. J Cell Biochem 2009; 107: 586-591.

[152] Selman M, Pardo A, Kaminski N. Idiopathic pulmonary fibrosis: Aberrant recapitulation of developmental programs? Plos Medicine 2008; 5: e62.

[153] Roh TS, Rah DK, Park BY. The fetal wound healing: a review. Yonsei Med J 2001; 42: 630-633.

[154] Blanpain C, Fuchs E. Epidermal homeostasis: a balancing act of stem cells in the skin. Nat Rev Mol Cell Biol 2009; 10: 207-217.

[155] Galli SJ, Kalesnikoff J, Grimbaldeston MA, Piliponsky AM, Williams CMM, Tsai M. Mast cells as "tunable" effector and immunoregulatory cells: recent advances. Ann Rev Immunol 2005; 23: 749-786.
[156] Ng MFY. The role of mast cells in wound healing. Int Wound J 2010; 7: 55-61.
[157] Baver O, Razin E. Mast cell-nerve interactions. News Physiol Sci 2000; 15: 213-218.
[158] Tore F, Tuncel N. Mast cells: target and source of neuropeptides. Curr Pharm Des 2009; 15: 3433-3445.
[159] Grützkau A, Krüger-Krasagakes S, Baumeister H, Schwartz C, Kögel H, Welker P, Lippert U, Henz BM, Möller A. Synthesis, storage and release of vascular endothelial growth factor/vascular permeability factor (VEGF/VPF) by human mast cells: Implications for the biological significance of VEGF. Mol Biol Cell 1998; 9: 875-884.
[160] Russo A, Russo G, Peticca M, Pietropaolo C, Dirosa M, Jovone T. Inhibition of granuloma-associated angiogenesis by controlling mast cell mediator release: role of mast cell protease-5. Br J Pharmacol 2005; 145: 24-33.
[161] Nienartowicz A, Sobaniec-Lotowska ME, Jarocka-Cyrta E, lemancewicz D. Mast cells in neoangiogenesis. Med Sci Monit 2006; 12: RA53-RA56.
[162] Soucek L, Lawlor ER, Soto D, Shchors K, Swigart LB, Evan GI. Mast cells are required for angiogenesis and macroscopic expansion of Myc-induced pancreatic islet tumors. Nat Med 2007; 13: 1211-1218.
[163] Galli SJ, Nakae S. Mast cells to the defense. Nat Immunol 2003; 4: 1160-1162.
[164] Nakaya Y, Sheng G. Epithelial to mesenchymal transition during gastrulation: an embryological view. Dev Growth Differ 2008; 50: 755-766.
[165] Doherty T, Broide D. Cytokines and growth factors in airway remodeling in asthma. Curr Opin Immunol 2007; 19: 676-680.
[166] Kato A, Schleimer RP. Beyond inflammation: airway epithelial cells are at the interface of innate and adaptive immunity. Curr Opin Immunol 2007; 19: 711-720.
[167] Holgate ST. Epithelium dysfunction in asthma. J Allergy Clin Immunol 2007; 120: 1233-1244.
[168] Aller MA, Arias JL, Arias J. The mast cell integrates the splanchnic and systemic inflammatory response in portal hypertension. J Transl Med 2007; 5: 44.
[169] Nathan C. Oxygen and the inflammatory cell. Nature 2003; 422: 675-676.
[170] Diegelmann RF, Evans MC. Wound healing: an overview of acute, fibrotic and delayed healing. Front Biosci 2004; 9: 283-289.
[171] Mori R, Shaw TJ, Martin P. Molecular mechanisms linking wound inflammation and fibrosis: knockdown of osteopontin leads to rapid repair and reduced scarring. J Exp Med 2008; 205: 43-51.
[172] Andre J, Gallini R, Betsholtz C. Role of platelet-derived growth factors in physiology and medicine. Genes Dev 2008; 22: 1276-1312.
[173] Hamilton TG, Klinghoffer RA, Corrin PD, Soriano P. Evolutionary divergences of platelet-derived growth factor α receptor signaling mechanisms. Mol Cell Biol 2003; 23: 4013-4025.
[174] Weisel-Eichler A, Libersat F. Venom effects on monoaminergic systems. J Comp Physiol A. Neuroethol Sens Neura Behav Physiol 2004; 190: 683-690.
[175] Chai OH, Kim EK, Lee Y-H, Kim J-G, Baik BJ, Lee MS, Han EH, Kim HT, Song CH. Histamine release induced by dendroaspis natriuretic peptide from rat mast cells. Peptides 2001; 22: 1421-1436.

[176] Toledo RC, Jared C. Cutaneous glanular glands and amphibian venoms. Comp Biochem Physiol 1995; 111A: 1-29.

[177] Brinkman DL, Burnell JN. Biochemical and molecular characterisation of cubozoan protein toxins. Toxicon 2009; 54: 1162-1173.

[178] Suput D. *In vivo* effects of cnidarian toxins and venoms. Toxicon 2009; 54: 1190-1200.

[179] Birsa LM, Verity PG, Lee RF. Evaluation of the effects of various chemicals on discharge of and pain caused by jellyfish nematocysts. Comp Biochem Physiol C Toxicol Pharmacol 2010; 151: 426-430.

[180] Flügge G, Van Kampen M, Mijnster MJ. Perturbations in brain monoamine system during stress. Cell Tissue Res 2004; 315: 1-14.

[181] Greaves MW. Pathogenesis and treatment of pruritus. Curr Allergy Asthma Rep 2010; 10:236-42.

[182] Matsue H, Kambe N, Shimada S. Murine fetal skin-derived cultured mast cells: A useful tool for discovering functions of skin mast cells. J Invest Dermatol 2009; 129: 1120-1125.

[183] Ruiz-Maldonado R, Orozco-Covarrubias ML. Postinflammatory hypopigmentation and hyperpigmentation. Semin Cutan Med Surg 1997; 16: 36-43.

[184] Lacz NL, Vafaie J, Kihiczak NI, Schwartz RA. Postinflammatory hyperpigmentation: a common but troubling condition. Int J Dermatol 2004; 43: 362-365.

[185] Engrav LH, Garner WL, Tredget EE. Hypertropic scar, wound contraction and hyper-hypopigmentation. J Burn Care Res 2007; 28: 593-597.

[186] Kragl M, Knapp D, Nacu E, Khattak S, Maden M, Epperlein HH, Tanaka EM. Cells keep a memory of their tissue origin during axolotl limb regeneration. Nature 2009; 460: 60-65.

[187] Kuroda Y, Kitada M, Wakao S, Nishikawa K, Tanimura Y, Makinoshima H, Goda M, Akashi H, Inutsuka A, Niwa A, Shigemoto T, Nabeshima Y, Nakahata T, Nabeshima Y-I, Fujiyoshi Y, Dezawa M. Unique multipotent cells in adult human mesenchymal cell populations. PNAS 2010; 107:8639-8643

[188] Li L, Clevers H. Coexistence of quiescent and active adult stem cells in mammals. Science 2010; 327: 542-545.

[189] Roszko I, Sawada A, Solnica-Krezel L. Regulation of convergence and extension movements during vertebrate gastrulation by the Wnt/PCP pathway. Semin Cell Develop 2009; 20: 986-997.

[190] Sethi JK, Vidal-Puig A. Wnt signalling and the control of cellular metabolism. Biochem J 2010; 427: 1-17.

Send Orders for Reprints to reprints@benthamscience.net
Surgical Inflammation, **2013**, 99-128

CHAPTER 4

Phases of the Acute Inflammatory Response to the Injury

Maria-Angeles Aller[1], Jose-Ignacio Arias[2], Isabel Prieto[3], Carlos Gilsanz[4], Jorge-Luis Arias[5], Heping Yang[6] and Jaime Arias[1,*]

[1]Surgery Department, School of Medicine, Complutense University of Madrid, Madrid, Spain; [2]General and Digestive Surgery Unit, Monte Naranco Hospital, Oviedo, Asturias, Spain; [3]General and Digestive Surgery Unit, La Paz Hospital, Autonoma University of Madrid, Madrid, Spain; [4]General Surgery Unit, Sudeste Hospital, Arganda del Rey, Madrid, Spain; [5]School of Psychology, University of Oviedo, Oviedo, Asturias, Spain and [6]Division of Gastroenterology and Liver Disease, USC Research Centre for Liver Diseases, Los Angeles, California, USA

Abstract: The surgical inflammatory response can be a type of high-grade acute stress response associated with an increasingly complex trophic functional system for using oxygen. This systemic neuro-immune-endocrine response seems to induce the re-expression of 2 extraembryonic-like functional axes, *i.e.* coelomic-amniotic and trophoblastic-yolk-sac-related, within the injured tissues and organs, thus favoring their re-development. Accordingly, through the up-regulation of two systemic inflammatory phenotypes, *i.e.* neurogenic and immune-related, a gestational-like response using embryonic functions would be induced in the patient's injured tissues and organs, which would therefore result in their repair. A comparison has been established between the pahtophysiological mechanisms that are produced during the inflammatory response and the physiological mechanisms that are expressed during early embryonic development. Surgical inflammation could be a high-grade stress response whose pathophysiological mechanisms would be based on the recapitulation of ontogenic and phylogenetic-related functions. Thus, the ultimate objective of surgical inflammation, as a gestational process, is creating new tissues/organs for repairing the injured ones. Since surgical inflammation and early embryonic development share common mechanisms of production, the factors that hamper the wound healing reaction in surgical patients could be similar to those that impair the gestational process.

Keywords: Coelomic-amniotic axis, trophoblastic-yolk sac axis, neuro-immune-endocrine response, gestation, surgical inflammation, poly-traumatized patient, macrophages, multiple organ dysfunction syndrome, systemic inflammatory response syndrome, hypercatabolism, ontogeny, phylogenetic evolution.

***Address correspondence to Jaime Arias:** Cátedra de Cirugía, Facultad de Medicina, Universidad Complutense, Pza. de Ramón y Cajal s.n., 28040 MADRID, Spain; Tel: +34 91 394 1389; Fax: +34 91 3947115; E-mail: jariasp@med.ucm.es

Jaime Arias, Maria-Angeles Aller and Jose-Ignacio Arias (Eds)

INTRODUCTION

Hans Selye described the stress response or General Adaptation Syndrome as a non-specific response to any stressor that occurs in three stages: general alarm reaction, resistance and exhaustion [1]. This syndrome was compared by Selye to other general defense reactions, such as the syndrome of inflammation, particularly in secondary to surgical injury [1, 2]. The considerable progress that has been made in discerning the cellular and molecular mechanisms of the stress-response [3-9] and the inflammatory response [10-15] enables establishing close links between both types of defense reactions [16-21]. All the new biochemical knowledge could also allow for a comprehensive interpretation of the complex interactions between the nervous, immune and endocrine responses triggered by a stressor during the evolution of both general reactions, and most especially when related to surgery.

SURGICAL INFLAMMATION

The inflammatory response related to surgery, either elective or anesthetized injury, or trauma-related, *i.e.* accidental or anaesthetized injury, could be a surgical inflammation [14]. Surgical inflammation usually triggered by psychophysiological stimuli occurs with pathophysiological changes associated with the stress response [22], which is why the stress response could have evolved from and is intricately linked to the surgical inflammatory response [16, 22]. From a general point of view, surgical inflammation is a systemic response of the body. Surgical inflammation varies in intensity, depending on the severity of the injury suffered. The pathophysiological characteristics of this systemic response are obvious in the cases of severe injury, as seen in polytraumatized patients [14, 23-25]. In the cases of mild injury, however, such as in skin wound healing, the systemic response is imperceptible or subtle [22]. Severe injury induces a systemic inflammatory response that seems to develop by expressing three successive and overlapping phenotypes: the neurogenic, immune and endocrine [12, 26] (Table **1**). The mechanisms that regulate the systemic surgical inflammatory response would be based on the body metabolic capacity for using oxygen through the three phases of its evolution towards repair. In turn, the diverse ways used for cellular energy production would define the metabolic ability of each phenotype [12, 26]. The above-mentioned phenotypes, which characterize the evolution of the systemic inflammatory response to the injury, have been represented as focused and integrated within an interstitial circular space restricted by the different types of the endothelium making up the microcirculatory system (Fig. **1**). This suggests that the systemic endothelial dysfunction, in its broadest sense, not only affects the three principal types of endothelium that are involved in the inflammatory response – the blood capillary, lymphatic and venous-, but also produces an endothelial-type redistribution with the progressive prominence of the venous and lymphatic endothelium at the expense of the blood capillary endothelium. When the systemic endothelium functions normally, the blood capillary endothelium would therefore recover its leading role mediating the exchange of oxygen, nutrients and waste catabolites. Meanwhile, the inflammatory activity mediated by the venous and lymphatic endothelium would be dramatically reduced [26] (Fig. **1**). The molecular and cellular mediators of the host stress response to the injury are therefore selected for passing through the heterogeneous endothelial barrier that limits the interstitium, where the inflammatory battle will be fought.

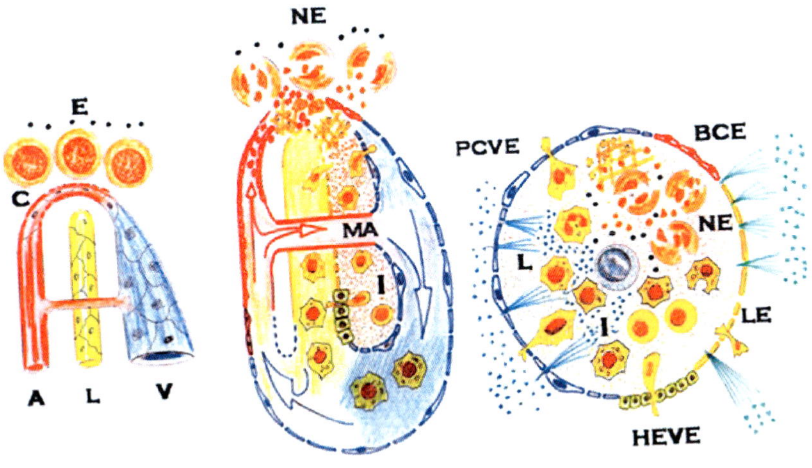

Figure 1: Schematic representation of microcirculation. In a steady state, the arterial blood flow moves through the capillaries, where it is deoxygenated before reaching the post-capillary venule. The lymphatic drainage from the interstitial space is reduced and there is a dynamic balance between the formation and the elimination of the interstitial fluid (left). When inflammation is produced, the arterial blood flow cannot be deoxygenated, firstly because the epithelium is necrosed and, secondly since capillaries are also necrosed and/or obstructed. Arterial blood flow bypass through metaarteriolas prevents the post-capillary vein from being exposed to

high oxygen levels. In addition, lymphatic flow gains an unusual prominence (middle). The inflamed interstitium could be represented as surrounded by the different types of endothelium that make up microcirculation, as an "endothelial egg". The venous and lymphatic endothelium acquires higher extension and functionality since the molecular and cellular exchange between the inflamed interstitium and the rest of the body, that is the host, is produced through them. A: artery; BCE: blood capillary endothelium; C: capillary; E: epithelium; HEVE: high endothelial venule endothelium; I: interstitium; L: lymphatic; LE: lymphatic endothelium; Leu: leukocytes; MA: meta-arteriole; NE: necrosed epithelium; PCVE: postcapillary venule endothelium; SC: stem cell.

Table 1: Surgical inflammation could be viewed as a high-degree stress response of the patient composed of three overlapping successive phenotypes

INFLAMMATORY PHENOTYPES IN SURGICAL INFLAMMATION	
NEUROGENIC IMMUNE	**ENDOCRINE**
- Stress sensation - Bone marrow-related response	- Epiblast-derived pluripotent stem cells
- Inflammatory pain - Hematopoietic stem cell activation	- Mesenchymal stem cell activation
- Fight-to-flight effect - Signaling molecules: - Fibrocytes	
- Analgesia * Chemokines - Endothelial progenitor cells	
- Hypothalamic-pituitary-adrenal cortical * Toll-like receptors - Signaling molecules:	
activation * Cytokines	* Chemokines and their receptors
- Sympatico-adrenal medullary activation - Leukocyte activation - Anabolic hormones	
- Tachycardia - Bacterial translocation	* Insulin
- Shock - Enzymatic stress	* GH
- Ischemia-reperfusion - Acute phase response	* IGF1
- Renin-angiotensin-aldosterone axis - Coagulaton/Complement system - CARS	
activation	- Resolution
- Hydroelectrolytic alterations - Coagulopathy	* Lipoxin
- Interstitial edema - Dyslipidemia	* Resolvins
- Increased lymph flow - SIRS / MODS	* Protectins
- Hypoxia - Lymph node activation	- Angiogenesis / vasculogenesis
- Anaerobic acidosis - Local stress response by leukocytes	- Blood capillaries
- Hypothermia - Local cholesterol-derived hormones - Specialezed epithelium	
- Hypercatabolism - Energetic stress	
- Hypermetabolism - Oxidative phosphorylation	
- Centralization of neuroendocrine functions	
- PTSD	

CARS:: Compensatory anti-inflammatory response syndrome. SIRS / MODS: Systemic inflammatory response syndrome / multiple organ dysfunction syndrome. PTSD: Post-traumatic stress disorder.

THE NEUROGENIC INFLAMMATORY PHENOTYPE

The systemic inflammatory response begins with an immediate pathological neuromuscular response that includes sensitive impairments like stress sensation, inflammatory pain, analgesia and motor alterations. In addition, skeletal muscle is also involved, *i.e.* the fight-to-fight effect, behavior and withdrawal reflexes, the myocardium-tachycardia- and the vascular smooth muscle with vasoconstriction and vasodilatation, which induce systemic and local hemodynamic impairments, *i.e.* blood flow redistribution and ischemia-reperfusion [25, 26]. A common and basic etiopathogenic mechanism of this complex neurogenic reaction would be sudden hydroelectrolytic alterations [26]. Consequently, there is increasing evidence that the systemic inflammatory response actually induces an impaired transport of electrolytes [27]. In this phase of surgical inflammation, interstitial hydroelectrolytic alterations therefore stand out and nutrition by diffusion predominates. The ischemia-reperfusion phenomenon, which causes oxidative and nitrosative stress, could be responsible for exudation and the progression of the interstitial edema. While edema is being produced, the lymphatic circulation is activated [22, 25]. Since the inflammatory interstitium is initially hypoxic and shows metabolic anaerobic acidosis, mainly due to the accumulation of acidic by-products including lactate, the hypoxic environment could represent an ideal stem cell niche [28, 29] (Fig. **2**). In the early evolutionary period of the stress neurogenic response, the hypothalamic-pituitary-adrenocortical, sympathetic-adrenal medullary and renin-angiotensin-aldosterone axes, with the secretion of catecholamines, glucocorticoids and mineralocorticoids in the circulation, are activated [5, 30-33]. Chromaffin vesicles in adrenal medullary chromaffin cells also store granins, which can function as prohormones giving rise to bioactive peptides, some with potent antimicrobial activity [34]. Consequently, these substances are selectively accumulated in the interstitial space of the tissues previously suffering from ischemia-reperfusion since endothelial permeability is increased, especially in the post-capillary venules [12, 22, 25]. The elevated central venous saturation of oxygen seen in many patients with multiple organ dysfunction may therefore be driven by the hyperdynamic state with shunting through the microcirculation and/or cellular dysoxia [35] (Fig. **2**).

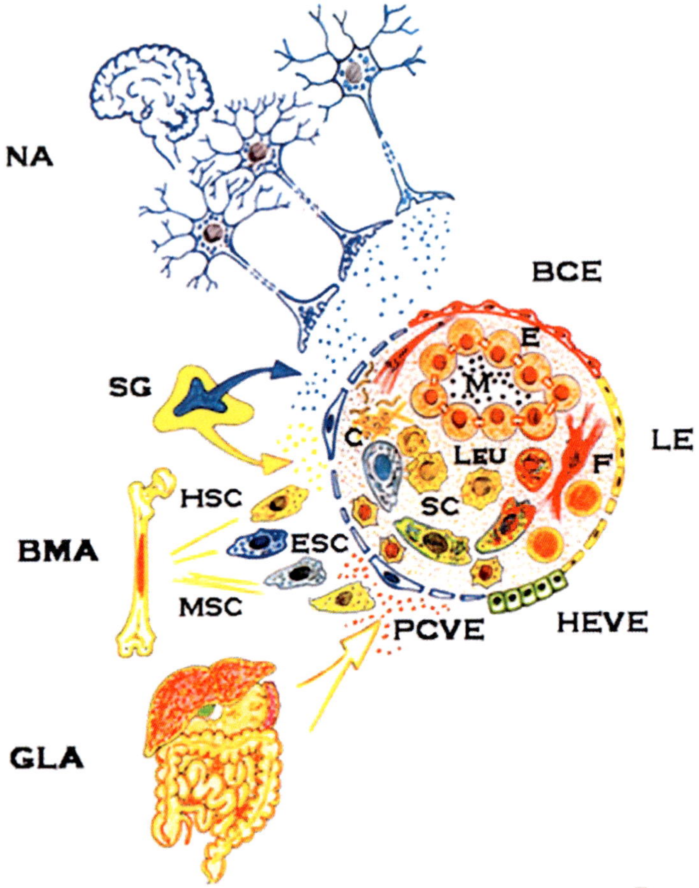

Figure 2: Surgical stressful inflammatory response. The host organism provides the inflamed interstitium molecules and cells by up-regulating a neurogenic-related axis (NA), a bone marrow-related axis (BMA) and a gut-liver axis (GLA). The molecular and cellular infiltration of the "endothelial egg" induces the development of a new tissue or organ using inflammatory mechanisms. BCE: blood capillary endothelium; C: coagulation; E: epithelium; ESC: endothelial precursor cell; F: fibroblast; HEVE: high endothelial venule endothelium; HSC: hemopoietic stem cell; LE: lymphatic endothelium; Leu: leukocytes; M: microbiome; MSC: mesenchymal stem cell; PCVE: postcapillary venule endothelium; SC: resident stem cell; SG: suprarenal gland.

THE IMMUNE INFLAMMATORY PHENOTYPE

The immune phenotype is the intermediate phase of the systemic inflammatory response to the stressor. In this phase, the interstitial space of the epithelial organs, which have previously suffered damage by ischemia-reperfusion, is occupied by leukocytes and bacteria. This recruitment happens in an edematous oxygen-poor environment [22, 25]. Today, the inflammatory bone-marrow-related response is considered both a key and complementary arm of the stress response [22]. The inflammatory activation of the bone marrow stem cell niche indicates the stimulation of the hematopoietic stem cells (HSCs) and the mesenchymal stem cells (MSCs), both multipotent stem cells [36]. HSCs are the progenitors of all blood and immune cells that infiltrate all the tissues and organs that have been previously primed by oxidative and nitrosative stress. Inflammatory signaling molecules, including leukotrienes, prostaglandins, interferons, tumor necrosis factor-alpha and toll-like receptors, appear to stimulate HSC proliferation in the short term [37]. In turn, interferon-gamma mediates HSC stimulation in response to chronic inflammation [38]. This immune phase represents enzymatic stress with processes related to intracellular digestion, *i.e.* autophagy, phagocytosis and antigen presentation, and extracellular digestion, *i.e.* fermentation, all of which favor tissue trophism [12, 26]. Macrophages and dendritic cells also use the lymphatic circulation for migration. In this way, macrophages are transported within the lymphatic circulation until reaching the lymph nodes where they activate lymphocytes by antigen presentation [26, 39] (Fig. **2**). The cells that infiltrate the interstitium in the inflamed tissues and organs, because of the open microcirculatory system, acquire metabolic characteristics that transform them into tissues with great functional autonomy. Thus monocytes, macrophages and lymphoid cells express β- and α_1-adrenoceptors and catecholamines [40-42]. Lymphocytes store and synthesize serotonin [43] and immune cell-derived cholinergic activity can modulate inflammation [44, 45]. Furthermore, the pro-opiomelanocortin (POMC)-peptides found in leukocytes, including adrenocorticotrophin (ACTH) exhibit the same structure of those present in the pituitary [46, 47]. POMC-derived peptides have a very ancient origin and an extremely high level of conservation [48]. They also play a critical role in regulating energy balance [49]. Maybe these are the reasons why the stress response axis can be retrieved by the immunocytes participating in the inflamed interstitium of tissues and organs, where the corticotropin-releasing hormone (CRH), ACTH-like and biogenic amines are present [47].

In this phase of the inflammatory response, the acute phase reaction becomes more prominent and exhibits diverse pathophysiological changes such as pyrexia, leukocytosis and dramatic changes in the plasmatic concentrations of acute phase proteins [50, 51]. Acute phase proteins are circulating biomarkers of inflammation and are defined as either positive or negative, depending on whether they increase or decrease during the inflammatory response [50, 52]. Albumin, transferrin and retinol-binding proteins are considered as negative acute phase proteins [51]. On the other hand, positive acute phase proteins are produced by hepatocytes when activated by IL-6 as part of the innate immune response [53]. The hepatic acute phase response uses skeletal muscle proteolysis as the main source for free amino acids [54]. Positive acute phase proteins include proteins of the coagulation-fibrinolysis system (fibrinogen, prothrombin, factor VIII, von-Willebrand factor, complement factors, plasminogen), protease inhibitors (alpha-1-antitrypsin, alpha-1-antichymotrypsin), transport proteins (ceruloplasmin, hemopexin, haptoglobin) and lipid transport proteins (serum amyloid A and serum amyloid P) [50, 51]. However, C-reactive protein is the main human acute phase protein and one of the most sensitive markers of inflammation, which is why biochemical tests are frequently requested [50, 55]. Trauma-induced coagulopathy is a biphasic process. Coagulopathy is initially related to excessive hyperfibrinolysis, hyperfibrinogenolysis, hypothermia, acidosis and hypometabolism. These changes affect the coagulation system and produce inappropriate anticoagulation with hemorrhagic tendency [56]. Then the acute post-traumatic stress correlates with pro-coagulant changes, such as increased levels of fibrinogen, clotting factors VII, VIII and XII and the von Willebrand factor [57]. Consequently, those patients which develop sepsis can suffer disseminated intravascular coagulation, with intravascular microcoagulation and subsequent consumption coagulopathy [56, 58]. Adrenal medullary epinephrine secretion exhibits robust hepatic glycogenolysis that rapidly elevates blood glucose concentrations, but also simultaneously stimulates lipolysis [59]. The major alterations in lipid metabolism during the systemic inflammatory response syndrome include increased lipolysis and fatty acid recycling, hypertriglyceridemia and hepatic steatosis. Hypocholesterolemia, however, is common in patients with critical illness and may be valuable for prognosis [58]. Serum amyloid A increases the ability of HDL to serve as an acceptor for cellular cholesterol efflux, promoting the removal of excess cholesterol from macrophages as well as increasing the availability of cellular free cholesterol [60]. In this way, acute-phase serum amyloid A belongs to a systemic response to injury in order of recycling cholesterol and lipoproteins from destroyed and damaged cells. If so, the reusing of cholesterol during severe injury could play a relevant survival role [61]. In fact, the predominance of the lipid metabolism with accumulation of cholesterol in the inflamed tissue could be attributed to its role as a precursor molecule of an array of hormones, including aldosterone, corticoids, progesterone, androgens and estrogen [62], and even vitamin D [63]. Major injury due to surgical or major trauma produces potentially severe immunological dysfunction resulting in the systemic inflammatory response syndrome (SIRS) and early multiple organ dysfunction syndrome (MODS), mediated primarily by the innate immune system [23-25, 64]. This is followed by a compensatory anti-inflammatory response syndrome (CARS) and late MODS, which are primarily mediated by the adaptive immune system [23, 24, 64]. Infection and sepsis may exhibit organ system dysfunction rather than its cause [65]. If so, gastrointestinal dysfunction and associated microbiome dysfunction may cause bacterial intestinal translocation to colonize the inflamed interstitium in the sickest patients with immunoparalysis [25, 65]. Hypercatabolism and hypermetabolism are both characteristic metabolic alterations of SIRS after polytrauma [24]. This metabolic association could suggest that, during the evolution of the immune response due to a severe injury, the body suffers a deconstruction process. The body would then obtain the substrates it needs to gestate new tissues and organs for self-repair.

THE ENDOCRINE INFLAMMATORY PHENOTYPE

Nutrition mediated by blood capillaries is established by angiogenesis. The main functional properties of the blood microcirculation are the exchange of oxygen as well as nutrients and waste substances. This oxygen support induces oxidative metabolism, but also causes oxidative stress. This is an effective way for obtaining ATP from blood substrates, which begins with the Krebs cycle and ends with oxidative phosphorylation [12, 25]. Oxygen and oxidative metabolism are an excellent combination through which cells can obtain an abundant energy supply for tissue and organ repair using specialized cells, although this combination also produces energetic stress [25].

Little is known, however, about the ability of eukaryotic cells to drive the redox state for supporting specialized functions [66]. Although NF-κB mainly triggers inflammation, it also resolves it [67]. Clearly, the mechanisms promoting tissue structuring and restoring of functions also include those involved in resolving inflammation [68]. In regards with endogenous pro-resolving lipid mediators, lipoxins, resolvins and protectins are the most studied. But in brief, these pro-resolving lipids return the pro-inflammatory phenotype to its prior physiological state and subsequently, the microcirculatory functions of tissues and organs return to homeostasis [69]. Inflammatory chemokines trigger the interstitial recruitment of leukocytes, but also signal the homing endothelial progenitor cells for migrating from the bone marrow to the sites of angiogenesis [70]. A novel mechanism has been identified in vasculature development known as vasculogenesis, a process in which new vessels form from bone marrow derived endothelial progenitor cells [71] rather than from sprouting or elongation of existing vessels [72, 73]. During vasculogenesis or neovascularization, precursor or stem cells from adult bone marrow are mobilized into circulation in response to various signals, including chemokines and their receptors, and are homed to the site where they differentiate into mature endothelial cells [74]. Although the key physiological role of circulating endothelial progenitor cells in adults is to ultimately maintain vascular integrity, they also home to and aid to revascularize ischemic inflammatory organs and tissues [71]. In repair, however, mesodermal-derived cells, particularly fibrocytes derived from the bone marrow stem cell niche, like MSC [75] or, alternatively epiblast-derived pluripotent stem cells that survive beyond embryonic development in adult tissues as so-called "hibernating backup" [76], play the leading role in the repair reaction. Fibrocytes can accelerate the recovery of homeostasis by the injured organism through stimulating proliferation and vessel remodeling. The recruitment of mural mesenchymal derived cells, *i.e.* pericytes and vascular smooth muscle cells, to nascent blood vessels, plays an important role in stabilizing and maturing new vascular networks [72, 73]. Nutrition supported by mature blood capillaries is established through the expression of this angiogenic and/or vasculogenic phenotype, which makes tissue and organ regeneration possible or, by default, their repair through fibrosis [22, 25].

In this final convalescence phase, the hypercatabolic syndrome is inhibited by down-regulation of catabolic hormones and cytokines, *i.e.* noradrenaline, adrenaline, pro-inflammatory cytokines, cortisol and glucagon and the release of anabolic hormones and molecules, *i.e.* insulin, growth hormones, insulin-like growth factor-1, anabolic steroids or anti-inflammatory cytokines, which are supported by tissues and organs through the new vessel arrangement and morphology [77].

Since the above-mentioned neurogenic and immune phenotypes become autonomous when expressed in the peripheral inflamed area, during the last endocrine phenotype expression, the body regains control over the neoformed tissue. This progressive centralization of the neuroendocrine functions, *i.e.* sympathetic and vagal nervous system- and endocrine- hypothalamic-pituitary-organ-hormonal axes, could be related to the progressive repair of the new tissues, controlled in turn by peripheral stimuli [78]. The failure to correctly centralize the neuroendocrine axes, however, would cause a chronic dysregulation with dysfunctional impairment and patients would suffer post-traumatic stress disorders in the long term [79, 80].

THE INFLAMMATORY "INTERSTITIUM" BEHAVES LIKE AN ENDOTHELIAL EGG

The "interstitium" is accepted as the space where the battle of inflammation develops. In particular, during the surgical inflammatory response, the interstitial space increases its size exceedingly as a consequence of the successive infiltration it suffers by molecules, cells and bacteria. Since these molecular, cellular and bacterial inflammatory mediators enter the interstitium through an endothelial pathway, the interstitial inflammatory space could be represented as an "endothelial egg". Thus this inflammatory endothelial egg would get cellular and bacterial substrates through the post-capillary venule endothelium, the high endothelial venule endothelium in the lymph nodes and, in lesser degree, through the capillary endothelium. In turn, the lymphatic endothelium could be equivalent to an excretory system of the endothelial inflammatory egg (Fig. **3**). Consequently, the successive phases of the inflammatory response, which ultimately would lead to the production of a new tissue formed by parenchyma and stroma, would be produced in the interior of this hypothetical endothelial egg.

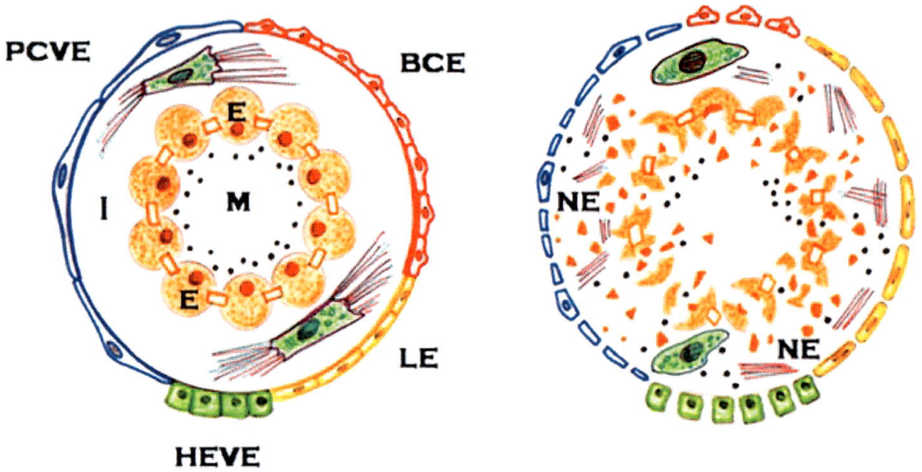

Figure 3: Schematic representation of normal tissue (left) and pathological (right) tissue when surgical inflammatory stress is developed. Epithelial necrosis triggers an inflammatory response in the interstitium that is restricted by an endothelial barrier made up of the different types of microcirculatory endothelium. BCE: blood capillary endothelium; E: epithelium; HEVE: high endothelial venule endothelium; I: interstitium; LE: lymphatic endothelium; M:microbiome; NE: necrosed epithelium; PCVE: post-capillary venule endothelium.

However, if harmful factors have an impact during the normal development of this hypothetical inflammatory egg, formation of a tissue similar to a pre-existing one by regeneration would be hindered, so the stromal component of the tissue would predominate and fibrosis would be induced. The deficit or excess of the above-mentioned molecular, cellular or bacterial mediator support also impairs the normal development of the inflammatory egg since it would prevent the development of a new tissue. Consequently, the inflammatory response would be chronic and finally, healing would fail. In surgical inflammation the "interstitium" is surrounded by a heterogenous endothelium. The different types of microcirculatory vascular endothelium that surround the inflammatory interstitium could function like an endothelial thermostat that auto-regulates bodily functions with the ability to return to normal in the short-term. However, when the auto-regulating ability of the interstitium is defective, an endothelial dysregulation inducing a chronic inflammatory pathology would be produced [26]. If we focus on the generic representation of the inflamed tissues and organs as an "endothelial egg", several hypothetical evolutive proposals could be considered during this egg development. The different types of evolution could range between its normal development and hitching, thanks to the influx of the mentioned inflammatory phenotypes induced by the host and the defective development due to noxious factors, which would involve endothelial egg development (intrinsic factors) and an effective response (by the host) to stress that induces normal gestation (extrinsic factors) (Fig. **3**).

RECAPITULATED EXTRAEMBRYONIC FUNCTIONS RELATED TO SURGICAL INFLAMMATORY PHENOTYPES

Surgical inflammation could recapitulate ontogeny by re-expressing two hypothetical extraembryonic trophic axes (amniotic and yolk sac or vitelline) in the interstitial space of the injured tissue [22, 78]. Thus surgical inflammation could represent the postnatal debut of ancestral biochemical mechanisms that were used for normal embryonic development. The re-expression of these old mechanisms is perhaps difficult to recognize during the adult life, since they are established in a very different environmental medium [22].

After fertilization, the first stage of embryogenesis is the zygote, which undergoes cleavage by mitosis. When the morula stage is reached, the embryo establishes polarity. The cells bind tightly to each other, forming a compact sphere (or blastocyst) with two different cell layers. The outermost layer becomes the trophoblast, giving rise to the placenta, and the inner cells become the inner cell mass, giving rise to the embryo and the remaining structures, including the amnion, yolk sac, and allantoids [81]. The extraembryonic "coelum" or exocoelomic cavity surrounds the blastocyst, which is formed of two structures, the amnion and the primary yolk sac. At the end of the fourth week of gestation, the developing exocoelomic cavity splits the extraembryonic mesoderm into two layers, the somatic mesoderm, lining the trophoblast, and the splanchnic mesoderm, covering the secondary yolk sac and the embryo [82] (Fig. **4**). Coelomic fluid results from the maternal serum to which placental and vitelline by-products are added [82, 83]. The hypothetical recapitulation of these phases of the embryonic development during the early surgical inflammatory response would imply the expression of functions similar to the extraembryonic "coelum" that surrounds the blastocyst. Accordingly, the phenotype could be adopted by the inflamed interstitium that subsequently induces the accumulation of fluid with similar characteristics to coelomic fluid in an environment with low pH and oxygen [82-84]. In essence, interstitial edema with high levels of proteins, in particular albumin, as well as electrolytes, metals, amino acids, antioxidants, cytokines and cholesterol-derived hormones would be produced in the inflammatory exudate [82-88]. This initial interstitial pro-inflammatory edema secondary to ischemia-reperfusion would play the leading role in the trophism of the injured tissue [12, 89]. The biological properties and the anatomical location of the exocoelomic cavity also suggest that it plays a major role as an essential nutritional pathway for the embryo and early fetus before placental circulation is fully established [83].

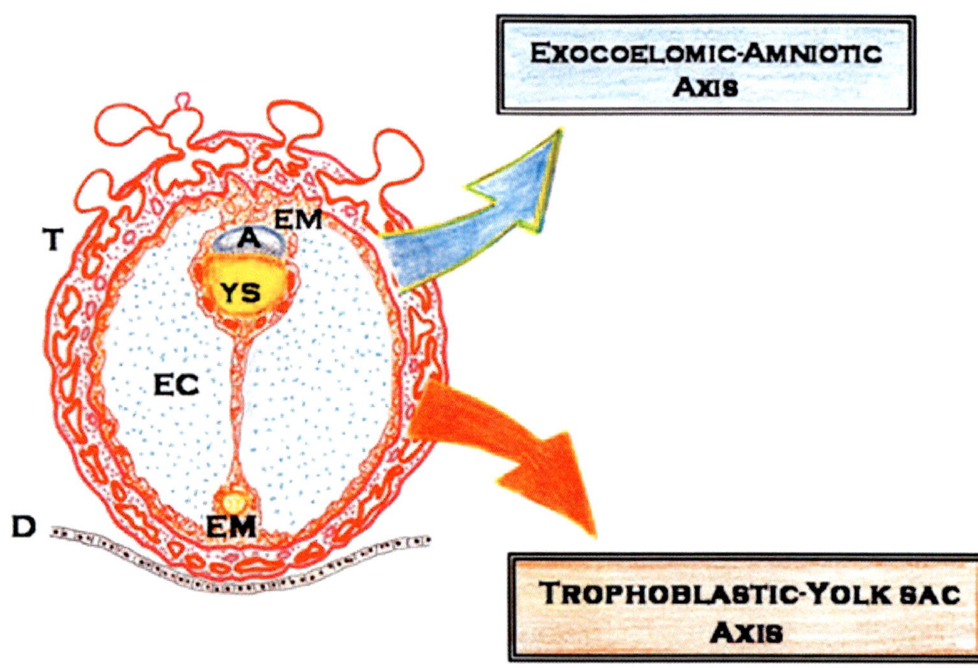

Figure 4: Schematic representation of early embryonic development. During early embryo development, the extraembryonic mesoderm and the exocoelomic cavity (EC) relate the trophoblast (T) to the amnion and the secondary yolk sac (YS). It could be proposed the existence of two extra-embryonic axes, an exocoelomic-amniotic axis and a trophoblastic-yolk sac axis, would enable the formation of the intraembryonic mesenchymal since they are integrated. These extraembryonic functions are expressed by the host organism when it suffers an injury and focus on the injured tissue or organ. After these functions are incorporated by the injured tissue or organ, this said tissue or organ acquires the embryonic functional autonomy needed to successfully repair itself. A: amnion; EC: exocoelomic cavity; EM: extraembryonic mesoderm; D: decidua; T: trophoblast; YS: secondary yolk sac.

The amnion is an embryonic functional axis with strong neurogenic potential [90]. Amnion-derived multipotent progenitor cells produce a unique mixture of cytokines and growth factors, called the "amnion-derived cellular cytokine solution", which achieves a close link between mesenchymal and epithelial cells during early embryo development [91]. The amniotic fluid surrounding the fetus may therefore be an extension of the extracellular space of the fetal tissues [92]. Furthermore, pluripotent stem cells within the amniotic fluid could be a new source for stem cell research [93, 94]. The amniotic-like phenotype could offer the stem cell a hypoxic and hydrated interstitial axis [92] with cytokines and growth factors [91] favoring not only nutrition by diffusion, but also transport, excretion and bacteriostatic and anti-inflammatory protection [92, 94] (Fig. **4**).

The wall of the secondary yolk sac in mammals is made up by an external mesothelial layer in relation with the exocoelomic cavity, a vascular interstitial mesenchyme and an endodermal layer surrounding the yolk sac cavity [82] (Fig. **4**). The formation of blood islands in the mesenchymal layer promotes the development of hematopoiesis and angiogenesis [95]. The endothelial and blood progenitors of blood islands develop independently from the epiblast before they migrate to the extraembryonic yolk sac. Hemangioblasts found in these blood islands could generate blood cells through intermediate progenitors called hemogenic endothelial cells [96]. From the sixth week of gestation, the secondary yolk sac develops as a cystic structure covered by a network of superficial small vessels [82]. The mesothelial and endodermal layers have absorptive functions and are active in endocytosis/digestion [95, 97]. In addition, the endodermal layer is the origin of several proteins including acute phase proteins such as prealbumin, albumin, transferrin and α_1-antitrypsin [93], as well as α-fetoprotein, which is produced by both, adult and fetal liver [82, 96].

A major function of the yolk sac is carbohydrate, protein and lipid accumulation for embryo nutrition. Because of that it is called "vitellum" [98]. The yolk sac therefore provides lipids and lipid-soluble nutrients to embryos when they begin to develop [98]. Particularly, the yolk sac endoderm is involved in the regulation of vascular integrity of developing embryos [99]. During the 10th week of gestation, however, the yolk sac starts to degenerate and quickly ceases to function [82]. The yolk sac-related phenotype could upregulate the lipid metabolism genes [99], the hematopoietic-cell derived control with recruitment of immune cells and the activation of an angiogenic switch [96] to enable new tissue immunological tolerance during the surgical inflammatory response. In addition, through the synthesis and release of acute phase proteins, this extraembryonic phenotype reduces oxidative, nitrosative and enzymatic stress and activates the Complement-coagulation system, regulates the lipid metabolism [50, 51] and favors phagocytosis [51], a specific form of endocytosis primarily associated with nutrition in unicellular organisms *i.e.* phagotrophic nutrition, and with innate and adaptive immunity in mammals [100].

During trophoblast differentiation, trophoblast cells also exhibit intense phagocytic activity leading to events as diverse as engulfment and destruction of extracellular material and the production of inflammatory mediators that may modulate both the immune response [100] and trophoblast invasiveness [101, 102].

THE RECAPITULATED AMNIOTIC-VITELLINE AXES AND THE INTERSTITIAL INFLAMMATORY ENDOTHELIAL EGG

The molecular and cellular contribution made by the above-mentioned extraembryonic membranes, *i.e.* exocoelomic cavity, amnion, yolk sac and trophoblast to the intraembryonic mesoderm, could be essential for embryo development and organogenesis [78]. Moreover, these primitive extraembryonic structures can be internalized by the embryo at early developmental stages [103]. Consequently, the hypothesized re-expression of these extraembryonic functions after injury during postnatal life could be a key process needed to repair the injured organism [22, 78]. In this way, both the amniotic and vitelline axes re-expressed during the interstitial inflammation would contribute to the "interstitial inflammatory endothelial egg" those molecules and cells that would be necessary during evolution of the wound healing response to form a new tissue by regeneration and/or by scarring. Therefore, these two axes act on the inflamed interstitium in a similar fashion as they act during embryonic development, although in this case an embryo is not created, but the injured tissue is repaired using similar mechanisms. The representation of the inflamed interstitial tissue like a sphere whose surface is covered by different types of endothelium-arterial capillary, venous and lymphatic- allows for a better understanding of the specific function of this endothelium in relationship with the embryo-like metabolism that is developed in this interstitium. In this way, it is possible to modify the type of substrates, cells or bacteria that the new developing tissue needs in each evolutionary phase of inflammation changing the venous incretory phenotype, and modifying the metabolism waste products using the different excretory functions of the lymphatic endothelium that surrounds it (Fig. **2**)

COUPLING THE RE-EXPRESSED EXTRAEMBRYONIC PHENOTYPES WITH POSTNATAL SURVIVAL

The systemic surgical inflammatory response is a complex process involving systemic alterations related to a stress response. The magnitude of this systemic response, however, could reflect the demands required for tissue and organ repair. Here we have been trying to establish similarities between the complex pathophysiological mechanisms developed in surgical inflammation and the pluripotential extraembryonic pathways during embryo development. While the surgical inflammatory response progresses, the re-expressed extraembryonic functions target the injured tissues and this would condition the evolution of the repair response. Embryonic programs adapted to the severity of the injury would then be activated to begin to repair. The recapitulation of the extraembryonic coelomic and amniotic functions could be represented by initially activating the systemic neurogenic axis, while the latter recapitulation of the trophoblast and yolk sac functions would be carried out by activating a systemic bone-marrow-related axis.

The activation of the pathological systemic axes, *i.e.* neurogenic and bone marrow-related, in the injured tissue could be completed in 2 steps. First, the upregulated amniotic phenotype would induce a sudden and early neurogenic response with systemic cardiovascular, hemodynamic, and hydroelectrolytic alterations. In this early response, cells that produce substances for export first synthesize and then store large amounts of molecules, such as biogenic amines [22], in secretory vesicles that are ready for rapid release [104]. In turn, the upregulated systemic vitelline phenotype could mediate the inflammatory bone marrow response through a lipid metabolic switch linked to steroid and acute phase response protein synthesis, respectively [22]. This slower response would therefore be developed by steroidogenic cells that store very little steroid hormones, in which case a rapid steroidogenic response would require immediate synthesis of new steroids, such as cortisol. The increase of the acute-phase protein synthesis, *i.e.* innate immunity, by the hepatocytes is linked with the acute phase response and follows the upregulation of pro-inflammatory cytokines and chemokines [50, 51].

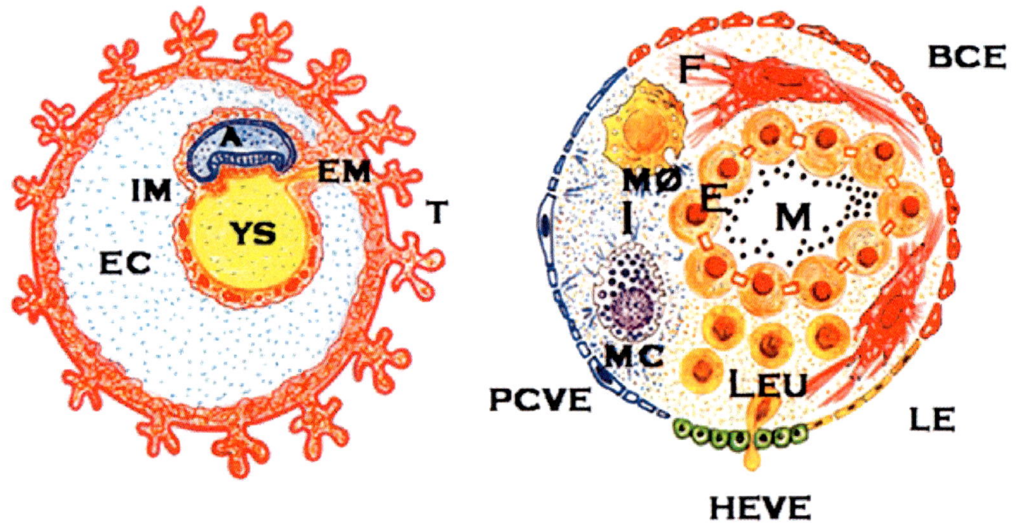

Figure 5: Comparative representation between the embryo, with its extra-embryonic membranes (left) and the inflamed tissue (right). Recapitulation of the extra-embryonic exocoelomic-amniotic (E-A)- axis and trophoblastic-yolk sac-related (T-YS) axis within the inflamed tissue would allow the development of a new tissue from the intra-embryonic mesoderm, like it occurs during embryonic development. BCE: blood capillary endothelium; E: epithelium; EC: exocoelomic cavity; EM: extra-embryonicmesoderm; F: fibroblast; HEVE: high endothelial venule endothelium; IM: intraembryonic mesenchyma; LE: lymphatic endothelium; Leu: leukocyte; M: microbiome; MC: mast cell; MØ: Macrophage; PCVE: postcapillary venule endothelium; YS: yolk sac.

Finally, the systemic pathological axes, *i.e.* neurogenic and bone-marrow related are focused and coupled in the interstitium of the injured tissues and organs. This interstitial integration of both pathological axes in the injured tissues and organs could finally induce a gastrulation-like process [78]. Gastrulation, which involves the *de novo* formation of reparative tissue, is based on the recapitulation of the intra-embryonic mesenchyme formation process [78, 81]. In essence, the integration of both extraembryonic-related phenotypes, coelomic-amniotic and trophoblast-vitelline, by the multipotent mesenchymal stem/stromal cells [105-107] would support the functional and metabolic heterogeneity needed to successively modulate their injured microenvironment through the evolution of the surgical inflammatory response [105, 107]. Therefore, the interaction of extraembryonic functional axes in the interstitium of the damaged tissue and organs allows for the recapitulation of the mechanisms characteristic of gastrulation, subsequently forming a mesenchyme similar to that present in the early development phases [22, 78].

Mesodermal-derived cells, particularly fibrocytes [108] or alternatively, epiblast-derived pluripotent stem cells that survive beyond embryonic development in adult tissues and known as the "hibernating backup" [109] play the leading role in the repair reaction. Fibrocytes are bone marrow-derived mesenchymal progenitors that express surface markers for leukocytes and mesenchymal cells [110]. In addition, fibrocytes can accelerate wound repair by activating epithelial and endothelial cells proliferation [111], although they can also be involved in inflammatory fibrotic processes [112, 113].

A PHYLOGENETIC POINT-OF-VIEW ABOUT SURGICAL INFLAMMATION

Since it has been hypothesized that during the surgical inflammatory response, extraembryonic axes *i.e.* coelomic-amniotic and trophoblastic-yolk sac-related, are systemically re-expressed and converge into the interstitium of injured tissues and organs, the final aim of this process could also be collaborating in some type of development similar to embryonic development during the postnatal life [22].

The repair process could therefore have properties comparable to an embryo. One of the main objectives of the upregulated extraembryonic axes could be the collaboration in the establishment of an open circulation in the injured tissues and organs when the inflammatory response begins. An open circulatory system could facilitate interstitial fluid diffusion and concomitantly tissue nutrition when the blood circulation loses its prominent role [22, 114]. Animals have adapted a circulatory system through evolution. Vertebrates have a closed circulatory system and a heart that drives blood through closed blood vessels [115], whereas in invertebrates, like insects, the body fluid (hemolymph) is pumped by a dorsal heart through the tissues with no closed vessels [116]. In the inflamed tissues and organs, the closed circulatory system could therefore suffer a switch to acquire some of the characteristics of the open circulatory system and possibly characteristics of the hemolymph [114]. The inflammatory exudates bathe the cells of the injured tissues and organs thanks to the quick infiltration of the extracellular matrix [22]. Consequently, through the activation of the postcapillary venules, the endothelium and the high endothelial venules, extravasation of plasma and blood cells is produced during the inflammatory response. An open pathway in the inflamed tissues and organs would therefore be established through the associated simultaneous activation of the lymphatic circulation [22, 114]. Thanks to this new open microcirculatory system, where hemo-lymphatic circulation becomes predominant, tissues and organs are provided with molecules and cells coming from the upregulated extraembryonic coelomic-amniotic (*i.e.* neurogenic-related axis) and the trophoblast-yolk sac (*i.e.* bone-marrow-related axis) axes. Perhaps through the upregulation of ancestral phylogenetic mechanisms, the plasma, the interstitial fluid and lymph compartments could become closely linked during inflammation, thus favoring the continuous flow of fluid and cells from one compartment to the next [22, 114] (Fig. **1**).

The venous endothelium acquires trophoblastic properties since it becomes an intermediary between the stressed host and the inflamed interstitium, playing the leading role in the host trophism [100, 101]. The inflammatory venous endothelium phenotype represents the immunological first line of recognition of damage- and pathogen-associated-molecular patterns (DAMPs and PAMPs) through the innate immune receptors, like the Toll-like receptors (TLRs) and Nod-like receptors (NLRs) [117]. The inflammasome, a multi-protein complex including an NLR, is activated in response to PAMP and DAMP signals, which mediate the processing of intracellular pro-interleukin (IL)-1β and pro-IL-8 into their active secreted forms [117, 118]. While DAMPs and PAMPs activate the inflammasomes, a variety of regulatory mechanisms minimize changes caused by the inflammatory activity, such as molecular chaperones and heat shock proteins [118].

Vertebrate cells possess cholesterol and although different tissues have specific patterns of cholesterol metabolism and functions, the basic pattern is common to all the cells [119]. During inflammation, cholesterol esters may be transferred from high density lipoproteins (HDL) to apolipoprotein E and apoliprotein B (apo B)-containing particles, such as low-density lipoproteins and very low density lipoproteins (LDL/VLDL). The trapping of apolipoproteins, particularly apo B containing particles, is an essential initiating event for the development of vascular inflammation [120]. Furthermore, the small non-coding RNA (microRNAs) could modulate the expression of key genes in cholesterol metabolism during inflammation [119]. Today, it is accepted that inflammation and the associated acute phase reaction cause severe impairments in the lipoprotein profile [121] and cholesterol metabolism [122]. The characteristics of the inflammatory acute phase response and the associated cholesterol traffic have been compared with those playing the lead role in the accumulation of yolk materials into oocytes during oogenesis and their mobilization during embryogenesis [114].

The hypothesized endothelial inflammatory egg would turn into a reservoir of nutrients, including albumin. Bird embryos also consume egg white as a supplementary nutrient to yolk proteins [123]. Ovalbumin, ovotransferrin, trypsin inhibitor and other egg white proteins are absorbed into the extraembryonic cavity, through the albumen sac, then into the amniotic cavity and finally, reach the yolk sac through the vitello-intestinal duct [123].

Both cholesterol acquisition and leukocytic infiltration by the inflamed tissue collaborate to establish its new neuro-endocrine autonomy. Cholesterol is used locally to synthesize glucocorticoids and mineralocorticoids, which could regulate microcirculatory functions and immune cell activation. More evidence demonstrates the novo synthesis of glucocorticoids and mineralocorticoids in primary lymphoid organs, skin, brain and intestine [124]. Perhaps this ability of local corticosteroid synthesis is upregulated in the inflamed tissue due to the metabolic and functional needs of the neoformed tissue [114]. The pro- and anti-inflammatory functions of androgens and estrogens and progesterone respectively, suggest that endogenous sex steroids may influence immune functions [125, 126]. Progesterone, for example, increases vascular permeability and local accumulation of inflammatory cells. Definitely, the role of progesterone in the inflammatory response merits future research [125]. In addition, leukocytes in the inflamed interstitium could develop neuroendocrine functions. Particularly, the pro-opiomelanocortin (POMC)-derived peptides found in leukocytes exhibit the same structure as those present in the pituitary [127]. Also, leukocyte-derived microparticles could harbor cytoplasmic proteins as well as bioactive lipids in the inflamed interstitium [128]. Inflamed tissues and organs acquire a progressive neuro-immune-endocrine autonomy through the previous recapitulation of extraembryonic functions. We have hypothesized that the phylogenetic evolution of our body is written in the successive phases making up the acute inflammatory response [129]. When the evolution of a severe traumatized patient is favorable, the patient could therefore undergo dedifferentiation followed by a process of differentiation (or specialization) representing a complete metamorphosis, just as it occurs with insects [128]. This specialization would need the return of oxidative metabolism and the development of a closed circulation, in which epithelial regeneration and angiogenesis are mainly involved, as well as the centralization of the neuro-immune-endocrine functions that are reduced to a symbolic presence in the periphery [22].

Angiogenesis allows for nutrition supported by the new formed vessels which acquire functional properties like the exchange of oxygen, nutrients and waste products. Thanks to this oxygen support, oxidative metabolism, an efficient method for extracting energy from blood substrates, is induced. Thus, oxygen and oxidative metabolisms make up an excellent combination through which cells can obtain a substantial energy supply for repairing tissues through specialized cells. This combination, however, produces energetic stress [12, 25]. Perhaps the persistence in the adult microcirculation of a hypoxic venous territory, key for recapitulating those ancestral functions enabling development, is our safe-conduit to pass without vital risk through a hyperoxygenated environment. If so, then the maintenance of this microcirculatory hypoxic world in mammals has been made at the expense of either diverting oxygen through meta-arterioles or consuming and removing it through the specialized epithelia. In this case, our energetic way of life would be no less than a system for scavenging toxins with the ultimate aim of achieving the survival of our true pluripotential and ancestral gestation mechanisms. The return to ancestral phylogenetic mechanisms of life during surgical inflammation therefore opens a splendid path for translational research, as it has been previously shown in remodeling wound healing and inflammation in Drosophila [130].

In summary, surgical inflammation could be considered a high-grade stress response associated with an increasingly complex trophic functional system for using oxygen [131]. These mechanisms triggered by an acute stressor could be based on the recapitulation of ontogenic and phylogenic-related functions. Thus, the injured organism suffers processes of dedifferentiation, catabolism and autophagy mediated by the neuro-immune-response to stress. Consequently, the different types of endothelium that make up the microcirculation of the injured tissues and organs suffer a switch to turn into a functional endothelial inflammatory egg, capable of re-expressing extraembryonic functions to create a new tissue or organ. The pathophysiological mechanisms that characterize the surgical inflammatory response could therefore be essential for the normal life of animals, such as invertebrates, far below mammals on the phylogenetic scale. In this paper, we have described those arguments that seem to demonstrate the existence of a recapitulation of ontogenic and phylogenetic mechanisms along the evolution of the surgical inflammatory response with an intensity related to the intensity and severity of the injury suffered by the body.

ACKNOWLEDGEMENTS

We would like to thank Maria Elena Vicente for preparing the manuscript, Elizabeth Mascola for translating it into English and librarians of Complutense University Medical School, particularly the Director, Francisco Javier Jorge García-Reyes, and Manuela Crego and María José Valdemoro and B. Braun Surgical S.A. for their technical assistance.

This study was carried out in part with grants from Mutua Madrileña Research Foundation (Ref. nº PA 3077/2008 and AP5966/2009), MICINN PSI2010-19348 and with the special collaboration of the INEUROPA (Instituto de Neurociencias del Principado de Asturias).

CONFLICT OF INTEREST

The author(s) confirm that this chapter content has no conflict of interest.

REFERENCES

[1] Selye H. A syndrome produced by diverse noxious agents. Nature 1936; 138:32.
[2] Selye H. Stress and Inflammation. In: Selye H, Ed. The Stress of Life. Revised Edition. New York Mc Graw-Hill Book Co., 1978; pp. 129-43.
[3] Van de Kar LD, Richarson-Morton KD, Rittenhouse PA. Stress: Neuroendocrine and pharmacological mechanisms. In: Jasmin G. and Cantin M. Eds. Stress Revisited. 1. Neuroendocrinology of stress. Basel, Karger. 1991; pp. 133-173.
[4] Laborit H. The major mechanisms of stress. In: Jasmin G, Proschek L. Eds. Stress revisited. 2. Systemic effects of stress. Methods and achivements in Experimental Pathology. Basel. Switzerland 1991; pp. 1-26.
[5] Pruett SB. Stress and the immune system. Pathophysiology 2003; 9: 133-53.
[6] Baumann N, Turpin J-C. Neurochemistry of stress. An overview. Neurochem Res 2010; 35:1875-9.
[7] Denadal E, Ammerer G, Posas F. Controlling gene expression in response to stress. Nat Rev Genet 2011; 12: 833-45.
[8] Popoli M, Yan Z, McEwen BS, Sanacara G. The stressed synapse: the impact of stress and glucocorticoids on glutamate transmision. Nat Rev Neurosci 2011; 13: 22-37.
[9] Mora F, Segovia G, Del Arco A, *et al.* Stress, neurotransmitters, corticosterone and body-brain integration. Brain Res 2012; Jan 3 [Epub ahead of print]
[10] Cone JB. Inflammation. Am J Surg 2001; 182: 558-62.
[11] Nathan C. Points of control in inflammation. Nature 2002; 420: 846-52.
[12] Aller MA, Arias JL, Nava MP, Arias J. Post-traumatic inflammation is a complex response based on the pathological expression of the nervous, immune and endocrine functional systems. Exp Biol Med (Maywood) 2004; 229: 170-81.
[13] Hotamisligil GS. Inflammation and metabolic disorders. Nature 2006; 444: 860-7.
[14] Kohl BA, Deutschman CS. The inflammatory response to surgery and trauma. Curr Opin Crit Care 2006; 12: 325-32.
[15] Eming SA, Krieg T, Davidson JM. Inflammation in wound repair: Molecular and Cellular mechanisms. J Invest Dermatol 2007; 127: 514-25.
[16] Black PH, Garbutt LD. Stress, inflammation and cardiovascular disease. J Psychosom Res 2002; 52: 1-23.
[17] Rosmond R. Role of stress in the pathogenesis of the metabolic syndrome. Psychoneuroendocrinology 2005; 30: 1-10.
[18] Arch PC, Slominski A, Theoharides TC, Peters EM, Paus R. Neuroimmunology of stress: Skin takes center stage. J Invest Dermatol 2006; 126: 1697-704.
[19] Hänsel A, Hong S, Camara RJA, Von Känel R. Inflammation as a psychophysiological biomarker in chronic psychosocial stress. Neurosci Biobehav Rev 2010; 35: 115-21.
[20] Rath E, Haller D. Inflammation and cellular stress: a mechanistic link between immune-mediated and metabolically driven pathologies. Eur J Nutr 2011; 50: 219-33.

[21] Gu H-F, Tang C-K, Yang Y-Z. Psychological stress, immune response and atherosclerosis. Atherosclerosis 2012; Jan 18 [Epub ahead of print]

[22] Aller MA, Blanco-Rivero J, Arias JI, Balfagon G, Arias J. The wound healing response and the upregulated systemic extraembryonic phenotypes: brothers-in-arms forever. Exp Dermatol 2012; 21:497-503.

[23] Lenz A, Franklin GA, Cheadle WG. Systemic inflammation after trauma. Injury 2007; 38: 1336-45.

[24] Stahel PE, Smith WR, Moore EE. Role of biological modifiers regulating the immune response after trauma. Injury (Int J Care Injured) 2007; 381: 409-22.

[25] Aller MA, Arias JI, Alonso-Poza A, Arias J. A review of metabolic staging in severely injured patients. Scand J Trauma Resusc Emerg Med 2010; 18: 27.

[26] Arias JI, Aller MA, Gilsanz C, Arias A, Arias J. The re-expression of amniotic and vitelline functions in carcinogenesis: the cancer cell-mast cell connection. In: Agutter PS ed. *Hypotheses in Clinical Medicine*. Nova Scientific 2012, *in press*.

[27] Eisenhut M. Changes in ion transport in inflammatory disease. J Inflammation 2006; 3: 5.

[28] Scadden DT. The stem-cell niches as an entity of action. Nature 2006; 441: 1075-9.

[29] Glotzbach JP, Wong VW, Gutner GC, *et al*. Regenerative medicine. Curr Probl Surg 2011; 48: 148-212.

[30] Chrousos GP. Stress and disorders of the stress system. Nat Rev Endocrinol 2009;5: 374-81.

[31] Szczepanska-Sadowska E, Cudnoch-Jedrzejewska M, Ufani T, *et al*. Brain and cardiovascular diseases: Common neurogenic background of cardiovascular metabolic and inflammatory diseases. J Physiol Pharmacol 2010; 61: 509-21.

[32] Aguilera G. HPA axis responsiveness to stress: implications for health aging. Exp Gerontol 2011; 46: 90-5.

[33] Groeneweg FL, Karst H, De Kloet ER, *et al*. Rapid non-genomic effects of corticosteroids and their role in the central stress response. J Endocrinol 2011; 209: 157-67.

[34] Crivellato E, Nico B, Ribatti D. The chromaffin vesicle: Advances in understanding the composition of a versatile, multifunctional secretory organelle. Anat Rec (Hoboken) 2008; 291: 1587-602.

[35] Wendon J. Critical care "normality": Individualized *vs*. protocolized care. Crit Care Med 2010; 38: S590-9.

[36] Ehninger A, Trumpp A. The bone marrow stem cell niche grows up: mesenchymal stem cells and macrophages move in. J Exp Med 2011; 208: 421-8.

[37] Balbridge MT, King KY, Goodell MA. Inflammatory signals regulate hematopoietic stem cells. Trends Immunol 2011; 32: 57-64.

[38] Balbridge MT, King KY, Boles NC, *et al*. Quiescent haematopoietic stem cells are activated by IFN-gamma in response to chronic infection. Nature 2010; 465: 793-7.

[39] Aller MA, Arias JI, Giner M, *et al*. Oxygen-related inflammatory wound phenotypes. In: Middelton JE. ed. Wound healing: Process, Phases and Promoting. N.Y. USA Nova Sciences Publishers-Huntington 2011; pp. 1-26.

[40] Flierl MA, Rittirsch D, Huber-Lang M, Sarma JV, Ward PA. Catecholamines-crafty weapons in the inflammatory arsenal of immune/inflammatory cells or opening Pandora's box? Mol Med 2008; 14: 195-204.

[41] Grisanti LA, Evanson J, Marchus E, *et al*. Pro-inflammatory responses in human monocytes are β_1-adrenergic receptor subtype dependent. Mol Immunol 2010; 47: 1244-54.

[42] Sarkar C, Basu B, Chakroborty D, Dasgupta PS, Basu S. The immunoregulatory role of dopamine: an update. Brain Behav Immun 2010; 24: 525-8.

[43] Marazzitti D, Consoli G, Masala L, Catena Dell'Osso M, Baroni S. Latest advancements on serotonin and dopamine transporters in lymphocytes. Mini Rev Med Chem 2010; 10: 32-40.

[44] Czura CJ, Tracey KJ. Autonomic neural regulation of immunity. J Intern Med 2005; 257: 156-66.

[45] Rosas-Ballina M, Olofsson PS, Ochani M, *et al.* Acetylcholine-synthesizing T cells relay neural signals in a vagus nerve circuit. Science 2011; 33: 498-101.

[46] Smith EM, Galin FS, Boeuf LE, *et al.* Nucleotide and amino acid sequence of lymphocyte-derived corticotropin: endotoxin induction of a truncated peptide. Proc Natl Acad Sci USA 1990; 87: 1057-60.

[47] Smith EM. Neuropeptides as signal molecules in common with leukocytes and the hypothalamic-pituitary-adrenal axis. Brain Behav Immun 2008; 22: 3-14.

[48] Malagoli D, Accorsi A, Ottaviani E. The evolution of pro-opiomelanocortin: looking for the invertebrate fingerprints. Peptides 2011; 32: 2137-40.

[49] Wardlan SL. Hypothalamic proopiomelanocortin processing and the regulation of energy balance. Eur J Pharmacol 2011; 660: 213-9.

[50] Gabay C, Kushner I. Acute-phase proteins and other systemic responses to inflammation. N Engl J Med 1999; 340: 448-54.

[51] Jain S, Gautam V, Naseem S. Acute-phase proteins: As diagnostic tool. J Pharm Bioallied Sci 2011; 31: 18-27.

[52] Kelly-Spratt KS, Pitteri SJ, Gurley KE, *et al.* Plasma proteome profiles associated with inflammation, angiogenesis and cancer. PLOS One 2011; 6: e19721.

[53] Mihara M, Hashizume M, Yoshida H, Suzuki M, Shiina M. IL-6/IL-6 receptor system and its role in physiological and pathological conditions. Clin Sci (Lond) 2012; 122: 143-59.

[54] Bonetto A, Aydogdu T, Kunzevitzky N, *et al.* STAT 3 activation in skeletal muscle links muscle wasting and the acute phase response in cancer cachexia. PLOS One 2011; 6: e22538.

[55] Correale M, Brunetti ND, De Gennaro L, Di Biase M. Acute phase proteins in atherosclerosis (acute coronary syndrome). Cardiovasc Hematol Agents Med Chem 2008; 62: 72-7.

[56] Sorensen B, Fries D. Emerging treatment strategies for trauma-induced coagulopathy. Br J Surg 2012; 99: 40-50.

[57] Von Kanel R, Kudielka BM, Haeberli A, *et al.* Prothrombotic changes with acute psychological stress: Combined effect of hemoconcentration and genuine coagulation activation. Thromb Res 2009; 123: 622-30.

[58] Mizock BA. The multiple organ dysfunction syndrome. Dis Mon 2009; 55:476-526.

[59] Ritter S, Li A-J, Wang Q, Dinh TT. The value of looking backward: The essential role of the hindbrain in counterregulatory responses to glucose deficit. Endocrinology 2011; 152: 4019-32.

[60] Lund-Katz S, Phillips MC. High density lipoprotein structure-function and role in reverse cholesterol transport. Subcell Biochem 2010; 51: 183-227.

[61] Kisilevsky R, Manley PN. Acute-phase serum amyloid A: Perspectives on its physiological and pathological roles. Amyloid 2012; 19: 5-14.

[62] Miller WL, Bose HS. Early steps in steroidogenesis: intracellular cholesterol trafficking. J Lipid Res 2011; 5:2111-35.
[63] Chagas CEA, Borges MC, Martin LA, Rogero MM. Focus on Vitamin D, inflammation and type 2 diabetes. Nutrients 2012; 4: 52-67.
[64] Kimura F, Shimizu H, Yoshidome H, Ohtsuka M, Miyazaki M. Immunosuppression following surgical and traumatic injury. Surg Today 2010; 40: 793-808.
[65] Marshall JC, Christou NV, Meakins JL. The gastrointestinal tract. The "undrained abscess" of multiple organ failure. Ann Surg 1993; 218: 111-9.
[66] Agarwal AK, Auchus RJ. Cellular redox state regulates hydroxysteroid dehydrogenase activity and intracellular hormone potency. Endocrinology 2005; 146: 2531-8.
[67] Ghosh S, Hayden MS. New regulators of NF-κB in inflammation. Nat Rev 2008; 8: 837-49.
[68] Serhan CN, Brain SD, Buckley CD, *et al.* Resolution of inflammation: State of the art, definitions and terms. FASEB J 2007; 21: 325-32.
[69] Lawrence T, Gilroy DW. Chronic inflammation: a failure of resolution? Int J Exp Path 2007; 88: 85-94.
[70] Raman D, Sobolik-Delmaire T, Richmond A. Chemokines in health and disease. Exp Cell Res 2011; 317: 575-89.
[71] George AL, Bangalore-Prakash P, Rajoria S, *et al.* Endothelial progenitor cell biology in disease and tissue regeneration. J Hematol Oncol 2011; 4: 24.
[72] Herbert SP, Stainier DYR. Molecular control of endothelial cell behaviour during blood vessel morphogenesis. Nat Rev Mol Cell Biol 2011; 12: 551-64.
[73] Potente MGerhardt, H, Carmeliet P. Basic and therapeutic aspects of angiogenesis. Cell 2011; 146: 87387.
[74] Masuda H, Asahara T. Postnatal endothelial progenitor cells for neovascularization in tissue regeneration. Cardiovasc Res 2003; 58: 390-8.
[75] De Miguel MP, Fuentes-Julián S, Blázquez-Martínez A, *et al.* Immunosuppressive properties of mesenchymal stem cells: advances and applications. Curr Mol Med. 2012; 12: 574-91.
[76] Kao H-K, Chen B, Murphy G, *et al.* Peripheral blood fibrocytes: Enhancement of wound healing by cell proliferation, re-epithelization, contraction and angiogenesis. Ann Surg 2011; 254: 1066-74.
[77] Van Der Berghe G. Neuroendocrine axis in critical illness. Curr Opin Endocrinol Diabetes 2011; 8: 47-54.
[78] Aller MA, Arias JI, Arias J. Pathological axes of wound repair: Gastrulation revisited. Theor Biol Med Model 2010; 7: 37.
[79] Bryant R. Post-traumatic stress disorder *vs.* traumatic brain injury. Dialogues Clin Neurosci 2011; 13: 251-60.
[80] Sherin JE, Nemeroff CB. Post-traumatic stress disorder: the neurobiological impact of psychological trauma. Dialogues Clin Neurosci 2011; 13: 263-78.
[81] De Miguel MP, Arnalich-Montiel P, Lopez-Iglesias A, Blazquez Martinez A, Nistal M. Epiblast-derived stem cells in embryonic and adult tissues. Int J Dev Biol 2009; 53: 1529-40.
[82] Jauniaux E, Gulbis B. Fluid compartments of the embryonic environment. Hum Reprod Update 2000; 6: 268-78.

[83] Jauniaux E, Gulbis B, Jurkovic D. Relationship between protein concentrations in embryological fluids and maternal serum and yolk sac size during human pregnancy. Hum Reprod 1994; 9: 161-6.

[84] Burton GJ, Hempstock J, Jauniaux E. Nutrition of the human fetus during the first trimester- A review. Placenta 2001; 22: S70-7.

[85] Jauniaux E, Sherwood RA, Jurkovic D, Boa FG, Campbell S. Amino acid concentrations in human embryological fluids. Hum Reprod 1994; 9: 1175-9.

[86] Wathen NC, Delves HT, Campbell DJ, Chard T. The coelomic cavity- A reservoir for metals. Am J Obstet Gynecol 1995; 173: 1884-8.

[87] Jauniaux E, Hempstock J, Teng C, Battaglia FC, Burton GJ. Polyol concentrations in the fluid compartments of the human conceptus during the first trimester of pregnancy: maintenance of redox potential in a low oxygen environment. J Clin Endocrinol Metab 2005; 90:1171-5.

[88] Calleja-Agius J, Jauniaux E, Muttukrishna S. Inflammatory cytokines in maternal circulation and placenta of chromosomally abnormal first trimester miscarriages. Clin Dev Immunol 2012; 2012: 175041.

[89] Aller MA, Arias JL, Sanchez-Patan F, Arias J. The inflammatory response: An efficient way of life. Med Sci Monit 2006; 12: RA225.

[90] Chang YJ, Huang SM, Tseng CP, *et al.* Isolation of mesenchymal stem cells with neurogenic potentials from the mesoderm of the amniotic membrane. Cell Tissues Organs 2010; 192: 93-105.

[91] Uberti MG, Pierpont YN, Ko F, *et al.* Amnion-derived cellular cytokine solution (ACCS) promotes migration of kertinocytes and fibroblasts. Ann Plast Surg 2010; 64: 632-5.

[92] Bellini C, Boccardo F, Bonioli E, Campisi C. Lymphodynamics in the fetos and newborn. Lymphology 2006; 39: 110-7.

[93] Siegel N, Rosner M, Hanneder M, Freilinger A, Hengstschläger M. Human amniotic fluid stem cells: a new perspective. Amino Acids 2008; 35: 291-3.

[94] Shaw SW, David AL, De Coppi P. Clinical applications of prenatal and postnatal therapy using stem cells retrieved from amniotic fluid. Curr Opin Obstet Gynecol 2011; 23: 109-16.

[95] Fraser ST, Baron MH. Embryonic fates for extraembryonic lineages: new perspectives. J Cell Biochem 2009; 107: 586-91.

[96] Ueno H, Weisman IL. The origin and fate of yolk sac hematopoiesis: application of chimera analysis to developmental studies. Int J Dev Biol 2010; 54: 1019-31.

[97] Gulbis B, Jauniaux E, Cotton F, Stordeur P. Protein and enzyme patterns in the fluid cavities of the first trimester gestational sac: relevance to the absorptive role of secondary yolk sac. Mol Hum Reprod 1998; 4: 857-62.

[98] Yoshida S, Wada Y. Transfer of maternal cholesterol to embryo and fetus in pregnant mice. J Lipid Res 2005; 46: 2168-74.

[99] Nakazawa F, Alev C, Jakt LM, Sheng G. Yolk sac endoderm is the major source for serum proteins and lipids and is involved in the regulation of vascular integrity in early chick development. Dev Dyn 2011; 240: 2002-10.

[100] Bevilacqua E, Hoshida M-S, Amarante-Paffaro A, Albieri-Borges A, Gomes S.Z. Trophoblast phagocytic program: roles in different placental systems. Int J Dev Biol 2010 54: 495-505.

[101] Knöfler M. Critical growth factors and signalling pathways controlling human trophoblast invasion. Int J Dev Biol 2010; 54: 269-80.

[102] Knöfler M, Pollheimer J. IFPA Award in Placentology Lecture: Molecular regulation of human trophoblast. Placenta 2012; 33: S55-62.
[103] Romen JW, Lütjen-Drecoll E. Introduction. Fundamental concepts. In: Funktionell Embryology. Sttutgart, Germany. Schattauer 2006; pp. 1-37
[104] Crivellato E, Nico B, Ribatti D. The chromaffin vesicle: Advances in understanding the composition of a versatile, multifunctional secretory organelle. Anat Rec (Hoboken) 2008; 291: 1587-602.
[105] Hocking AM, Gibran NS. Mesenchymal stem cells: Paracrine signaling and differentiation during cutaneous wound repair. Exp Cell Res 2010; 316: 2213-9.
[106] Dazzi F, Krampera M. Mesenchymal stem cells and autoimmune diseases. Best Pract Res Clin Haematol 2011; 24: 49-57.
[107] Otto WR, Wright NA. Mesenchymal stem cells: from experiment to clinic. Fibrogenesis Tissue Repair 2011; 4: 20.
[108] Kao H-K, Chen B, Murphy G, *et al.* Peripheral blood fibrocytes: Enhancement of wound healing by cell proliferation, re-epithelization, contraction and angiogenesis. Ann Surg 2011; 254: 1066-74.
[109] Ratajczak MZ, Liu R, Ratajczak, Kucia M, Shin DM. The role of pluripotent embryonic-like stem cells residing in adult tissues in regeneration and longevity. Differentiation 2011; 81:153-61.
[110] Ekert JE, Murray LA, Das AM *et al.* Chemokine (C-Cmotif) ligand 2 mediates direct and indirect fibrotic responses in human and murine cultured fibrocytes. Fibrogenesis Tissue Repair 2011; 4: 23.
[111] Jones CP, Rankin SM. Bone marrow-derived stem cells and respiratory disease. Chest 2011; 140: 205-11.
[112] Wasmuth HE, Tacke F, Trautwein C. Chemokines in liver inflammation and fibrosis. Semin Liver Dis 2010; 30: 215-25.
[113] Meran S, Steadman R. Fibroblasts and myofibroblasts in renal fibrosis. Int J Exp Pathol 2011; 92: 158-67.
[114] Aller MA, Arias N, Fuentes-Julian S, *et al.* Coupling inflammation with evo-devo. Med. Hypotheses 2012; 78: 721-31.
[115] Aird W.C. Discovery of the cardiovascular system: from Galen to William Harvey. J Thromb Haemost 2011 9: 118-29.
[116] Eble JA, Nilands S. The extracellular matrix of blood vessels. Curr Pharm Des 2009; 15: 1385-400.
[117] Abrahams VM. The role of the Nod-like receptor family in trophoblast innate immune responses. J Reprod Immunol 2011; 88: 112-7.
[118] Dunn JH, Ellis LZ, Fujita M. Inflammasomes as molecular mediators of inflammaton and cancer: potential role in melanoma. Cancer Letters 2012; 314: 24-33.
[119] Goedeke L, Fernandez-Hernando C. Regulation of cholesterol metabolism. Cell Mol Life Sci. 2012; 69: 915-30.
[120] Sniderman A, Couture P, De Graaf J. Diagnosis and treatment of apolipoprotein B dyslipoproteinemias. Nat Rev Endocrinol 2010; 6: 335-46.
[121] Jahangiri A. High-density lipoprotein and the acute plasma response. Curr Opin Endocrinol Diabetes Obest 2010; 17: 156-60.
[122] Targher G, Day CP, Bonora E. Risk of cardiovascular disease in patients with nonalcoholic fatty liver disease. N Engl J Med 2010; 363: 1341-50.

[123] Yoshizaki N, Ito Y, Hori H, Saito H, Iwasawa A. Absorption, transportation and digestion of egg white in quail embryos. Dev Growth Differ 2002; 44: 11-22.
[124] Taves MD, Gomez-Sanchez CE, Soma KK. Extra-adrenal glucocorticoids and mineralocorticoids: evidence for local synthesis, regulation and function. Am J Physiol Endocrinol Metab 2011; 301: E11-24.
[125] Gilliver SC. Sex steroids as inflammatory regulators. J Steroid Biochem Mol Biol 2010; 120: 105-15.
[126] Cunningham M, Gilkeson G. Estrogen receptors in immunity and autoimmunity. Clin Rev Allergy Immunol 2011; 40; 66-73.
[127] Malagoli D, Accorsi A, Ottaviani E. The evolution of pro-opiomelanocortin: Looking for the invertebrate finger prints. Peptides 2011; 32: 2137-40.
[128] Angelillo-Scherrer A. Leukocyte-derived microparticles in vascular homeostasis. Circ Res 2012; 110: 356-69.
[129] Aller MA, Arias JL, Nava MP, Arias J. Evolutive trophic phases of the systemic acute inflammatory response, oxygen use mechanisms and metamorphosis. Psicothema 2004; 16: 369-72.
[130] Razzell W, Wood W, Martin P. Swatting flies: modelling wound healing and inflamation in Drosophila. Dis Model Mech 2011; 4: 569-74.
[131] Arias JI, Aller MA, Arias J. Surgical inflammation: a pathophysiological rainbow. J Transl Med 2007; 5: 44.

Send Orders for Reprints to reprints@benthamscience.net
Surgical Inflammation, 2013, 129-153

CHAPTER 5

The Wound Healing Reaction

María-Angeles Aller[1], Isabel Prieto[2], Javier Blanco-Rivero[3], Jose-Ignacio Arias[4], Gloria Balfagon[3] and Jaime Arias[1,*]

[1]Department of Surgery, School of Medicine, Complutense University of Madrid, Madrid, Spain; [2]General and Digestive Surgery Unit, La Paz Hospital, School of Medicine, Autonoma University of Madrid, Madrid, Spain; [3]Department of Physiology, School of Medicine, Autonoma University of Madrid, Madrid, Spain and [4]General Surgery Unit, Monte Naranco Hospital, Oviedo, Asturias, Spain

Abstract: The cutaneous wound healing reaction occurs in overlapping but inter-related phases which finally involves fibrosis. The pathophysiological mechanisms involved in fibrotic diseases, including those organ-related or even systemic, like systemic sclerosis, could represent the successive systemic upregulation of extraembryonic-like phenotypes, *i.e.*: amniotic and vitelline. These two extraembryonic-like phenotypes would focus on the injured tissue to induce a process similar to that occurs in the early phases of embryo development, which is gastrulation. The amniotic-like phenotype would play a leading role in the development of a neurogenic response with noteworthy hydroelectrolytic alterations that essentially would represent the creation of an open microcirculation in the injured tissue. In turn, through the overlapped expression of a vitelline-like phenotype, a bone-marrow-related response is produced. The interstitial infiltration by molecular and cellular mediators contributed by the amniotic- and vitelline-like functions provides the functional and metabolic autonomy which is needed for inducing the formation of a new tissue by using mechanisms similar to those expressed in gastrulation during the early phases of the embryo development. Thus, a new tissue is formed but unfortunately it quickly evolves by premature senescence to fibrosis. The hypothesized use of mechanisms is related to extraembryonic-like functions in the three following physiological and pathological processes: the embryonic development; the wound healing reaction during adult life and, finally in senescence, where the existence of a basic self-organizing fractal-like functional pattern as an essential characteristic of our way of life is suggested.

Keywords: Wound healing, embryo development, vitelline, clot, coagulation, hemostasis, re-epithelization, amniotic fluid, extraembryonic functions, intraembryonic mesenchyma, leukocytes, microcirculation, senescence, interstitium.

***Address correspondence to Jaime Arias:** Cátedra de Cirugía, Facultad de Medicina, Universidad Complutense, Pza. de Ramón y Cajal s.n., 28040 MADRID, Spain; Tel: +34 91 394 1389; Fax: +34 91 3947115; E-mail: jariasp@med.ucm.es

INTRODUCTION

Nowadays, it is accepted that the cause-effect relationship between inflammation and the fibrotic processes is so narrow that the term "inflammatory fibrosis" [1] seems to be very appropriate for multiple fibrotic diseases, either local, including wound healing [1, 2], or organ-related, *i.e.* pulmonary fibrosis [3], liver cirrhosis [4], renal fibrosis [5], myocardial infarction [6] or even systemic, *i.e.* systemic sclerosis affecting the skin and internal organs [7]. Actually, the fibrotic tissue disease related to inflammation is a major unresolved problem in clinical medicine because its pathophysiology is not completely understood and because of the lack of effective therapeutic strategies [8].

With this aim in mind, in the current article we are focusing on an integrative perspective about physiological, *i.e.* aging, and pathological, fibrotic diseases, conditions in the adult life in which inflammatory fibrosis adopts a key role. In this way, the link between these apparently different processes could be the use in postnatal life of many pathways that play an ancestral essential role during embryologic development [9, 10]. Maybe this is the reason why aberrant activation of these ontogenic pathways when we suffer an acute or chronic injury could also lead from the formation of new tissues, either normal by regeneration [10] to pathological ones, *i.e.* fibrosis [9, 10] and tumors [11]. Therefore, these complex mechanisms are critical to maintain and restore the tissue structure and function whether they occur during development or under pathological conditions.

After a brief introduction of the wound healing reaction in two of the most frequent and relevant clinical presentations, like the skin and the liver, we emphasize the usually forgotten associated systemic involvements. What is the reason why we highlight these underestimated systemic disorders? Perhaps, since these systemic changes are in fact masked functions of embryonic development whose objective would be to repeat the generation of a new tissue, but in this case it would be for supplying the dead one. Then, what could be the new clinical perspectives derived from this comparison? The patients could gain great benefits in the resolution of their fibrotic diseases if these upregulated embryonic systemic functions could undergo therapeutic modulation. This proposition could be a valid alternative to the actual ineffective anti-fibrotic therapies.

CUTANEOUS WOUND HEALING: THE LOCAL INFLAMMATORY PHENOTYPES

The wide range of pathophysiological mechanisms that overlap along the evolution of the skin wound healing reaction is possibly the reason that there is no consensus among authors in terms of the number and characteristics of the phases that integrate this reaction. For some authors, wound healing involves three phases: inflammation, proliferation or tissue formation, and tissue remodeling or tissue organization [2, 12-14]. However, other authors consider that the response to injury occurs in four stages: hemostasis, inflammation, proliferation or tissue formation and tissue remodeling [15-17]. However, and regardless of the number of phases, all authors agree that these phases are interrelated [2, 12, 15, 16], thus suggesting that the wound healing process is a *continuum*.

If three stages of the wound healing process are accepted, inflammation includes coagulation with the formation of a fibrin rich clot and recruitment of inflammatory cells [2]. During the subsequent proliferative phase, granulation tissue deposition, consisting of endothelial cells, macrophages and fibroblasts [12], provides a provisional wound bed for re-epithelization [2]. The final stage involves the contraction and reorganization of the newly synthesized matrix and finally, apoptosis of unneeded fibroblasts and blood vessels [13] (Table **1**).

Table 1: Overlapping but interrelated proposed phases during the wound healing process.

* **Inflammation** - Coagulation - Recruitment of inflammatory cells * **Proliferation or tissue formation** - Granulation tissue * **Tissue remodelling or tissue organization** - Contraction - Extracellular matrix reorganization [2, 12, 13]	* **Hemostasis** * **Inflammation** * **Proliferation** * **Tissue remodelling** [14-16]	* **Ischemia-reperfusion** - Interstitial edema * **Immune or Leukocytic infiltration** - Interstitial infiltration by inflammatory cells * **New tissue formation and remodelling** - Mesenchymal-derived tissue - Fibrosis - Dysfuncional parenchyma [17-19]

However, in a broader integrating way, the inflammatory response would include all the phases that constitute wound healing, instead of being considered as only one of its stages [18-20]. Thus, the inflammatory response induced in the wounded skin could be a succession of three overlapping phases during which phenotypes of metabolic progressive complexity in using oxygen are expressed [20]. These phases emphasize the trophic role of the mechanisms developed in the damaged tissue [18, 19].

Hence, in the first or immediate phase of the inflammatory response, interstitial hydroelectrolytic alterations stand out and nutrition by diffusion predominates. The ischemia-reperfusion phenomenon, which in turn causes oxidative and nitrosative stress, is responsible for the progression of the interstitial edema [14]. As edema is produced, the lymphatic circulation is activated at the same time [20]. Furthermore, since active wounds are initially anoxic or near anoxic and chronic ischemic wounds are essentially hypoxic [21, 22], both the anoxic and the severe hypoxic environment in the injured tissue could represent an ideal stem cell niche [23, 24].

In the following intermediate or immune phase, interstitial infiltration by inflammatory blood-born cells is produced. This phase represents enzymatic stress with intracellular (autophagy, phagocytosis, antigen presentation) and extracellular (fermentation) digestion, which favors tissue trophism [19, 20, 25]. Wound metabolism during this phase could be able to manage the increased oxidative and nitrosative stress by the hypermetabolism imposed by reoxygenation. Furthermore, macrophages and dendritic cells take advantage of the lymphatic circulation activation, migrating through it until reaching the lymph nodes, where they activate lymphocytes [20].

During the third phase, or endocrine, angiogenesis enables numerous substances including hormones, to be transported by the blood circulation. Angiogenesis could also have antioxidant and anti-enzymatic properties, favoring resolution as well as wound repair by defective epithelial regeneration and scarring. Blood capillaries could supply oxygen, which induces oxidative metabolism with oxidative phosphorylation [10]. Consequently, in this long-term phase, the new tissue is structured, specialized and matured by remodeling [18-20] (Table **1**).

However, since the successive phases of the inflammatory response are overlapped, maybe the different evolutive metabolism types, which depend on the growing presence of oxygen, are also overlapped and complementary. If so, a metabolic chain of different staging, from anaerobic glycolysis (Pasteur Effect), through aerobic glycolysis (Warburg effect), to the oxidative metabolism, would be developed in wounds. This metabolic chain would use the electron chain transport to maximize obtaining energy in an efficiently growing manner. Therefore, wounds could have the ability to change their metabolism and, consequently their inflammatory phenotypes during their evolution. These properties enable wounds to resemble the malignant tumors, which in turn reinforced Dvorak´s prediction twenty six years ago, suggesting that *"tumors are wounds that cannot be healed"* [11].

THE EXTRAEMBRYONIC RECAPITULATED FUNCTIONS AND THE INDUCTION OF A REPARATIVE GASTRULATION-LIKE PROCESS

It has been proposed that the inflammatory response associated with wound healing in the skin could recapitulate ontogeny through the re-expression of two hypothetical extraembryonic trophic axes, that are, amniotic and yolk sac or vitelline, in the interstitial space of the injured tissue [10]. Likewise, the body could be repaired according to embryonic biochemical patterns through the expression of extraembryonic functions after injury. If so, inflammation could represent the debut during postnatal life of ancestral biochemical mechanisms that were used for normal embryonic development. The re-expression of these ancient mechanisms, with a prenatal solvent path, is perhaps inappropriate and hard to recognize since they are anachronistic during postnatal life and because they are established in a different environmental medium [10, 11]. Embryogenesis starts after fertilization with the zygote, which undergoes cleavage or division by mitosis. When the morula stage is reached, the embryo establishes polarity. The cells bind tightly to each other forming a compact sphere in which there are two different cell layers. The outermost layer becomes the trophoblast, that gives rise to the placenta; and the inner cells become the inner cell mass that gives rise to the embryo and the remaining structures, such as amnion, yolk sac and allantoids [26] (Fig. **1**).

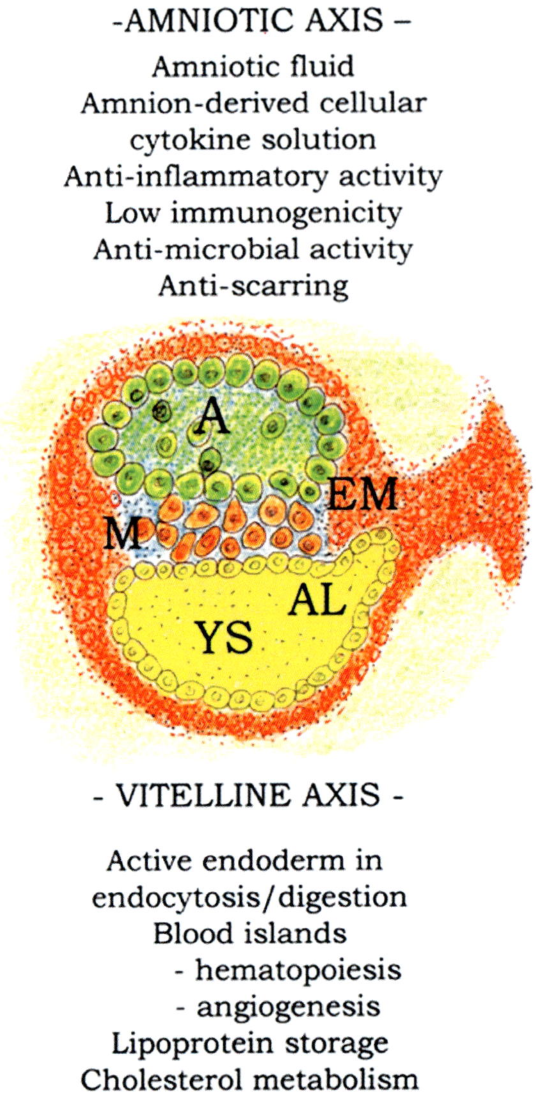

Figure 1: Representative drawing of the early mammalian embryo during gastrulation. A: Amnion; YS: Yolk sac; M: Mesoderm; EM: Extraembryonic mesoderm; AL: Allantoids.

The molecular and cellular contribution made by the two extraembryonic tissues that surround the fetus, the amnion and yolk sac, to the interstitial space located between them, namely, the mesoderm, is essential for organogenesis. In fact, the nascent mesoderm generated during gastrulation could involve an internalization process of extraembryonic, *i.e.* amniotic and vitelline, functions [26] (Fig. **1**).

The amnion is an embryonic functional axis with strong neural potential [27, 28]. Amnion-derived multipotent progenitor cells secrete a unique combination of cytokines and growth factors, known as the "amnion-derived cellular cytokine solution," which establishes a communication network between mesenchymal and epithelial cells during embryo development [29]. The amniotic fluid that surrounds the fetus may therefore be considered an extension of the extracellular space of the fetal tissues [30]. Furthermore, pluripotent stem cells can be isolated from amniotic fluid, which suggests that amniotic fluid represents a new and very promising source for stem cell research [31, 32] (Fig. **1**).

The yolk sac in mammals is composed of two layers: the visceral endoderm, which is active in endocytosis/digestion with larger lysosomes, and the underlying mesoderm layer, in which "blood islands" develop supporting hematopoiesis and angiogenesis [33]. The endothelial and blood progenitors of blood islands arise independently from the epiblast before they migrate to the extraembryonic yolk sac [34]. Then hemangioblasts in the blood islands could generate blood cells through specialized intermediate progenitors known as the hemogenic endothelium [34]. Also, a major function of the yolk sac is the accumulation of carbohydrates, proteins and lipids for embryo nutrition (*vitellum*) [35]. Therefore, the yolk sac plays a vital role in providing lipids and lipid-soluble nutrients to embryos during the early phases of development [35]. In particular, the yolk sac endoderm plays an important role in the regulation of vascular integrity in developing embryos [36] (Fig. **1**).

The molecular and cellular contribution made by both extraembryonic structures, *i.e.* the amnion and the yolk sac, to the interstitial space located between them, namely, the mesoderm, is essential for organogenesis. Therefore, it could be suggested that these primitive extraembryonic functions are internalized during gastrulation in order to be integrated in the intraembryonic mesoderm [10] (Fig. **1**), which in turn could explain the greater postnatal plasticity of the mesodermal derived cells [5]. Consequently, the re-expression of extraembryonic functions after injury during the post-natal life could be a key process needed to repair the injured tissue.

That is why we have hypothesized that wound repair would require the upregulation of signaling pathways characteristic of the extraembryonic, amniotic and vitelline, functions during embryo development [10]. In this way, the pathophysiological mechanisms involved in the inflammatory response could represent the recapitulation of the above-mentioned extraembryonic functions, *i.e.* amniotic and vitelline ones, to collaborate together in making an embryo-like tissue. The amniotic-like phenotype could offer the stem cells a hypoxic and hydrated interstitial axis [30], with cytokines and growth factors [29], favoring nutrition by diffusion, transport, excretion and bacteriostatic and anti-inflammatory protection [29, 31, 32]. The vitelline phenotype could in turn favor the regulation of lipid metabolism genes [36]; the hematopoietic-cell derived control with recruitment of immune cells and, at last, the induction of an angiogenic switch [34] to permit the new tissue immunological tolerance. The integration of both extraembryonic phenotypes, amniotic and vitelline, by the multipotent mesenchymal stem/stromal cells (MSC) [37-39] would support the functional and metabolic heterogeneity needed to successively modulate their microenvironment during their development in the wounded tissue [37, 39] (Table **2**). The fibroblasts form a heterogeneous collection of mesenchymal cells and they are the principal cellular constituents of connective tissues. The major role of the mesodermal cells and their ability to differentiate from the first stage of embryonic development enables considering them as the cell prototype that should be resorted to when the repair of any tissue in the body is needed [10]. And for this reason, perhaps the post-traumatic inflammatory response after a skin wound has the same intention, namely, to use the embryonic mesodermal phenotype with a therapeutic objective [31, 32].

Table 2: The upregulation of extraembryonic phenotypes could be involved in the different types of inflammatory diseases affecting the adult body, and this fact, in turn, upregulates gastrulation, a basic embryonic phenotype that ultimately induces fibrosis.

Phenotypes	**Embryonic**	**Development**	**Inflammatory Response in Wound Repair**	
Extra-embryonic Phenotypes (Extra-embryonic mesoderm-related)	Amniotic	- Neural potential - Amnion-derived cellular Cytokine solution. - Anti-inflammatory	Neuromuscular response	- Stress response - Biogenic amines release. - Sensitive and motor alteration - Ischemia-reperfusion - Local oxidative and nitrosative stress

				- Hydroelectrolytic alterations - Edema
	Vitelline	- Endocytosis/Digestion - Vitellum - Hematopoiesis - Angiogenesis	Bone-marrow Related response	- Inflammation blood cells - Coagulation. - Enzymatic stress - Corticosuprarenal hormones – Local storage - Hematopoietic stem cells - Mesenchymal stem cells - Endothelial progenitor cells
Embryonic Phenotypes	Gastrulation	Mesoderm (26, 34-36, 38, 40)	Wound healing Response	- Fibrocytes - Myofibroblasts - Fibroblasts - Vasculogenesis - Angiogenesis - Re-epithelization - Fibrosis (2, 11-19, 42, 44-51)

Politrauma		**Chronic Liver Disease**	
Neurogenic phase	- Sensitive and motor alterations - Blood flow redistribution - Ischemia-reperfusion - Shock - Hydration	Amniotic-like axis	- Autonomic dysfunction - Hemodynamic alterations * Portal hypertension * Hyperactive circulation - Hydroelectrolytic de-compensation * Sodium and water retention * Hepatorenal syndrome * Ascites
Inmune phase	- Acute phase response - Cholesterol-derived hormones systemic inflammatory - Disseminated Intravascular coagulation response syndrome - Multi-organ failure - Hypercatabolic syndrome	Vitellogenic like axis	- Splanchnic infiltration by inflammatory cells - Dyslipidemia - Estrogenization - Impaired splenic function - Splenomegaly - Splanchnic and systemic excessive angio-genesis

Endocrine phase	- Neuroendocrine centralized control - Convalescence - Anabolism - Systemic tissue remodelling (17, 18, 52)	Gastrulation-like	- Hepatic fibrosis - Cirrhosis (4, 76, 77, 80-84, 87, 90, 91, 93, 98-100)

THE CUTANEOUS WOUND HEALING REACTION: FROM LOCAL TO SYSTEMIC INFLAMMATORY PHENOTYPES

Cutaneous wound healing is a complex process involving systemic inflammatory alterations related to a stress response. The magnitude of this systemic response could reflect the demands required for wound repair. Establishing certain similarities between the complex pathophysiological mechanisms of the systemic inflammatory response developed in normal healing and the pluripotent extraembryonic pathways during embryo development has been attempted. During wound healing, the body could induce a systemic recapitulation of vitelline and amniotic functions which would then be selectively integrated into the injured area. Thus, embryonic programs with a repairing aim would be activated. In this way, the recapitulation of amniotic functions would be represented by the activation of a systemic neurogenic axis, while the recapitulation of vitelline functions would be played by the activation of a systemic bone marrow-related axis.

The Neurogenic Systemic Axis

Wounds produce a pathological neuromuscular response that includes sensitive alterations like stress sensation, inflammatory pain, analgesia and motor alterations. These alterations include skeletal muscle (fight-to-flight effect and withdrawal reflexes), the miocardium (tachycardia) and the vascular smooth muscle, with vasoconstriction and vasodilation, which induce systemic and local hemodynamic impairments, *i.e.* ischemia-reperfusion [10]. A common and basic pathogenic mechanism of this complex neuromuscular response would be the sudden hydroelectrolytic alterations. There is increasing evidence that the conditions characterized by intense local or systemic inflammatory response are actually associated with abnormal ion transport [40, 41] (Fig. **2**).

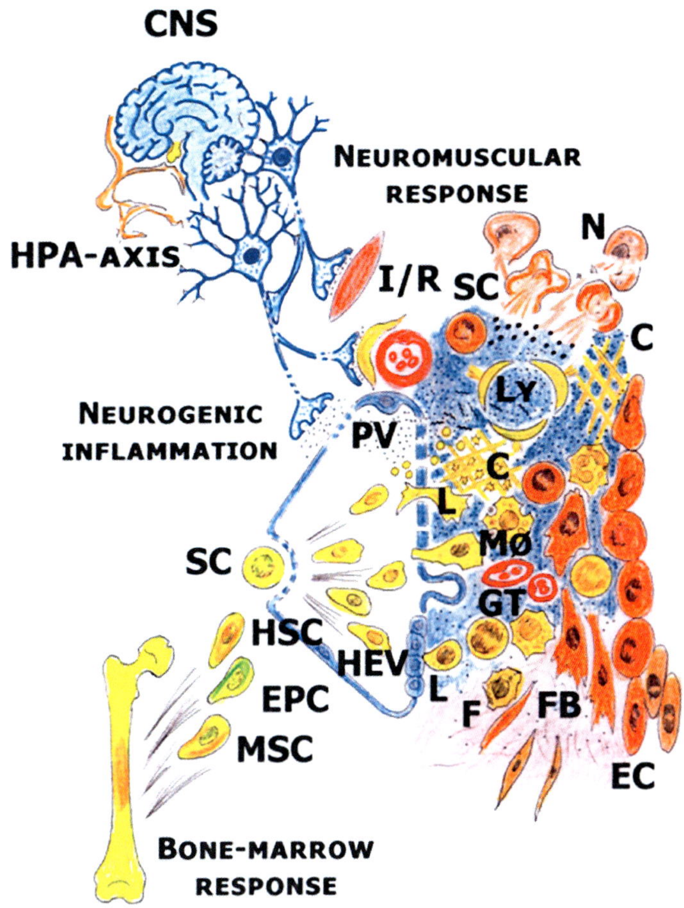

Figure 2: In the wound healing reaction, the extraembryonic axes could be upregulated. Thus, the amniotic axis, represented by the neurogenic response, induces a neuromuscular reaction associated with Ischemia-Reperfusion (I/R), increase of the postcapillary vein permeability and interstitial edema. In turn, the vitelline axis, represented by the bone-marrow response, could be responsible of the interstitial infiltration of those cells that will participate in the creation of the new tissue. These systemic upregulated extraembryonic axes converge in the *interstitium* of the injured tissue favoring the induction of a gastrulation-like phenotype, which evolves in the adult organism towards fibrosis. C: coagulation; CNS: Central nervous system; EC: epithelial cells; EPC: epithelial-derived stem cell; F: fibrocytes; FB: fibroblasts; GT: granulation tissue; HEV: high endothelial venule; HPA-axis: Hypothalamic-pituitary-adrenal-axis; HSC: hematological stem cell; L: lymphocytes; Ly: lymphatic vessel; MØ: macrophages; MSC: mesenchymal-derived stem cell; N: necrosis; PV: postcapillary vein; SC: stem cell.

In the early stress neurogenic response, the activation of the hypothalamo-pituitary-adrenocortical, sympathetic-adrenal medullary and renin-angiotensin-aldosterone axes occurs, with the secretion of catecholamines, glucocorticoids and mineralocorticoids in the circulation [42-45]. Consequently, a selective accumulation of these substances in the interstitial space of the tissues that suffer ischemia-reperfusion is produced because endothelial permeability is increased, especially in the post-capillary venules [18, 19]. In particular, considerable evidence suggests that stress, both acute and chronic, induces the elevation of catecholamines, especially epinephrine [46, 47]. This is why beta blockers are considered a new therapeutic approach to treat chronic, non-healing wounds [48, 49].

The Systemic Bone-Marrow-Related Axis

Nowadays, the inflammatory bone-marrow related response induced by wounds must be considered as a key and complementary arm of the stress response. The inflammatory activation of the bone marrow stem cell niche would imply the stimulation of its principal cellular components, like the hematopoietic stem cell (HSC) and the MSC, both considered as multipotent stem cells [23, 50] (Fig. **2**).

HSCs are the progenitors of all blood and immune cells. Recent studies suggest that inflammatory signaling molecules, including interferons, tumor necrosis factor-alpha and Toll-like receptors, appear to stimulate HSC proliferation in the short term [51]. In turn, interferon-gamma mediates the HSC stimulation in response to chronic inflammation [52] (Fig. **2**).

Macrophages generated from HSC are the dominant phagocytes at sites of wound healing and the presence of activated platelets may exacerbate pro-inflammatory macrophage activation [53]. Progressive fibrotic diseases, such as hepatic fibrosis, pulmonary fibrosis and systemic sclerosis, are tightly regulated by macrophages [54, 55]. In particular, pro-fibrotic macrophages, through the production of mediators that directly activate fibroblasts, including transforming growth factor (TGF)-β_1, platelet derived growth factor (PDGF) and insulin-like growth factors (IGF)-1, are intimately involved in wound healing [15, 54, 55]. Nevertheless, although macrophages are clearly required for the initiation and maintenance of fibrosis, they are also involved in its suppression, resolution and reversal [54-57]. Since these extreme phenotypes are not expressed in pure form *in vivo*, recent publications have embraced the view that macrophage activation is best derived from a continuous spectrum of phenotypic characteristics [56].

Angiogenesis is needed during embryonic development while it also plays important roles throughout postnatal life in wound healing and tissue ischemia [58, 59]. Recent research, however, has identified a novel mechanism in vasculature development known as vasculogenesis, or new vessels that form from bone marrow derived endothelial progenitor cells [58], rather than from sprouting or the elongation of existing vessels [59]. During vasculogenesis or neovascularization, precursor cells from adult bone marrow are mobilized into circulation in response to various signals, including chemokines and their receptors and are homed to the source where they differentiate into mature endothelial cells [60]. Although the major physiological role of circulating endothelial progenitor cells is to maintain vascular integrity, they can also home to and aid in revascularization of ischemic tissues [58] (Fig. **2**).

The Interstitial Integration of the Neurogenic and Bone-Marrow-Related Axes into the Injured Area

The activation of the pathological systemic axes, *i.e.* neurogenic and bone-marrow-related, in the injured tissue could be produced in two-steps. Thus, the upregulated amniotic phenotype would be responsible for a sudden and early neurogenic response with systemic cardiovascular, hemodynamic and hydroelectrolytic alterations. In this early response, those cells that produce substances for export, first synthesize and then store large amounts of molecules in secretory vesicles that are ready for rapid release, *i.e.* catecholamines, which play the leading role [61]. In turn, the upregulated systemic vitelline phenotype could mediate the inflammatory bone marrow response with a lipid metabolic switch linked to steroid synthesis. Therefore, this slower response would be developed by steroidogenic cells that store very little steroid hormones, so that a rapid steroidogenic response would require rapid synthesis of new steroids, *i.e.* cortisol [62] (Fig. **2**).

Finally, the polarization of the mentioned systemic pathological axes, *i.e.* neurogenic and bone-marrow-related, in the injured tissue would condition the evolution of the repair response. Gastrulation, with neoformation of a reparative tissue, is based on the recapitulation of the formation process of the intraembryonic mesenchymal. In essence, the interaction of the extraembryonic functional axes in the interstitium of the damaged tissue allows for recapitulating the mechanisms characteristic of gastrulation and, subsequently forms the intraembryonic mesenchyma, during the early phases of development. Mesodermal derived cells, in particular fibrocytes [63], or alternatively, epiblast-derived pluripotent stem cells that survive beyond embryonic development in adult tissues as a "hibernating backup" [64], play the leading role in the repair reaction. Fibrocytes are bone marrow-derived mesenchymal progenitors that have been reported to express surface markers for leukocytes and mesenchymal cells [65]. In addition, fibrocytes have ambivalent repair functions so they can accelerate wound healing by stimulating cell proliferation, re-epithelization and angiogenesis [63], in contrast, however, they can also be involved in inflammatory fibrotic processes, such as hypertrophic scarring, keloid formation, asthma, atherosclerosis and systemic fibrosis [65-67] (Table **2**).

In contrast to adult wound healing, the early gestation fetus has the remarkable ability to heal skin wounds without scarring [68]. There are numerous intrinsic and extrinsic differences between the fetus and adult that may influence wound healing. In particular, the fetal wound is continuously bathed in amniotic fluid rich in growth factors and extracellular matrix components, such as hyaluronic acid, type III collagen and matrix metalloproteinases. In addition, fetal wound healing is characterized by a rapid upregulation of genes in progenitor cells involved in cell growth and proliferation, with decreased platelet aggregation and degranulation, compared to adult wound healing [68]. One intrinsic difference also includes fetal tissue oxygenation. The fetus has a very low pO_2 since there is a large transplacental oxygen gradient between maternal arterial and umbilical venous blood. Consequently, the fetus can heal in a relatively hypoxemic environment [69]. However, during fetal development, they begin to heal with significant inflammation and scarring as the skin becomes more mature. In particular, mast cells may mediate this transition from scarless to fibrotic healing [70]

THE SYSTEMIC UPREGULATION OF EXTRAEMBRYONIC PHENOTYPES IN THE LIVER WOUND HEALING REACTION

The wound healing reaction could represent the polarization in the injured tissue of the upregulated systemic extraembryonic phenotypes. The hypothetical ability of the adult body for the systemic recapitulation of extraembryonic functions related to wound healing could explain the homogeneity of this response whatever its etiology and location. Thus, other organic locations of the wound healing reaction, aside from the cutaneous, not only have similar mechanisms related to fibrosis development, but also similar associated systemic impairments.

The liver stands out among other organs as the one whose persistent injury usually results in the chronic activation of inflammation and the wound healing response [4, 71-73]. Development of the liver during early embryogenesis may share similarities with pathophysiological processes seen in adulthood, such as acute liver injury and liver regeneration, but also in liver fibrosis [73, 74]. The hypothetical ability of the liver during the evolution of the inflammatory response to involute or dedifferentiate could constitute an effective defense mechanism against injury since it could make retracing a well-known route possible, which is the prenatal specialization phase [73]. This specialization would require the return to the prominence of oxidative metabolism, and thus angiogenesis, to create a capillary bed that would make regeneration possible or alternately, for carrying out the repair through fibrosis or scarring [4, 72].

The increasing knowledge on the extra-hepatic involvement typical of this fibrotic liver disease, however, suggests that this wound healing process is associated with a complex systemic pathogenesis [75]. Portal hypertension is the major hemodynamic complication of a variety of diseases that obstruct portal blood flow, including liver cirrhosis [76]. Portal hypertension in the cirrhotic patient could be associated with autonomic dysfunction [77], hyperdynamic circulation, increased total blood volume by sodium and water retention [75], decreased splanchnic and systemic vascular resistance [75], endothelial dysfunction in the extrahepatic *i.e.* splanchnic and systemic, circulation [75], cirrhotic cardiomyopathy, hepatopulmonary syndrome, portopulmonary hypertension [78, 79], coagulopathy [80], esophageal varices [81], ascites, hepatic encephalopathy and hepatorenal syndrome [82, 83].

These severe systemic complications of the portal hypertension syndrome accompanying the wound healing liver reaction could be based on some metabolic similarities that can be established with the extraembryonic amniotic and vitelline functions playing the leading role during embryonic development [84]. In brief, the impairments related to hydroelectrolytic decompensation like the hyperactive splanchnic and systemic circulation [75], sodium and water retention with expansion of the plasma volume [75], increased interstitial hepato-intestinal lymph flow [85], ascites [85] and hepatorenal syndrome [83] could be attributed to the upregulation of a systemic amniotic-like axis [84, 85]. In turn, the immune response with interstitial splanchnic infiltration by inflammatory cells, including mast cells [86], the impaired splenic function with splenomegaly [87], the changes of the hepatic lipid metabolism with dyslypidemia [84], the male hypogonadims [88] and an excessive angiogenic splanchnic and systemic response [89], could represent the upregulation of a systemic vitellogenic-like axis [84]. Finally, the confluence of both systemic extraembryonic axes in the injured liver could favor a gastrulation-like response in which fibrogenesis would predominate [84] (Table **2**).

THE BASICS OF WOUND HEALING: A BRIEF JOURNEY FROM EMBRYO TO PREMATURE SENESCENCE

Since it has been hypothesized that during wound healing extraembryonic functions are systemically re-expressed and converge into the injured tissue, it seems appropriate to propose that the final aim of this process could also be collaborating in some type of development similar to embryonic development during the postnatal life. This is why we have considered that the upregulated systemic extraembryonic functions would have the objective of stimulating the development of a new repairing tissue after tissue injury during adult life [10]. Thus the wound healing reaction could have properties comparable to an embryo. If so, one of the main objectives in which the above-mentioned upregulated extraembryonic phenotypes could collaborate during the early phase of wound healing is in the establishment of an open circulation in the injured area. Thus an open circulatory system could facilitate the interstitial fluid diffusion and, concomitantly tissue nutrition when the blood circulation losses its prominent role.

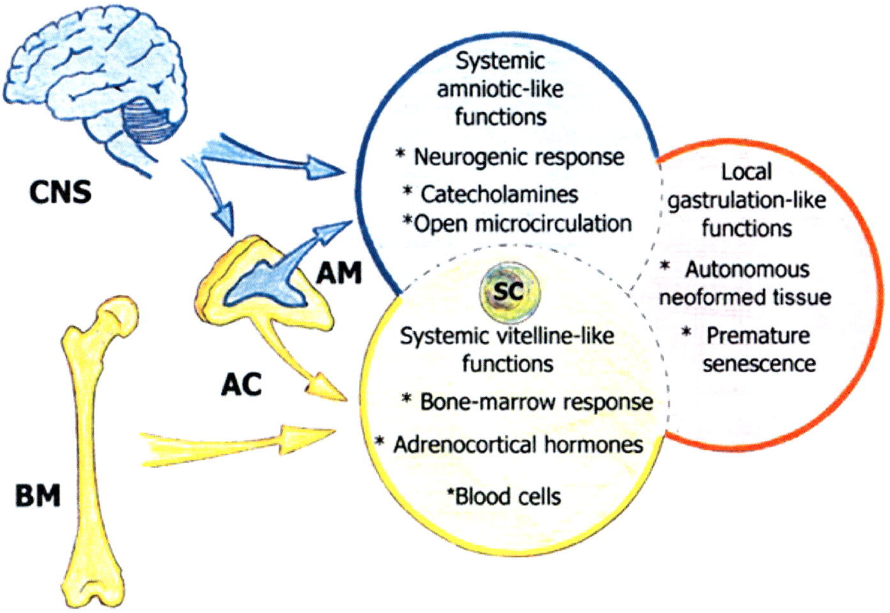

Figure 3: Wound healing would involve the re-expression of systemic extraembryonic-like phenotypes, *i.e.* amniotic and vitelline. The interstitial overlapping of these extraembryonic phenotypes in the injured tissue would allow for the stem or progenitor cells (SC) to induce the expression of a gastrulation-like phenotype with production of new tissue with a dysfunctional parenchyma and an exuberant stroma or fibrosis because of its premature transition to senility. AC: adrenal cortex; AM: adrenal medulla; BM: bone marrow; CNS: central nervous system.

Animals have adapted a circulatory system during evolution. Vertebrates, the most advanced deuterostome animals, have a closed circulatory system and a heart that drives blood through closed blood vessels [90], whereas in insects- the most developed protostomes- the body fluid called hemolymph is pumped by a dorsal heart through the tissue without closed vessels [91]. Therefore, inflammation in mammals converts a closed microcirculation into an open microcirculation in the injured tissue. Thus through the post-capillary venule, which is the preferred extravasation site of plasma and blood cells during the inflammatory response [17, 18] and by means of the associated simultaneous activation of the lymphatic circulation [92], an open microcirculatory pathway in the injured tissue would be established. This new open microcirculation would be thus provided with molecules and cells coming from the upregulated extraembryonic amniotic and vitelline axes. So, maybe through the upregulation of ancestral phylogenetic mechanisms, the plasma, the interstitial fluid and lymph compartments are closely linked during inflammation, favoring then the continuous flow of fluid from one compartment to the next [92, 93]. In essence, an open microcirculation during the wound healing reaction favors the integration into the injured tissue of the systemic molecular and cellular mediators coming from the upregulated extraembryonic phenotypes that, in turn, would control the tissue repair.

The collection of cells that infiltrates the *interstitium* in the inflamed tissue, thanks to the open microcirculatory system, acquires metabolic characteristics that transform them into a tissue with great functional autonomy. Thus, monocytes, macrophages and lymphoid cells have been shown not only to express β-and α_1-adrenoceptors, but also synthesize catecholamines [94, 95]. Lymphocytes also have been shown to store and synthesize serotonine [96]. In addition, immune cell-derived cholinergic activity can modulate inflammation [97]. Furthermore, the pro-opiomelanocortin (POMC)-peptides, including adrenocorticotrophin (ACTH), found in leukocytes show the same structure of those present in the pituitary [98]. POMC-derived peptides have a very ancient origin and an extremely high level of conservation [99]. They also play a critical role in regulating energy balance [100]. Maybe these are the reasons why the stress response axis can be retrieved by the immunocytes participating in the wound healing reaction, where the corticotropin-releasing hormone (CRH), ACTH-like and biogenic amines are present [99-101].

It's possible that the procurement of this functional and metabolic autonomy for expressing extraembryonic phenotypes by the new formed tissue favors its early development. Nonetheless, its inappropriate persistence could produce the characteristic imbalance in the fibrotic diseases between parenchyma and stroma in favor of this last component [2-5]. Therefore, the prompt termination of this autonomic stress response could be essential to prevent the negative effects of inappropriate levels of stress hormones over the neoformed tissue, and in a similar way, the excessive or persistent action of the stress hormones in the adult organism inevitably leading to sclerosis, that is, to a rapid aging [44]. The mechanisms that underlie the age-dependent risk of fibrosis are unknown. However, the aging tissue is more susceptible to injury and fibrosis associated with endoplasmic reticulum stress, apoptosis and activation of pro-fibrotic pathways. Progressive fibrosis is a hallmark of aging in various organs such as kidney, liver, pancreas and lung, as well as in the cardiovascular system [102]. In particular, with accelerating age, skin functions deteriorate due to structural and morphological changes and the incidence of chronic non-healing is increased. Multiple pathways are involved in the pathogenesis of aged skin, including alterations in DNA repair and stability, mitochondrial function, cell cycle and apoptosis, extracellular matrix and cellular metabolism [103].

However, cellular senescence might participate in complex biological processes, including tumor suppression or promotion, tissue repair and aging, some of which have apparently opposing effects [104]. This duality of complex effects associated with the age-phenotypes could be attributed to the dedifferentiating property that the persistent recapitulation of extraembryonic functions would provide to the aged tissues. Consequently, with advanced age, chronic low-grade inflammation may lead to cell dedifferentiation which, in turn, induces mechanisms in the senescent tissues that drive a wide variety of morphogenetic and functional changes typical of early embryonic development, but in an inappropriate environment. Cellular senescence might therefore be antagonistically pleiotropic and display multiple phenotypes [104, 105].

The ancestral character of the inflammatory mechanisms involved during the wound healing response to injury suggests the great relevance its phylogenetic preservation should have had. The link between these mechanisms, whether with physiological processes (embryo development) or with pathological conditions (fibrotic diseases) could also explain the impossibility of individualizing both types of responses as in aging. In turn, this similarity among the mechanisms that drives embryo development, wound healing reaction and senility, suggests the existence of a basic functional pattern that repeats itself at different magnifications, like fractals [106-108]. In theory, a perfect fractal is self-similar at all scales; it can be scaled up and down to infinity [108]. Because of these limits of self-similarity, it is preferable, as advised by Brown *et al.* [108], to refer to this biological system as fractal-like. This self-organizing fractal hypothesis applied to wound healing research could allow for the generation of knowledge through the comparison and complementing of empirical data across different disciplines [108-110].

ACKNOWLEDGEMENTS

We would like to thank Maria Elena Vicente for preparing the manuscript, Elizabeth Mascola for translating it into English and librarians of Complutense University Medical School, particularly the Director, Francisco Javier Jorge García-Reyes, and Manuela Crego and María José Valdemoro and B. Braun Surgical S.A. for their technical assistance.

This study was carried out in part with grants from Mutua Madrileña Research Foundation (Ref. nº PA 3077/2008 and AP5966/2009), MICINN PSI2010-19348 and with the special collaboration of the INEUROPA (Instituto de Neurociencias del Principado de Asturias).

CONFLICT OF INTEREST

The author(s) confirm that this chapter content has no conflict of interest.

REFERENCES

[1] Hunt TK, Andrew WS, Halliday B, *et al.* Coagulation and macrophage stimulation of angiogenesis and wound healing. In: *The Surgical Wound. Chapter 1.* Edited by Dineen P, Hildick-Smith G. Philadelphia: Ed. Lea & Febiger; 1981; 1-18.

[2] Lau K, Paus R, Tiede S, *et al.* Exploring the role of stem cells in cutaneous wound healing. Exp Dermatol 2009; 18: 921-933.

[3] Wynn TA. Integrating mechanisms of pulmonary fibrosis. J Exp Med 2011; 208: 1339-1350.

[4] Pinzani M, Roselli M, Zuckermann M. Liver cirrhosis. Best Pract Res Clin Gastroenterol 2011; 25: 281-290.

[5] Meran S, Steadman R. Fibroblasts and myofibroblasts in renal fibrosis. Int J Exp Pathol 2011; 92: 158-167.

[6] Frantz S, Bauersachs J, Ertl G. Post-infarct remodelling: contribution of wound healing and inflammation. Cardiovasc Res 2009; 81: 474-481.

[7] Romano E, Manetti M, Guiducci S, *et al.* The genetics of systemic sclerosis: an update. Clin Exp Rhematol 2011; 29(2 suppl. 65): S75-S86.

[8] Li Z, Xie WB, Escawo CS, *et al.* Response gene to complement 32 is essential for fibroblast activation in renal fibrosis. J Biol Chem 2011; 286:41323-30.

[9] Selman M, Pardo A, Kaminski N. Idiopathic pulmonary fibrosis: Aberrant recapitulation of developmental programs? PLoS Medicine 2008; 5: e62.

[10] Aller MA, Arias JI, Arias J. Pathological axes of wound repair: Gastrulation revisited. Theor Biol Med Model 2010; **7:** 37.

[11] Arias JI, Aller MA, Prieto I, *et al.* The amazing power of cancer cells to recapitulate extraembryonic functions: The Cuckoo's tricks. J Oncol 2012; 2012: 521284.

[12] Eming SA, Krieg T, Davidson JM. Inflammation in wound repair: Molecular and Cellular mechanisms. J Invest Dermatol 2007; 127: 514-525.

[13] Macri L, Clark RAF. Tissue engineering for cutaneous wounds: Selecting the proper time and space for growth factors, cells and the extracellular matrix. Skin Pharmacol Physiol 2009; 22: 83-93.

[14] Schreml S, Landthaler M, Schäferling M, *et al.* A new state on the H_2Orizon of wound healing? Exp Dermatol 2010; 20: 229-231.

[15] Goldberg SR, Diegelmann RF. Wound healing primer. Surg Clin North Am 2010; 90: 1133-1146.

[16] Delavary RM, Van der Veer WM, Van Egmond M, *et al.* Macrophages in skin injury and repair. Immunobiology 2011; 216: 753-762.

[17] Yates CC, Bodnar R, Wells A. Matrix control of scarring. Cell Mol Life Sci 2011; 68: 1871-1881.

[18] Aller MA, Arias JL, Nava MP, *et al.* Post-traumatic inflammation is a complex response based on the pathological expression of the nervous, immune and endocrine functional systems. Exp Biol Med (Maywood) 2004; 229: 170-181.

[19] Aller MA, Arias JL, Sanchez-Patan F, *et al.* The inflammatory response: an efficient way of life. Med Sci Monit 2006; 12: RA225-RA234.

[20] Aller MA, Arias JI, Giner M, *et al.* Oxygen-related inflammatory wound phenotypes. In: *Wound Healing: Process, Phases and Promoting. Chapter 2.* Edited by J.E. Middleton. N.Y. USA: Nova Sciences Publishers-Huntington Ed; 2011; 1-26.

[21] Bishop A. Role of oxygen in wound healing. J Wound Care 2008; 17: 399-402.

[22] Schreml S, Szeimies RM, Prantl L, *et al.* Oxygen in acute and chronic wound healing. Br J Dermatol 2010: 163: 257-268.

[23] Scadden DT. The stem-cell niches as an entity of action. Nature 2006; 441: 1075-1079.

[24] Glotzbach JP, Wong VW, Gurtner GC, *et al.* Regenerative medicine. Curr Probl Surg 2011; 48: 148-212.

[25] Harris J. Autophagy and cytokines. Cytokine 2011; 56:140-144.

[26] De Miguel MP, Arnalich-Montiel P, Lopez-Iglesias A, *et al.* Epiblast-derived stem cells in embryonic and adult tissues. Int J Dev Biol 2009; 53: 1529-1540.

[27] Acloque H, Adams MS, Fishwick K, *et al.* Epithelial-mesenchymal transitions: the importante of changing cell state in development and disease. J Clin Invest 2009; 119:1438-1449.

[28] Chang YJ, Hwang SM, Tseng CP, *et al.* Isolation of mesenchymal stem cells with neurogenic potentials from the mesoderm of the amniotic membrane. Cell Tissues Organs 2010; 192:93-105.

[29] Ubertu MG, Pierpont YN, Ko F, *et al.* Amnion-derived cellular cytokine solution (ACCS) promotes migration of keratinocytes and fibroblasts. Ann Plast Surg 2010; 64: 632-635.

[30] Bellini C, Boccardo F, Bonioli E, *et al.* Lymphodynamics in the fetos and newborn. Lymphology 2006; 39: 110-117.

[31] Siegel N, Rosner M, Hanneder M, *et al.* Human amniotic fluid stem cells: a new perspective. Amino Acids 2008; 35: 291-293.

[32] Shaw SW, David AL, De Coppi P. Clinical applications of prenatal and postnatal therapy using stem cells retrieved from amniotic fluid. Curr Opin Obstet Gynecol 2011; 23: 109-116.

[33] Fraser ST, Baron MH. Embryonic fates for extraembryonic lineages: new perspectives. J Cell Biochem 2009; 107: 586-591.
[34] Ueno H, Weissman IL. The origin and fate of yolk sac hematopoiesis: application of chimera analyses to developmental studies. Int J Dev Biol 2010; 54: 1019-1031.
[35] Yoshid S, Wada Y. Transfer of maternal cholesterol to embryo and fetus in pregnant mice. J Lipid Res 2005; 46: 2168-2174.
[36] Nakazawa F, Alev C, Jakt LM, *et al.* Yolk sac endoderm is the major source for serum proteins and lipids and is involved in the regulation of vascular integrity in early chick development. Dev Dyn 2011; 240: 2002-2010.
[37] Hocking AM, Gibran NS. Mesenchymal stem cells: Paracrine signaling and differentiation during cutaneous wound repair. Exp Cell Res 2010; 316: 2213-2219.
[38] Dazzi F, Krampera M. Mesenchymal stem cells and autoimmune diseases. Best Pract Res Clin Haematol 2011; 24: 49-57
[39] Otto WR, Wright NA. Mesenchymal stem cells: from experiment to clinic. Fibrogenesis Tissue Repair 2011; 4: 20.
[40] Eisenhut M. Changes in ion transport in inflammatory disease. J Inflammation 2006; 3: 5.
[41] Eisenhut M, Wallace H. Ion channels in inflammation. Pflugers Arch 2011; 461:401-421.
[42] Arck PC, Slominski A, Theoharides TC *et al.* Neuroimmunology of stress: skin takes center stage. J Invest Dermatol 2006; 126: 1697-1704.
[43] Szczepanska-Sadowska E, Cudnoch-Jedrzejewska M, Ufnal T, *et al.* Brain and cardiovascular diseases: Common neurogenic background of cardiovascular, metabolic and inflammatory diseases. J Physiol Pharmacol 2010; 61: 509-521.
[44] Aguilera G. HPA axis responsiveness to stress: implications for health aging. Exp Gerontol 2011; 46: 90-95.
[45] Groeneweg FL, Karst H, De Kloet ER *et al.* Rapid non-genomic effects of corticosteroids and their role in the central stress response. J Endocrinol 2011; 209: 157-167.
[46] Pullar CE, Grahn JC, Liu W, *et al.* Beta-2-adrenergic receptor activation delays wound healing. FASEB J 2006; 20: 76-86.
[47] Romana-Souza B, Otranto M, Vieira AM *et al.* Rotational stres-induced increase in epinephrine levels delays cutaneous wound healing in mice. Brain Behav Immun 2010; 24: 427-437.
[48] Sivamani RK, Pullar CE, Manabat-Hidalgo CG, *et al.* Stress-mediated increases in systemic and local epinephrine impair skin wound healing: Potential new indication for beta blockers. PLoS Med 2009; 6: e12.
[49] Romana-Souza B,Porto LC, Monte-Alto-Costa A. Cutaneous wound healing of chronically stressed mice is improved through catecholamine blockade. Exp Dermatol 2010; 19: 821-829.
[50] Ehninger A, Trumpp A. The bone marrow stem cell niche grows up: mesenchymal stem cells and macrophages move in. J Exp Med 2011; 208: 421-428.
[51] Balbridge MT, King K, Goodell MA. Inflammatory signals regulate hematopoietic stem cells. Trends Immunol 2011; 32: 57-64.
[52] Balbridge MT, King KY, Boles NC, *et al.* Quiescent haematopoietic stem cells are activated by IFN-gamma in response to chronic infection. Nature 2010; 465: 793-797.
53] Scull CM, Hays WD, Fischer TH. Macrophage pro-inflammatory cytokine secretion in enhanced following interaction with autologous platelets. J Inflamm (Lond) 2010; **7: 53.**

[54] Mosser DM, Edwards JP. Exploring the full spectrum of macrophage activation. Nat Rev Immunol 2008; 8: 958-969.
[55] Murray PJ, Wynn TA. Protective and pathogenic functions of macrophage subsets. Nat Rev Immunol 2011; 11: 723-737.
[56] Brancato SK, Albina JE. Wound macrophages as key regulators of repair. Origin, phenotype and function. Am J Pathol 2011; 178: 19-25.
[57] Koth TJ, Di Pietro LA. Inflamamtion and wound healing: the role of the macrophage. Expert Rev Mol Med 2011; 13: e23.
[58] George AL, Bangalore-Prakash P, Rajoria S, *et al.* Endothelial progenitor cell biology in disease and tissue regeneration. J Hematol Oncol 2011; 4: 24.
[59] Bayless JK, Johnson GA. Role of the cytoskeleton in formation and maintenance of angiogenic sprouts. J Vasc Res 2011; 48: 369-385.
[60] Masuda H, Asahara T. Post-natal endothelial progenitor cells for neovasularization in tissue regeneration. Cardiovasc Res 2003; 58: 390-398.
[61] Grieb G, Steffens G, Pallua N, *et al.* Circulating fibrocytic-biology and mechanisms in wound healing and scar formation. Int Rev Cell Mol Biol 2011; 291: 1-19.
[62] Ratajczak MZ, Liu R, Ratajczak J *et al.* The role of pluripotent embryonic-like stem cells residing in adult tissues in regeneration and longevity. Differentiation 2011; 81: 153-161.
[63] Ekert JE, Murray LA, Das AM, *et al.* Chemokine (C-C motif) ligand 2 mediates direct and indirect fibrotic responses in human and murine cultured fibrocytes. Fibrogenesis Tissue Repair 2011; 4: 23.
[64] Kao H-K, Chen B, Murphy G, *et al.* Peripheral Blood Fibrocytes: Enhancement of Wound Healing by Cell Proliferation, Re-Epithelialization, Contraction, and Angiogenesis. Ann Surg 2011; 254:1066-1074.
[65] Jones CP, Rankin SM. Bone marrow-derived stem cells and respiratory disease. Chest 2011; 140: 205-211.
[66] Miller WL, Bose HS. Early steps in steroidogenesis: intracellular cholesterol trafficking. J Lipid Res 2011; Oct 5 [Epub ahead of print.
[67] Arima Y, Hayashi H, Kamata K, *et al.* Decreased expression of neurofibromin contributes to epithelial-mesenchymal transition in neurofibromatosis type 1. Exp Dertamol 2009; 19: e136-e141.
[68] Larson BJ, Longaker MT, Lorenz HP. Scarless fetal wound healing: a basic science review. Plast Reconstr Surg 2010; 126: 1172-1180.
[69] Roh TS, Rah DK, Park RY. The fetal wound healing: a review. Yonsei Med J 2001; 42: 630-633.
[70] Wulf BC, Parent AE, Meleski MA, *et al.* Mast cells contribute to scar formation during fetal wound healing. J Invest Dermatol 2011; doi:10.1038/j.d. 2011: 324).
[71] Wasmuth HE, Tacke F, Trautwein C. Chemokines in liver inflammation and fibrosis. Semin Liver Dis 2010; 30: 215-225.
[72] Forbes SJ, Parola M. Liver fibrogenic cells. Best Pract Res Clin Gastroenterol 2011; 25: 207-217.
[73] Aller MA, Arias JL, Garcia-Dominguez J. *et al.* Experimental obstructive cholestasis: the wound-like inflammatory liver response. Fibrogenesis Tissue Repair 2008; 1: 6.
[74] Aller MA, Arias JL, Prieto I, *et al.* Bile duct ligation: step-by-step to cholangiocyte inflammatory tumorigenesis. Eur J Gastroenterol Hepatol 2010; 22: 651-661.

[75] Iwakiri Y. Endothelial dysfunction in the regulation of cirrhosis and portal hypertesion. Liver Int 2011; 32:199-213.
[76] Møller S, Hobolth, L, Winkler C, *et al.* Determinants of the hyperdynamic circulation and central hypovolaemia in cirrhosis. Gut 2001; 60: 1254-1259.
[77] Frith J, Newton JL. Autonomic dysfunction in chronic liver disease. Hepat Med 2011: **3**: 81-87.
[78] Giusca S, Jinga M, Jurcut C, *et al.* Portopulmonary hypertension: from diagnosis to treatment. Eur J Inter Med 2011; 22: 441-447.
[79] Sawant PS, Vashishtha C, Nasa M. Management of cardiopulmonary complications of cirrhosis. Int J Hepatol 2011; 2011: 280569.
[80] Tripodi A, Mannucci PM. The coagulopathy of chronic liver disease. N Engl J Med 2011; 365: 147-156.
[81] Mahl TC, Groszmann RJ. Pathophysiology of portal hypertension and variceal bleeding. Surg Clin North Am 1990; 70: 251-266.
[82] Bosch J, Garcia-Pagan JC. Complications of cirrhosis. I. Portal hypertension. J Hepatol 2000; 32: 141-156.
[83] Sola E, Gines P. Renal and circulatory dysfunction in cirrhosis: Current management and future perspectives. J Hepatol 2010; 53: 1135-1145.
[84] Aller MA, Heras N, Blanco-Rivero J, *et al.* Portal hypertensive cardiovascular pathology: The rescue of ancestral survival mechanisms? Clin Res Hepatol Gastroenterol 2011; DOI 10.1016/j.clinre.2011.07.017.
[85] Aller MA, Prieto I, Argudo S, *et al.* The interstitial lymphatic peritoneal mesothelium axis in portal hypertension ascites: when in danger go back to the sea. Int J Inflam 2010; 2010: 148689.
[86] Aller MA, Arias JL, Arias J. The mast cell integrates the splanchnic and systemic inflammatory response in portal hypertension. J Transl Med 2007; 5: 44.
[87] Tarantino G, Savastano S, Capone D, *et al.* Spleen: A new role for an old player? World J Gastroenterol 2011; 17: 3776-3784.
[88] Foresta C, Schipilliti M, Ciarleglio FA *et al.* Male hypogonadism in cirrhosis and after liver transplantation. J Endocrinol Invest 2008; 31: 470-478.
[89] Coulon S, Heindryckx F, Geerts A, *et al.* Angiogenesis in chronic liver disease and its complications. Liver Int 2011; 31: 146-162.
[90] Aird WC. Discovery of the cardiovascular system: from Galen to William Harvey. J Thromb Haemost 2011; 9: 118-129.
[91] Eble JA, Nilands S. The extracellular matrix of blood vessels. Curr Pharm Des 2009; 15: 1385-1400.
[92] Wilting J, Papoutsi M, Becker J. The lymphatic vascular system: secondary or primary? Lymphology 2004; 37: 98-106.
[93] Levick JR, Michel CC. Microvascular fluid exchange and the revised Starling principle. Cardiovasc Res 2010; 87: 198-210.
[94] Grisanti LA, Evanson J, Marchus E *et al.* Pro-inflammatory responses in human monocytes are β_1-adrenergic receptor subtype dependent. Mol Immunol 2010; 47: 1244-1254.
[95] Sarkar C, Basu B, Chakroborty D *et al.* The immunoregulatory role of dopamine: an update. Brain Behav Immun 2010; 24: 525-528.
[96] Marazziti D, Consoli G, Masala L *et al.* Latest advancements on serotonin and dopamine transporters in lymphocytes. Mini Rev Med Chem 2010; 10: 32-40.

[97] Rosas-Ballina M, Olofsson PS, Ochani M *et al.* Acetylcholine-synthesizing T cells relay neural signals in a vagus nerve circuit. Science 2011; 334: 98-101.

[98] Smith EM, Galin FS, Le Boeuf RD *et al.* Nucleotide and amino acid sequence of lymphocyte-derived corticotropin: endotoxin induction of a truncated peptide. Proc Natl Acad Sci U S A. 1990; 87:1 057-1060.

[99] Malagoli D, Accorsi A, Ottaviani E. The evolution of pro-opiomelanocortin: looking for the invertebrate fingerprints. Peptides 2011; 32: 2137-2140.

[100] Wardlan SL. Hypothalamic proopiomelanocortin processing and the regulation of energy balance. Eur J Pahrmacol 2011; 660: 213-219.

[101] Crivellato E, Nico B, Ribatti D. The chromaffin vesicle: Advances in understanding the composition of a versatile, multifunctional secretory organelle. Anat Rec (Hoboken) 2008; 291: 1587-1602.

[102] Biernacka A, Frangogiannis NG. Aging and cardiac fibrosis. 2011; 2: 158-173).

[103] Zouboulis CC, Makrantonaki E. Clinical aspects and molecular diagnostics of skin aging. Clinics in Dermatology 2011; 29: 3-14).

[104] Rodier F, Campisi J. Four faces of cellular senescence. J Cell Biol 2011; 192: 547-556.

[105] Lepperdinger G. Inflammation and mesenchymal stem cell aging. Curr Opin Immunol 2011; 23: 518-524.

[106] Mandelbrot BB. Stochastic models for the Earth´s relief, the shape and the fractal dimension of the coastlines, and the number-area rule for islands. Proc Natl Acad Sci USA 1975; 72: 3825-3828.

[107] Cross SS. Fractals in pathology. J Pathol 1997; 182:1-8.

[108] Brown JM, Gupta VX, Li B-L *et al.* The fractal nature of nature: power laws, ecological complexity anfd biodiversity. Philos Trans R Soc Lond B Biol Sci 2002; 357: 619-626.

[109] Kurakin A. The self-organizing fractal theory as a universal discovery method: the phenomenon of life. Theor Biol Med Model 2011; 8: 4.

[110] Aller MA, Blanco-Rivero J, Arias JI, Balfagon G, Arias J The wound healing response and upregulated embryonic mechanisms: brothers-in-arms forever. *Exp Dermatol, in press*

Surgical Inflammation, 2013, 154-179

CHAPTER 6

The Polytraumatized Patient

Maria-Angeles Aller[1], Jose-Ignacio Arias [2], Laureano Lorente[1], Isabel Prieto[3] Alfredo Alonso-Poza[4] and Jaime Arias[1,*]

[1]Surgery Department, School of Medicine, Complutense University of Madrid, Madrid, Spain; [2]General and Digestive Surgery Unit, Monte Naranco Hospital, Asturias, Oviedo, Spain; [3]General and Digestive Surgery Unit, La Paz Hospital, Autonoma University of Madrid, Madrid, Spain and [4]General and Digestive Surgery Unit, Sudeste Hospital, Arganda del Rey, Madrid, Spain

Abstract: An interpretation of the metabolic response to injury in patients with severe accidental or surgical trauma is made. In the last century, various authors attributed a meaning to the post-traumatic inflammatory response by using theleological arguments. Their interpretations of this response, not only facilitate integrating the knowledge, but also their flow from the bench to the bedside, which is the main objective of modern translational research. The goal of the current review is to correlate the metabolic changes with the three phenotypes -ischemia-reperfusion, leukocytic and angiogenic that the patients express through the evolution of the systemic inflammatory response. The sequence in the expression of multiple metabolic systems that becomes progressively more elaborate and complex in severe injured patients urges for more detailed knowledge in order to establish the most adequate metabolic support according to the evolutive phase.

Keywords: Inflammation, trauma, metabolic response, shock, hypothalamic-pituitary-adrenal axis, ebb phase, flow phase, acidosis, immunonutrition, metabolic staging, anaerobic glycolysis.

INTRODUCTION

Inflammation is a complex, multiscale biologic response to stress that is also required for repair and regeneration after injury [1]. Particularly, in patients with severe accidental or surgical trauma, the inflammatory response shows its multifaceted and actually soundless capacity [2-5].

***Address correspondence to Jaime Arias:** Cátedra de Cirugía, Facultad de Medicina, Universidad Complutense, Pza. de Ramón y Cajal s.n., 28040 MADRID, Spain; Tel: +34 91 394 1389; Fax: +34 91 3947115; E-mail: jariasp@med.ucm.es

Jaime Arias, Maria-Angeles Aller and Jose-Ignacio Arias (Eds)

In the last century, David P. Cuthbertson [6], Hans Selye [7] and Francis D. Moore [8] attributed a meaning to the post-traumatic inflammatory response accordingly with previous discoveries and the knowledge of the time. By using theological arguments, these extraordinary authors tried to make inroads into the understanding of the metabolic response of the body to the injury [6-8]. Their interpretations of this response, not only facilitate integrating the knowledge, but also their flow from the bench to the bedside, which is the main objective of modern translational research [1, 9, 10].

Thus this would justify the contribution of new interpretations of the metabolic response to injury, in an attempt to facilitate incorporating the newly acquired knowledge of these conditions, in addition to other apparently disparate diseases that have common biological pathways and therapeutic approaches [9].

TROPHIC MECHANISMS LINKED TO THE EVOLUTION OF THE INFLAMMATORY RESPONSE

We have formulated the hypothesis that both acute local and systemic inflammatory responses to injury are based on the successive pathologic functional predominance of three systems referred to as the nervous, immune and endocrine systems. These names are based on the idea that the final and prevalent functions traditionally attributed to these systems may represent the consecutive response phases to stress [11-13].

This hypothesis implies that the successive pathophysiological mechanisms developed by the body when they undergo inflammation are considered increasingly complex trophic functional systems for using oxygen [12, 13].

The first or immediate phase has been referred to as the nervous phase, because the sensory (pain and analgesia) and motor (contraction and relaxation) alterations respond to the injury. The nervous or immediate functional system presents ischemia-revascularization and edema, which favor nutrition by diffusion through the tissues and organs. This trophic mechanism has a low energy requirement that does not require oxygen (ischemia) or in which the oxygen is not correctly used, with the subsequent development of oxidative and nitrosative stress. In this phase, while the progression of the interstitial edema increases the space between the parenchymal cells and the capillaries, the lymphatic circulation is simultaneously activated (circulatory switch). Thus, tissues and organs adopt an ischemia-revascularization phenotype [12, 13] (Fig. **1**).

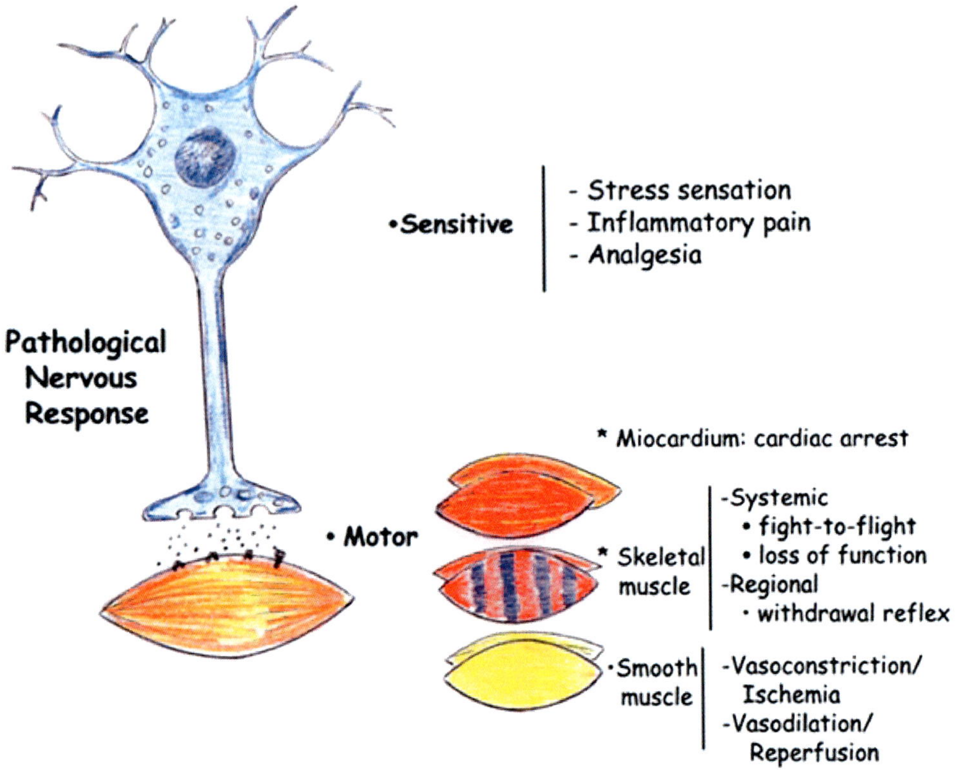

Figure 1: Schematic representation of the Pathological Nervous Response in the severe traumatized patient

In the following immune or intermediate phase of the inflammatory response, the tissues and organs which have suffered ischemia-reperfusion are infiltrated by inflammatory cells and bacteria. Symbiosis of these cells and bacteria for extracellular digestion by enzyme release (fermentation) and by intracellular digestion (phagocytosis) could be associated with a hypothetical trophic capacity. Improper use of oxygen persists in this immune phase and is also associated with enzymatic stress. Furthermore, lymphatic circulation plays a major role while macrophages and dendritic cells migrate to lymph nodes where they activate lymphocytes. As a result, tissues and organs adopt a leukocytic phenotype [12, 13].

Angiogenesis characterizes the last or endocrine phase of the inflammatory response, so nutrition mediated by the blood capillaries is established. However, the angiogenic process becomes active early and excessive proliferation of endothelial cells occurs which in turn, develops a great density of endothelial sprouts [14]. Though this initial and excessive proliferation, the endothelial cells could successively perform antioxidant and antienzymatic functions. These functions would favor the evolution of the inflammatory response towards tissue repair through specialized capillary development. If so, it would be in this last phase of the inflammatory response when the process of angiogenesis would be responsible for tissue nutrition through capillaries. Oxygen and oxidative metabolisms are an excellent combination through which cells can obtain abundant energy (energetic stress) for tissue repair by regeneration or wound healing. As a result, tissues and organs adopt an angiogenic phenotype [13, 14].

The sequence in the expression of progressively more elaborated and complex nutritional systems could hypothetically be considered the essence of the inflammation regardless of its etiology (traumatic, hypovolemic or infectious) or localization. Therefore, the incidence of harmful influences during their evolution could involve regression to the most primitive trophic stages, in which nutrition by diffusion (ischemia-reperfusion phenotype) takes place. Moreover, the incidence of noxious factors during the evolution of the systemic inflammatory response produces severe hemodynamic alterations again, and lastly, vasodilatory shock with tissue hypoxia, hypothermia and acidosis is established. This mechanism of metabolic regression is simple, and also less costly. It facilitates temporary survival until a more favorable environment makes it possible to initiate more complex nutritional ways to survive (leukocytic and angiogenic phenotypes) [12, 13].

PHASES OF THE METABOLIC RESPONSE TO THE INJURY

Severe injury induces a systemic inflammatory response in the body that could be developed through the expression of three successive phenotypes: Ischemia-reperfusion phenotype, leukocytic phenotype and angiogenic phenotype. In turn, it has already been proposed that these phenotypes could represent the expression of trophic functional systems of increasing metabolic complexity [12, 13]. This hypothetical approach to the mechanisms that govern the systemic inflammatory response could be based on the increasing metabolic ability of the body to use oxygen over the successive phases of its evolution towards the tissue repair. Therefore, in the severe injury trauma regardless of the energy type involved in its production (mechanical, thermic, electric or nuclear), it could be considered that the body adapts the support (trophic system) to the metabolic needs characteristic of each inflammatory phenotype. In turn, the metabolic ability of each phenotype would be determined by the mechanisms used for cellular energy production.

Metabolism Related to Ischemia-Reperfusion Phenotype

This phenotype would characterize the immediate or nervous phase of the systemic response to the injury. The nervous alterations in this phase, both sensitive (sensation of stress, inflammatory pain and analgesic response) and motor (contraction and relaxation) predominate. The latter alterations would correspond to both the myocardium (arrhythmias, cardiac arrest), and either the skeletal or voluntary muscle (fight-or-flight response, withdrawal reflexes, loss of motor function) or the smooth involuntary muscle (vasoconstriction with ischemia-reperfusion) related to vasodilation, shock and reperfusion injury [13].

A common pathogenic mechanism of this neuromuscular response would be the sudden alteration of the cellular membrane potential with depolarization. Thus, there is increasing evidence that conditions characterized by an intense local or systemic inflammatory response are associated with abnormal ion transport [15]. Early and pathological changes in ion transport in neuromuscular cells could therefore initiate the inflammatory response. In addition, disturbances of ion transport have been associated with intra and extracellular edema [13, 15] (Fig. **2**).

It has been proposed that both cellular as well as interstitial edema could represent an ancestral mechanism to feed cells by diffusion [12, 13]. Consequently small fluctuations in cell hydration can act as separate and potent signals for cellular metabolism and gene expression. Most importantly, cell volume changes can be secondary to cumulative substrates and hormones uptake [16]. Based on this idea, activation of the hypothalamic-pituitary-adrenal axis and the adrenomedullary system with glucocorticoid secretion and release of epinephrine into the circulation, which occurs in the early evolutionary period [17], causes the selective accumulation of these substances in the interstitial space of the tissues and organs that suffer ischemia-reperfusion because their endothelial permeability is increased [13].

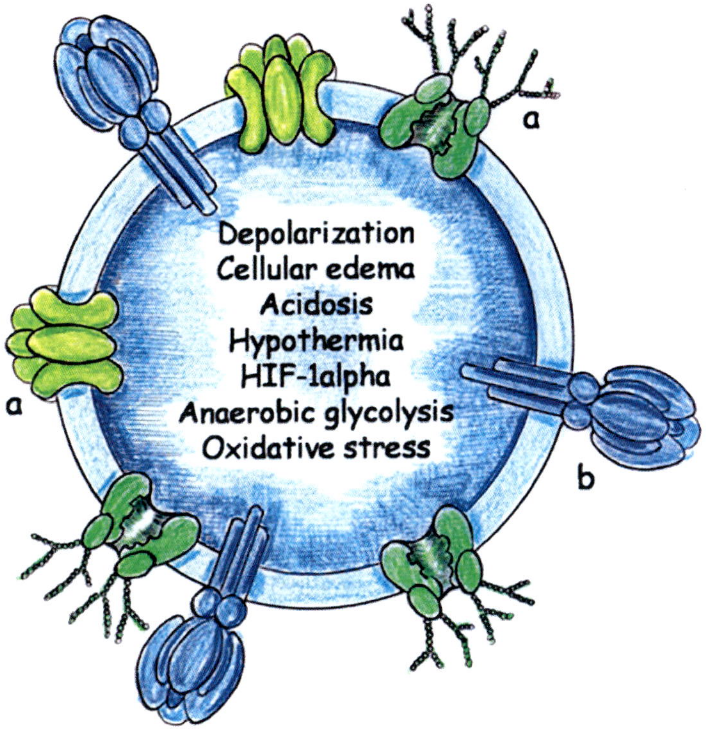

Figure 2: Cellular phenotype of Ischemia/Reperfusion. a: Sodium-Potassium pump. b: Calcium-ATPase pump.

In this initial phase of the inflammatory response, it could be considered that hypometabolism, anaerobic glycolysis with lactate production, low temperature, and a decrease in energy expenditure could be related to a primitive cellular trophic mechanism that may be favored by neuro-endocrine stress-response substances. Interestingly enough, the functional impotence of the somatic motor system, which controls voluntary movements, favors blood stasis and interstitial edema [13].

The edema associated with a depression of the metabolism has been termed by David Cuthbertson, the "ebb phase" [6, 18]. This phase is characterized by hemodynamic instability [19] and is described in classical literature on trauma as the period of shock [6].

The direct mitochondrial inhibition by nitrogen and oxygen species coupled with reduced hormonal stimulation and decrease positive feedback from decreased metabolic demands, all combine to reduce energy production. It is supposed that through this mechanism the affected cells enter in a dormant stage analogous to hibernation or aestivation [20]. That is why this metabolic pathway is considered a potentially protective mechanism because the reduced cellular metabolism could increase the chance of survival of cells, and thus organs, in the face of an overwhelming injury [20].

Hibernation is considered to be a retained ancestral trait in modern mammals. Whether hibernation is inherited or is a newly developed trait, the widespread distribution of mammalian species that hibernate suggests that the genes required to specify the hibernating phenotype are common among the genomes of all mammals [21]. Therefore "cell hibernation" or "cell stunning" during ischemia could be a situation of dedifferentiation, with an intention to adapt to the imposed changes. In this situation, specialized functions would not be expressed, although primitive metabolic pathways and the corresponding primitive trophic functions would be maintained [13].

In essence, the objective of the alterations produced during the expression of the ischemia-reperfusion phenotype could be to induce the highest metabolic autonomy of tissues and organs. Thus the swollen interstitial space would become the storage area for those substances that are suddenly released into the blood circulation during the response to stress [7]. In this way, raised blood concentrations of catecholamines and stress hormones, such as cortisol [7, 17, 22] and glucagon [23], growth hormone and prolactin [24], glucose and glycolytic intermediates *i.e.* lactate and pyruvate [6], triglycerides, free fatty radicals and glycerol [6, 24], amino acids as alanin, nitrogen [8, 25] and sulfur [6, 25] have been described. These substances stored in the interstitial space would facilitate the survival of the hypofunctional cells, allowing for their metabolic autonomy, so a normal state can be restored.

Anoxic environments have occurred throughout the Earth's history. The anoxic atmosphere of the primitive earth probably contained water vapor, N_2, H_2, hydrogen sulfide (H_2S), CO, CO_2, HCN and CH_4. However, as the level of O_2 increased, so did the toxic effects of its one-electron reduction products, its highly reactive singlet from reached proportions that necessitated the development of efficient scavenging and protection systems [26]. Sulfhydryl compounds (H_2S, CH_3, SH, cysteine, glutathione), antioxidants (carotenoids, vitamins C, A and E), an array of enzymes (catalase, superoxide dismutase, peroxidases) and thiol-rich proteins (thioredoxin, glutaredoxin) all became necessary as defenses against damage by reactive oxygen and nitrogen species [26]. H_2S must have been the predominant antioxidant early in prokaryotic evolution [26, 27].

Perhaps, by knowing these precedents it is not surprising that H_2S may play a beneficial role in conditions associated with the increased generation of reactive oxygen and nitrogen species [28]. In particular H_2S may be useful to prevent damage associated with hypoxia. Therefore mice exposed to H_2S enter into a physiological state similar to that observed when animals initiate hibernation, daily torpor or estivation that allows them to endure periods of low metabolic rate and decreased core body temperature without apparent ill effects [29, 30].

After a severe injury the cardiovascular response can move from cardiac arrest to shock. Since cardiac arrest is an evolutive injury, it has been suggested that the optimal treatment is phase-specific and includes: the electrical phase (0-4 minutes), the circulatory phase (4-10 minutes) and the metabolic phase (beyond 10 minutes after cardiac arrest) [31]. In any case, early initiation of cardiopulmonary resuscitation is the most effective measure [32].

Other metabolic, *i.e.* hypothermia, and biochemical interventions, however, are likely to be effective in the metabolic phase of cardiac arrest. Two complementary ways are considered to cover the management of the metabolic phase of cardiac arrest. The first phase consists in reducing the adverse effects of metabolic cardiac arrest promoting basic research on prolonged global whole-body ischemia. The second phase aims at diminishing the tissue injury from reperfusion related to cardiopulmonary resuscitation, studying the optimal metabolic conditions of reperfusion, *i.e.* restoring oxygen and substrates [31].

Shock, regardless of etiology, is characterized by decreased delivery of oxygen and nutrients to the tissues. Our therapeutic interventions are directed toward reversing the cellular ischemia and preventing its consequences [33, 34].

Reperfusion injury starts with the simple reoxygenation of tissues after ischemic insult [35]. Damage control resuscitation [33-36] and damage control surgery [36-39] are used in this early evolutive phase, in accordance with the patient's physiologic tolerance [39]. The principles of damage control have led to improved survival and have stopped bleeding until the physiologic derrangement has been restored and the patient could undergo a prolonged operation for definitive repair [5, 36-38]. Damage control avoids the "lethal triad" of hypothermia, acidosis and coagulopathy resulting in a vicious cycle that often cannot be interrupted [39, 40].

It is currently accepted that the pathophysiological processes in the first days after injury seem to be important for the development and final outcome in patients with early multiple organ failure [41]. That is why reducing initial damage caused by the ischemia and/or the reperfusion would determine a more favorable evolution. Therefore, the two hit hypothesis for the development of multi-organ dysfunction syndrome has been described to be caused either by the first hit, including organ and soft tissue injuries, as well as hypoxia and ischemia, or later due to a second or multiple hits, such as ischemia-reperfusion or surgical procedures [4, 38, 42].

Oxygen deprivation is an important determinant of cellular function during the expression of the ischemia-reperfusion phenotype [43]. The transcriptional response to hypoxia relies on multi-protein complexes to regulate several transcription factors, the best studied being hypoxia inducible factor (HIF). HIF is a heterodimer which enhances the expression of hypoxia responsive genes and therefore allows improved cell survival in situations of limited oxygen availability [43-45]. As a result, injured cells could turn to glycolysis to meet their energetic demands in hypoxia. Although glycolysis is less efficient than oxidative phosphorylation for producing ATP, the presence of sufficient glucose can sustain ATP production due to increased activity of glycolytic enzymes [46].

Post-traumatic hyperglycemia induced by catecholamines, among other factors [6, 19] would also favor the selective support of glucose and therefore the "glycolytic switch" in order to obtain ATP. In turn, glycolytic metabolism end products, *i.e.* pyruvate and oxaloacetate, can promote HIF-1α protein stability and activate HIF-1 inducible gene expression [45]. In addition to impairing cellular energy metabolism, hypoxia leads to differentiation inhibition and maintains the undifferentiated cell state [47].

Furthermore, the excess production of reactive oxygen and nitrogen species in this phase would cause oxidative stress, which would in turn result in bond cleavage and lipid and protein molecular breakdown, whose final products would become substrates in cases of extreme need [12, 13]. Lastly, oxidative stress is one of the principal factors inducing the expression of the nuclear factor Kappa B (NF-κB) [44].

Tissue reoxygenation is mediated by oxygenases. In particular, carbon monoxide (CO) is one of the three products of heme degradation by heme oxygenase (HO)-1. Essentially nothing is known about local concentrations of CO that are achieved *in vivo* and whether that CO produced endogenously has a therapeutic effect [48]. Another gas, nitric oxide (NO) has been involved as a tissue protective agent during ischemia-reperfusion. NO seems to protect cells by attenuating the oxidant stress that occurs during ischemia by inhibiting an oxidase system initiated during ischemia which becomes amplified during the reperfusion phase. In addition, NO can lessen oxidative injury by scavenging reactive oxygen molecules [49].

Resuscitation is related to microcirculatory distress. Microcirculatory failure can occur in the presence of normal or supranormal systemic hemodynamic- and oxygen-derived variables, with microcirculatory distress being masked from the systemic circulation by shunting pathways [50]. In particular, splanchnic microcirculatory dysfunction can produce gastrointestinal tract hypoxia or dysoxia, a state in which the O_2 supply is inadequate to meet tissue metabolic needs [51]. So by the great vulnerability of splanchnic blood flow [52], the first hit, usually ischemia, results in a gastrointestinal tract priming, rendering it more susceptible to a secondary challenge *i.e.* reoxygenation, that stimulates an inappropriate inflammatory response [53]. Therefore, the changes in the intestinal microcirculation are in concert with the “two-hit” theory for multiple organ failure [53, 54], which would at the same time confirm the proposal by Metchnikoff that the engine behind multiple-organ-failure syndrome is the gastrointestinal tract [55].

Metabolism Related to Leukocytic Phenotype

This phenotype would characterize the intermediate or immune phase of the systemic response to the injury. In this phase the tissues and epithelial organs, which have previously suffered ischemia-reperfusion, are infiltrated by inflammatory cells and bacteria. This infiltration occurs in an edematous oxygen-poor environment [13].

In these tissues and organs, which show oxidative and nitrosative stress, symbiosis of the inflammatory cells and bacteria for extra- and intra-cellular digestion could be associated with a hypothetical trophic capacity [12, 13] which is why their metabolic autonomy would persist in this phase.

The metabolic response to injury in this immune phase of the inflammatory response is characterized by hypercatabolism and hypermetabolism [8, 19, 24, 56]. This phase corresponds to the post-shock catabolic response or hypermetabolic flow phase of Cuthbertson [6, 18, 23].

The hypermetabolic response after a severe injury has been described as a hyperdynamic response with increased body temperature, oxygen and glucose consumption, CO_2 production, glycogenolysis, lipolysis, proteolysis and futile substrate cycling [18, 23, 24, 56-58]. The consequences of hypermetabolism are a great loss of body weight associated with a tremendous loss in essential body structures [58].

However, hypermetabolism is further associated with immunologic [2, 4, 38, 59] and endocrinologic responses [2, 59, 60]. The immuno-inflammatory response is initiated immediately following injury and is mainly regulated by cytokines, which act as communication mediators between leukocytes, bridging the innate and adaptive immune response [38]. The immune response leads to systemic inflammatory response syndrome or SIRS, followed by a period of recovery mediated by counter-regulatory anti-inflammatory response (CARS) [2, 4,38, 59, 61].

Activated phagocytes, *i.e.* granulocytes and monocytes, would require anaerobic glycolysis as the main source of ATP for their functions [62]. This suggests that activated leukocytes are able to metabolically adapt to the hypoxia environment in this evolutionary phase of inflammation. Thus, it was shown that HIF-1α is essential for the upregulation of enzymes of the glycolytic pathway to supply phagocytes with enough levels of ATP [62]. Also the oxidative burst is part of the physiological function of phagocytes connected to massive production and release of reactive oxygen species and respiratory burst [63]. Inability of the mitochondria to use oxygen due to the uncoupling of the electron chain transport is a focus of ongoing research [35] (Fig. **3**).

Depression of leukocyte mitochondrial respiration secondary to the decrease in oxygen metabolism could induce obtaining energy by other mechanisms. For example, phagocytes could generate sufficiently reduced nicotinamide dinucleotide phosphate (NADPH) for their biological functions, through the continuous replenishment of Krebs cycle intermediates [64]. Through these anaplerotic mechanisms, phagocytes could obtain sufficient energy not only for the new functions acquired but also for proliferation. These mechanisms, similar to those used by cancer cells, would also allow leukocytes to maintain a metabolic phenotype of biosynthesis aside from the normal physiological constrains and therefore, would acquire an increased metabolic autonomy [65].

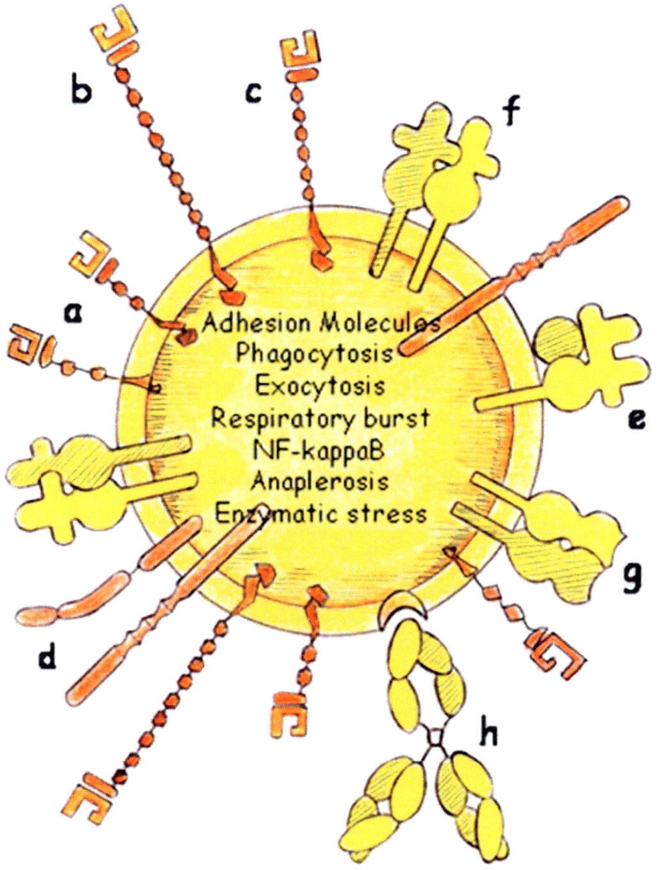

Figure 3: Leukocytic Phenotype. a: L-Selectin; b: P-Selectin; c: E-Selectin; d: Integrin; e: HLA-Class I molecule; f: HLA-Class II molecule; g: HLA-Class II receptor; h: Immunoglobulin.

Based on this metabolic similarity to cancer cells, glutamine, the most abundant amino acid in mammals, could be used to replenish the tricarboxylic acid cycle of leukocytes during this immune phase of the systemic inflammatory response [64]. It would then be explained that the administration of this non-essential amino acids induces an immunostimulatory effect [38] in these severe injured patients with a marked acute and prolonged depletion of intracellular glutamine [66]. Thus, NF-κB is known to be a redox sensitive transcription factor with regard to the production of proinflammatory molecules including chemokines, cytokines and adhesion molecules, which allow leukocytes to attach themselves to the endothelium and facilitate their extravasation to the interstitial space of tissues and organs [35, 67].

The metabolic autonomy of leukocytes would also be reflected in its ability for pro-opiomelanocortin (POMC) production [64]. POMC is processed in the anterior lobe of the pituitary gland into an N-terminal fragment, corticotropin (ACTH) and β-lipotrophic hormone (LPH), while the intermediate lobe produces γ-melanocyte-stimulating hormone (MSH), α-MSH, corticotropin-like intermediate lobe peptide (CLIP), γ-lipotropin (LPH) and β-endorphin. An interesting aspect of leukocyte POMC production is that, while the same peptides are produced as in the pituitary, the pattern varies, and some are unique to leukocytes [68].

Corticotropin releasing factor (CRF), which is released from the hypothalamus during stress, is also produced by leukocytes and within its action, proinflammation through the enhancement of the NF-κB intracellular signaling pathway stands out [69].

Immune cells are also considered a new, diffusely expressed adrenergic organ, and they have the ability to generate release and degradate catecholamines. It seems that catecholamines use intracellular oxidative mechanisms to exert autoregulatory functions on immune cells [70]. The physiological counterpart of the adrenergic system, the cholinergic system, is also known to be an integral part of human macrophage and lymphocyte regulation and is termed as the "cholinergic anti-inflammatory pathway". In this pathway, the efferent activity in the vagus nerve releases acetylcholine (ACh), which interacts specifically with macrophage α_7 subunits of nicotinic ACh receptor, leading to cellular deactivation and inhibition of proinflammatory cytokine release [71].

Therefore, leukocytes through their neurohormonal capacity could modulate the immunological response inducing even hyperinflammation or inmmunoparalysis [2, 61, 72, 73]. In essence, leukocytes seem to become a peripheral neuroendocrine system, with autocrine and paracrine functions. This would constitute an alternative to the central neuroendocrine system, with a predominantly endocrine function, represented by the hypothalamic-pituitary-organ hormonal axes. These are suppressed in prolonged critical illness and contribute to the general wasting syndrome [74, 75] (Fig. **4**).

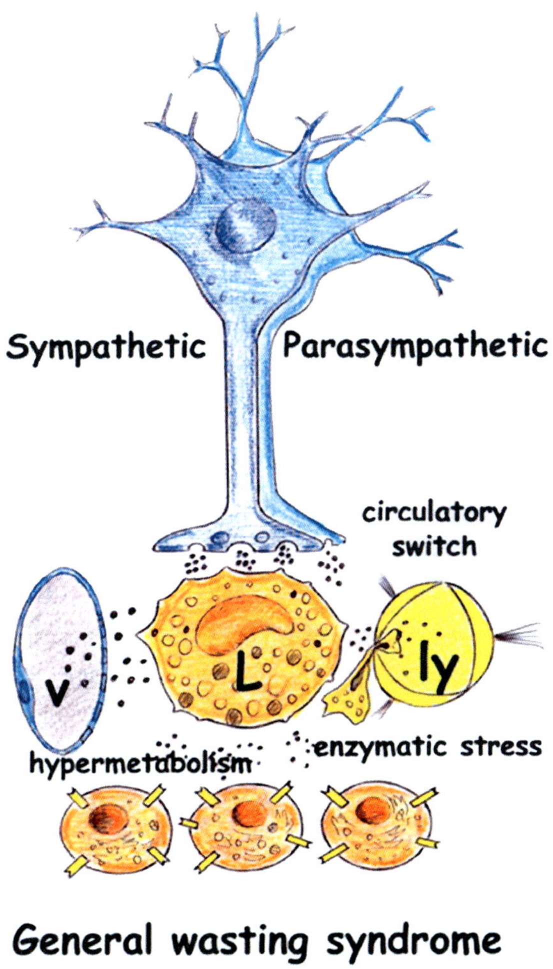

Figure 4: Schematic representation of the neuro-immune-endocrine capacity of the leukocytic (L) phenotype; a: autonomic nervous system; b: venous vascular system; c: lymphatic vascular system; d: parenchymal cells.

The immune response underlying the expression of the leukocyte phenotype could also have a gastrointestinal origin. The gastrointestinal tract mucosa contains the largest reservoir of macrophages in the body. As effector cells, intestinal macrophages, together with mast cells are first-line defense mechanisms [76]. If this defense capacity is overtaken, the intestine in the critically ill surgical patient becomes an "un-drained abscess" [77] and the pathological gastrointestinal colonization is associated with the development of infection and sepsis with late multiorgan failure [78]. Also, during the expression of this immune response, the lymphatic splanchnic circulation would acquire increasing importance [79, 80]. Therefore, the expression of the leukocyte phenotype in the intestine could possibly change this organ into the most important peripheral autonomous neuroendocrine system, in view of the large accumulation of leukocytes with metabolic autonomy and neuroendocrine capacity.

Metabolism Related to Angiogenic Phenotype

This phenotype would characterize the late or endocrine phase of systemic response to injury. In this phase, a return to the prominence of oxidative metabolism would be produced, and therefore angiogenesis, in the affected tissues and organs to create the capillary bed that would make regeneration possible or to carry out repair through fibrosis or scarring [12, 13].

The endocrine functional system facilitates the arrival of oxygen transported by red blood cells and capillaries. It is considered that angiogenesis characterizes this last phase of the inflammatory response, in which nutrition mediated by the blood capillaries is established. The ability to use oxygen in the oxidative metabolism is restored when patients recover their capillary function and, as a result, nutrition mediated by the capillaries is also restored (endocrine or late phase).

This type of metabolism is characterized by a large production of ATP (coupled reaction) which is used to drive multiple specialized cellular processes with limited heat generation that would induce the onset of healing. In the convalescent phase, the previous dedifferentiated epithelia specializes again, the energy stores that supply the substrate necessary for this demanding type of metabolism are repleted, and complete performance is reached, thus making active normal life possible [13, 14].

Angiogenesis is defined as the growth of new vessels from preexisting ones [81]. Although the final objective of endothelial growth is to form new vessels for oxygen, substrates and blood cells transport (vascular phase), other functions could also be carried out before the new vessels are formed (pre-vascular phase). In the initial phases of the inflammatory response, the new endothelial cells formed could have a function associated with anti-inflammatory effects. That is, with anti-oxidative and anti-enzymatic stress properties, favoring the progression of the inflammation as well as its resolution [14].

Angiogenesis is critically dependent on vascular endothelial growth factor (VEGF) action. HIF-1α upregulates a number of factors involved in cytoprotection, including angiogenic growth factors such as VEGF, endothelial progenitor cell recruitment *via* the endothelial expression of stromal-derived factor SDF-1, heme-oxygenase 1 (HO-1) and erithropoietin [82]. Furthermore, VEGF promotes monocyte chemotaxis and the expression of adhesion molecules [43]. Also, when this last phase of inflammation begins, macrophages and lymphocytes become the predominant cell types within the injured tissue. Macrophages, in particular, adopt a potentially angiogenic phenotype [83-85]. Moreover, peripheral blood mononuclear cells can be differentiated into monocytes, lymphocytes and endothelial cells. Therefore, endothelial progenitor cells in the circulation may promote neoangiogenesis and produce the spontaneous regeneration of the endothelium in the injured tissue [86].

In contrast to their role in promoting inflammation, the ability of alarmins to promote tissue repair and regeneration is of increasing interest. Importantly high mobility group box-1 (HMGB 1) induces migration of stem cells towards inflamed regions to promote repair and regeneration [87]. Furthermore it has the ability to stimulate angiogenesis. Interestingly enough, many of these restorative effects are mediated through the same receptors that mediate the proinflammatory properties of the molecule [88].

Obviously, the mechanisms that promote tissue structure and function restoration also include the mechanisms involved in the resolution of inflammation [89]. In particular endogenous pro-resolving lipid mediators, *i.e.* lipoxins, resolvins and protectins have been the most studied [88, 89]. In essence, pro-resolution factors revert back to the proinflammatory phenotype to its prior physiological state and therefore the microcirculatory functions of tissues and organs return to homeostasis [90].

Nutrition mediated by blood capillaries is established because of angiogenesis. The new functional properties of microcirculation include the exchange of oxygen, nutrients and waste products. This oxygen support induces oxidative metabolism, an efficient method for extracting energy from food molecules, which begins with the Krebs cycle and ends with oxidative phosphorylation [12, 13]. Oxygen and oxidative metabolism is an excellent combination through which cells can obtain an abundant energy supply (energetic stress) for tissue repair by specialized cells [12]. Nonetheless, little is known about the capacity of eukaryotic cells to monitor the redox state for supporting specialized functions [91]. Although NF-κB acts mainly as an initiator of inflammation, recent studies suggest that it also functions in the equally complex process of resolution of inflammation [92] (Fig. **5**).

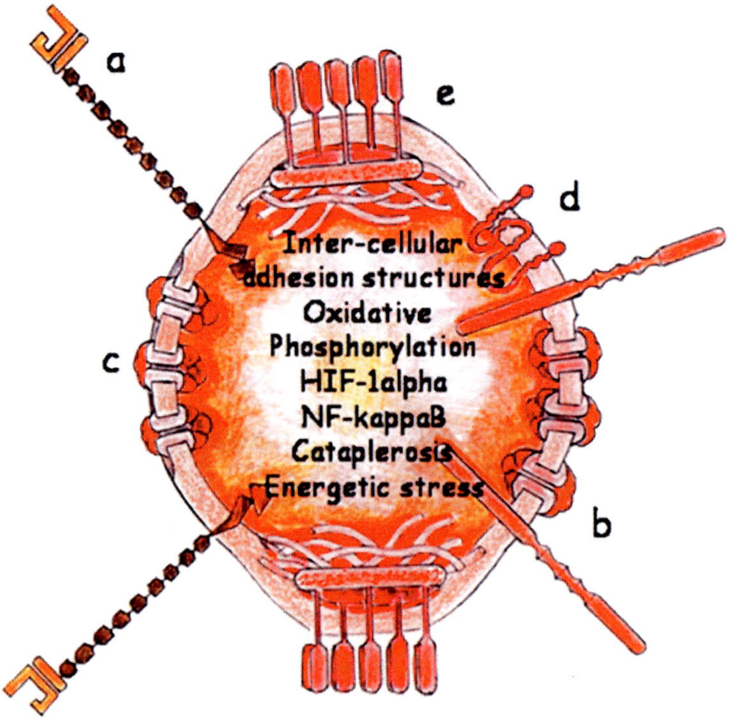

Figure 5: Angiogenic phenotype. a: P-Selectin; b: Integrin; c: Gap-junction; d: Claudin (tight junction protein); e: desmosome.

In this convalescence phase, the hypercatabolic syndrome is progressively down-regulated with the reduction of catabolic hormones and/or molecules (*e.g.*, catecholamines, proinflammatory cytokines, cortisol, glucagon) and the increase of anabolic hormones (*e.g.*, insulin, growth hormones, insulin-like growth factor-1 or anabolic steroids) [74, 93] that are supported by tissues and organs through the new vessel arrangement and morphology. Consequently, this anabolic response counteracts the catabolic stimuli and reverses the muscular, both skeletal and cardiac, wasting and impaired energetic metabolism with its consequent functional damage [93]. Clinical studies in recent years have supported the concept of "immunonutrition" for severely injured patients which takes into account the supplementation of omega-3 fatty acids and essential amino acids, such as glutamine [94].

The progressive recovery of the hypothalamic centralization of the autonomous neurofunctions (sympathetic and vagal nervous system) and endocrine (hypothalamic-pituitary-organ-hormonal axes) possibly corresponds to the progressive remodeling of the tissues and organs controlled by hemodynamic and metabolic stimuli. On the contrary, leukocytes during the transition to resolution would progressively inhibit the neuroendocrine functional capacity found in the previous phases [68-70]. In turn, they would modulate this last phase of the inflammatory response when leukocytes express a lymphocytic phenotype [95]. In particular, regulatory T (Treg) cells safeguard the tissues restored against autoimmunity and immune pathology [96].

The behavior of the gastrointestinal tract under normal conditions mainly depends on the morphology and function of its microcirculation. Thus, the trophic function of the intestine is coupled with the metabolic needs of the body. In particular lymph vessels in the mucosal and submucosal layers, or initial lymphatics, recover their ability to absorb dietary fat and fat soluble vitamins, which are secreted by enterocytes in the form of lipid particles or chylomicrons [97, 98].

In conclusion, the hypothetical capacity of the body to involute or dedifferentiate after a severe injury could mean an effective defense mechanism because it would make it possible to retrace a well-known metabolic route to the specialization of the systemic inflammatory response during the endocrine phase. This specialization would require the return of the prominence of oxidative metabolism and angiogenesis in the affected tissues and epithelial organs to create the capillary bed that would make the repair possible [12-14].

THE NEED OF A METABOLIC STAGING AFTER SEVERE TRAUMA

Elaborating a detailed metabolic staging after severe injury should be a preferential objective today in order to obtain a correct treatment for these patients. One requirement would be for the staging system to have a clinical significance and as a result, for it to allow for establishing the correct metabolic support.

In the current revision, it has been considered that while the systemic inflammatory response develops after a severe injury, the body would successively express phenotypes of increasing metabolic complexity.

The increasing metabolic complexity of the systemic acute post-traumatic inflammatory response also shares some similarities with the successive metabolic stages that eukaryotic cells develop to obtain energy from food [99]. Therefore, in a first stage (nervous phase) macromolecules (polysaccharides, proteins and fats) are broken down by oxidative stress to smaller molecules (glucose, amino acids, triglycerides and free fatty acids). Cells with an ischemia-reperfusion phenotype would base its metabolism on anaerobic glycolysis. The most important part of the second catabolic stage would be headed by enzymatic stress that produces the symbiosis of the inflammatory cells and bacteria (immune phase). Also the cells with leukocytic phenotype could use anaplerotic precursors (glutamine) to obtain energy (NADPH production) that would be employed in biosynthesis pathways (cataplerosis). The addition of an oxygen-requiring stage to the catabolic process provides cells with successively more powerful and efficient methods for extracting energy (electron transport chain). The ability to use oxygen in oxidative metabolism (oxidative phosphorylation) is recovered when the patients recover their capillary function (angiogenic phenotype) and therefore the nutrition mediated by them (endocrine or late phase). This type of metabolism is characterized by a large production of ATP (energetic stress) which is used to drive specialized multiple cellular processes with limited generation of heat.

In summary, the sequence in the expression of metabolic systems that becomes progressively more elaborate and complex could be considered the essence of the metabolic evolution of severe injured patients. In the successive metabolic switches or metamorphoses that patients undergo, possibly they would retrace a well-known embrionary-fetal route. If this is not properly executed, homeostasis is not recovered which is why the patient can suffer a post-traumatic stress syndrome.

The hypothesis that atmospheric oxygen concentration affected the timing of the evolution of cellular compartmentalization by constraining the size of domains necessary for communications across membranes has been suggested [100]. Thus, the relatively rapid changes in the size of the oxygen-rich external domains coincide with increasing organism complexity. This points towards a key role in the increase in abundance and size of receptors over time [100] and adds to a growing body of literature that most recently connects atmospheric oxygen levels and macroevolutionary changes with the complexity of metabolic networks and cell types [100, 101]. Therefore, a correlation between increased organism complexity and the development of the use of the atmospheric oxygen could be established [102-104].

ACKNOWLEDGEMENTS

We would like to thank Maria Elena Vicente for preparing the manuscript, Elizabeth Mascola for translating it into English and librarians of Complutense University Medical School, particularly the Director, Francisco Javier Jorge García-Reyes, and Manuela Crego and María José Valdemoro and B. Braun Surgical S.A. for their technical assistance.

This study was carried out in part with grants from Mutua Madrileña Research Foundation (Ref. nº PA 3077/2008 and AP5966/2009), MICINN PSI2010-19348 and with the special collaboration of the INEUROPA (Instituto de Neurociencias del Principado de Asturias).

CONFLICT OF INTEREST

The author(s) confirm that this chapter content has no conflict of interest.

REFERENCES

[1] Vodovotz Y, Csete M, Bartels J, Chang S, An G. Translocational systems biology of inflammation. PLOS Comput Biol 2008; 4: 1-6.

[2] Kohl BA, Deutschman CS. The inflammatory response to surgery and trauma. Curr Opin Crit Care 2006; 12: 325-332.

[3] Choileain NN, Redmond HP: Cell response to surgery. Arch Surg 2006, 141: 1132-1140.

[4] Lenz A, Franklin GA, Cheadle WG: Systemic inflammation after trauma. Injury 2007; 38: 1336-1345.

[5] Gebhard F, Huber-Lang M: Polytrauma-phatophysiology and management principles. Langenbecks Arch Surg 2008; 393: 825-831.

[6] Cuthbertson DP: The metabolic response to injury and other related explorations in the field of protein metabolism: An autobiographic account. Scot Med J 1982; 27: 158-171.

[7] Selye H: The part of inflammation in the local adaptation syndrome. Rev Can Biol 1953; 12: 155-175.

[8] Moore FD: Bodily changes in surgical convalescence. I – The normal sequence-Observations and interpretations. Ann Surg 1953; 137: 289-315.

[9] Zerhouni E: The NIH roadmap. Science 2003; 302: 63-72.

[10] Gittes GK: The surgeon-scientist in a new biomedical research era. Surgery 2006; 140: 123-131.

[11] Aller MA, Arias JL, Lorente L, Nava MP, Durán HJ, Arias J: Neuro-immune-endocrine functional system and vascular pathology. Med Hypotheses 2001; 57: 561-569.

[12] Aller MA, Arias JL, Nava MP, Arias J: Post-traumatic inflammation is a complex response based on the pathological expression of the nervous, immune, and endocrine functional systems. Exp Biol Med (Maywood) 2004; 229: 170-181.

[13] Aller MA, Arias JL, Sánchez-Patán F, Arias J: The inflammatory response: An efficient way of life. Med Sci Monit 2006; 12: RA225-234.

[14] Aller MA, Arias JL, Cruz A, Arias J: Inflammation: a way to understanding the evolution of portal hypertension. Theor Biol Med Model 2007; 4: 44.

[15] Eisenhut M: Changes in ion transport in inflammatory disease. J Inflamm 2006; 3: 5.

[16] Häussinger D: The role of cellular hydration in the regulation of cell function. Biochem J 1996; 313: 697-710.

[17] O'Connor TM, O'Halloran DJ, Shanahan F: The stress response and the hypothalamic-pituitary-adrenal axis: from molecule to melancholia. QJM 2000; 93: 323-333.

[18] Cuthbetson DP: Alterations in metabolism following injury: Part I. Injury 1980, 11: 175-189.

[19] Hill AG, Hill GL: Metabolic response to severe injury. Br J Surg 1998; 85: 884-890.

[20] Singer M, De Santis V, Vitale D Jeffcoate W: Multiorgan failure is an adaptative, endocrine-mediated, metabolic response to overwhelming systemic inflammation. Lancet 2004; 364: 545-548.

[21] Schaller B, Graf R: Hypothermia and stroke: the pathophysiological background. Pathophysiology 2003; 10: 7-35.

[22] Selye H: Stress and the general adaptation syndrome. Br Med J 1950; 1: 1383-1392.
[23] Cuthbertson DP: Alterations in metabolism following injury: part II. Injury 1980; 11: 286-303.
[24] Douglas RG, Shaw JH: Metabolic response to sepsis and trauma. Br J Surg 1989; 78: 115-122.
[25] Cuthbertson DP: The distribution of nitrogen and sulphur in the urine during conditions of increased catabolism. Biochem J 1931; 25: 236-244.
[26] Lloyd D: Hydrogen sulfide: clandestine microbial messenger? Trends Microb 2006; 14: 456-462.
[27] Kwak W-J, Kwon GS, Jin I, Kuriyama H, Sohn HY: Involvement of oxidative stress in the regulation of H_2S production during circadian metabolic oscillation of Saccharomyces cerevisae. FEMS Microbiol Lett 2003; 219: 99-104.
[28] Lowicka E, Bettowski J: Hydrogen sulfide (H_2S)- the third gas of interest for pharmacologists. Pharmacol Rep 2007; 59: 4-24.
[29] Blackstone E, Morrison M, Roth MB: H_2S induces a suspended animation-like state in mice. Science 2005; 308: 518.
[30] Blackstone E, Roth MB: Suspended animation-like state protects mice from lethal hypoxia. Shock 2007; 27: 370-372.
[31] Weisfeldt ML, Becker LB: Resuscitation after cardiac arrest: A 3-phase time-sensitive model. JAMA 2002; 288: 3035-3038.
[32] Ali BA, Zafari AM: Cardiopulmonary resuscitation and emergency cardiovascular care: Review of the current guidelines. Ann Intern Med 2007; 147: 171-179.
[33] Krausz MM: Initial resuscitation of hemorrhagic shock. World J Emergency Surg 2006; 1: 14.
[34] Velmahos GC, Alam HB: Advances in surgical critical care. Curr Probl Surg 2008; 45: 453-516.
[35] Rushing GD, Britt LD: Reperfusion injury after hemorrhage. A collective review. Ann Surg 2008; 247: 929-937.
[36] Flores HA, Stewart RM: The multiply injured patient. Semin Thorac Cardiovasc Surg 2008; 20: 64-68.
[37] Rotondo MF, Schwab CW, McGonigal MD: Damage control: an approach for improved survival in exanguinating penetrating abdominal injury. J Trauma 1993; 35: 375-383.
[38] Stahel PF, Smith WR, Moore EE: Role of biological modifiers regulating the immune response after trauma. Injury 2007; 38: 1409-1422.
[39] Germanos S, Gourgiotis S, Villias C, Bertucci M, Dimopoulos N, Salemis N: Damage control surgery in the abdomen: An approach for the management of severe injured patients. Intern J Surg 2008; 6: 246-252.
[40] Gentilello LM, Pierson DJ: Trauma critical care. Am J Respir Crit Care Med 2001; 163: 604-607.
[41] Lausevic Z, Lausevic M, Trbojevic-Stankovic J, Krstic S, Stojimirovic B: Predicting multiple organ failure in patients with severe trauma. Can J Surg 200; 51: 97-102.

[42] Moore FA, Sauaia A, Moore EE, Norris JM, Lezotte DC, Hamman RF: Postinjury multiple organ failure. A bimodal phenomenon. J Trauma 1996; 40: 501-512.

[43] Legrand M, Mik EG, Johannes T, Payen D, Ince C: Renal hypoxia and dysoxia after reperfusion of the ischemic kidney. Mol Med 2008; 14: 502-516.

[44] Haddad JJ: Oxygen sensing and oxidant/redox-related pathways. Biochem Biophys Res Comm 2004; 316: 969-977.

[45] Lopez-Lazaro M: HIF-1: hypoxia-inducible factor or dysoxia-inducible factor? FASEB J 2006; 20: 828-832.

[46] Michiels C: Physiological and pathological responses to hypoxia. Am J Pathol 2004; 164: 1875-1882.

[47] Gustafsson MV, Zheng X, Pereira T, Gradin K, Jin S, Lundkvist J, Ruas JL, Poellinger L, Lendahl U, Bondesson M: Hypoxia requires notch signaling to maintain the undifferentiated cell state. Develop Cell 2005; 9: 617-628.

[48] Bach FH: Carbon monoxide: from the origin of life to molecular medicine. TRENDS Mol Med 2006; 12: 348-350.

[49] Iwase H, Robin E, Guzy RD, Mungai PT, Vanden Hoek TL, Chandel NS, Levraut J, Schumacker PT: Nitric oxide during ischemia attenuates oxidant stress and cell death during ischemia and reperfusion in cardiomyocytes. Free Rad Biol Med 2007; 43: 590-599.

[50] Ince C: The microcirculation is the motor of sepsis. Crit Care 2005; 9: S13-S19.

[51] Fisher EM, Lamanna JC: Gut dysoxia: comparison of sites to detect regional gut dysoxia. Adv Exp Med Biol 200, 566: 151-157.

[52] Foëx A: Systemic response to trauma. Br Med Bull 1999; 55: 726-743.

[53] Garrison RN, Spain DA, Wilson MA, Keelen PA, Harris PD: Microvascular changes explain the “two-hit” theory of multiple organ failure. Ann Surg 1998; 227: 851-860.

[54] Meldrum DR, Cleveland JC, Moore EE, Partrick DA, Banerjee A, Harken AH: Adaptative and maladaptative mechanisms of cellular priming. Ann Surg 1997; 226: 587-598.

[55] Carrico CJ, Meakins JL, Marshall JC, Fry D, Maier RV: Multiple-Organ-Failure Syndrome. Arch Surg 1986; 121: 196-208.

[56] Stoner HB: Interpretation of the metabolic effects of trauma and sepsis. J Clin Pathol 1987; 40: 1108-1117.

[57] Atiyeh BS, Gunn WA, Dibo SA: Metabolic implications of severe burn injuries and their management: A systematic review of the literature. World J Surg 2008; 32: 1857-1869.

[58] Jeschke MG, Chinkes DL, Finnerty CC, Kulp G, Suman OE, Norbury WB, Branski LK, Gauglitz GG, Mlcak RP, Herndon DN: Pathophysiologic response to severe burn injury. Ann Surg 2008; 248: 387-401.

[59] Keel M, Trentz O: Pathophysiology of polytrauma. Injury 2005; 36: 691-709.

[60] Vanhorebeek I, Langouche L, Van den Berghe G: Endocrine aspects of acute and prolonged critical illness. Nat Clin Pract Endocrinol Metab 2006; 2: 20-31.

[61] Moore FA, Moore EE: Evolving concepts in the pathogenesis of post-injury multiple organ failure. Surg Clin North Am 1995; 75: 257-277.

[62] Sitkovsky MV, Lukashev D, Apasov S, Kojima H, Koshiba M, Caldwell C, Ohta A, Thiel M: Physiological control of immune response and inflammatory tissue damage by hypoxia-inducible factors and adenosine A_2 receptors. Ann Rev Immunol 2004; 22: 21.1-21.26

[63] Splettstoesser WD, Schuff-Werner P: Oxidative stress in phagocytes. "The enemy within". Microsc Res Tech 2002; 57: 441-455.
[64] Brunengraber H, Roe CR: Anaplerotic molecules: Current and future. J Inherit Metab Dis 2006; 29: 327-331.
[65] DeBerardinis RJ, Lum JJ, Hatzivassiliou G, Thompson CB: The biology of cancer: Metabolic reprogramming fuels cell growth and proliferation. Cell Metab 2008; 7: 11-20.
[66] Griffiths RD, Hinds CJ, Little RA: Manipulating the metabolic response to injury. Br Med Bull 1999; 55: 181-195.
[67] Hanada T, Yoshimura A: Regulation of cytokine signaling and inflammation. Cytokine Growth Fact Rev 2002; 13: 413-421.
[68] Smith EM: Neuropeptides as signal molecules in common with leukocytes and the hypothalamic-pituitary-adrenal axis. Brain Behav Immun 2007; 22: 3-14.
[69] Stephanou A, Jessop DS, Knight RA, Lightman SL: Corticotrophin-releasing factor-like immunoreactivity and mRNA in human leukocytes. Brain Behav Immun 1990; 4: 67-73.
[70] Flierl MA, Rittirsch D, Huber-Lang M, Sarma JV, Ward PA: Catecholamines-crafty weapons in the inflammatory arsenal of immune/inflammatory cells or opening Pandora's box? Mol Med 2008; 14: 195-204.
[71] Czura CJ, Tracey KJ: Autonomic neural regulation of immunity. J Intern Med 2005; 257: 156-166.
[72] Menger MD, Vollmar B: Surgical trauma: hyperinflammation *vs.* immunosuppression? Langenbecks Arch Surg 2004; 389: 475-484.
[73] Tschoeke SK, Ertel W: Immunoparalysis after multiple trauma. Injury 2007; 38: 1346-1357.
[74] Van Der Berghe G: Neuroendocrine axis in critical illness. Curr Opin Endocrinol Diabetes 2001; 8: 47-54.
[75] Vanhorebeek I, Langouche L, Van Der Berghe G: Endocrine aspects of acute and prolonged critical illness. Nat Clin Pract Endrocrinol Metab 2006; 2: 20-31.
[76] Smith PD, Ochsenbauer-Jambor C, Smythies LE: Intestinal macrophages: unique effector cells of the innate immune system. Immunol Rev 2005; 206: 149-159.
[77] Marshall JC, Christou NV, Meakins JL: The gastrointestinal tract. The "undrained abscess" of multiple organ failure. Ann Surg 1993; 218: 111-119.
[78] Suliburk J, Helmer K, Moore F, Mercer D: The gut in systemic inflammatory response syndrome and sepsis: Enzyme system/fighting multiple organ failure. Eur Surg Res 2008; 40: 184-189.
[79] Deitch EA: Bacterial translocation or lymphatic drainage of toxic products from the gut: What is important in human beings? Surgery 2002; 131: 241-244.
[80] Fanous MYZ, Phillips AJ, Windsor JA: Mesenteric lymph: The bridge to future management of critical illness. J Pancreas 2007; 8: 374-399.
[81] Puxeddu I, Ribatti D, Crivallato E, Levi-Schaffer F: Mast cells and eosinophis: A novel link between inflammation and angiogenesis in allergic diseases. J Allergy Clin Immunol 2005; 116: 531-536.

[82] Haase VH: Hypoxia-inducible factors in the kidney. Am J Physiol Renal Physiol 2006; 291: F271-F281.

[83] Lingen MW: Role of leukocytes and endothelial cells in the development of angiogenesis in inflammation and wound healing. Arch Pathol Lab Med 2001; 125: 67-71.

[84] Conway EM, Collen D, Carmeliet P: Molecular mechanisms of blood vessel growth. Cardiovasc Res 2001; 49: 507-521.

[85] Avraamides CJ, Garay-Susini B,Varner JA: Integrins in angiogenesis and lymphangiogenesis. Nature Rev Cancer 2008; 8:604-617.

[86] Abedin M, Tintut Y, Demer LL: Mesenchymal stem cells and the artery wall. Circ Res 2004; 95: 671-676.

[87] Palumbo R, Bianchi ME: High mobility group box 1 protein, a cue for stem cell recruitment. Biochem Pharmacol 2004; 68: 1165-1170.

[88] Klune JR, Dhupar R, Cardinal J, Billiar TR, Tsung A: HMGB1: Endogenous danger signaling. Mol Med 2008; 14: 476-484.

[89] Serhan CN, Brain SD, Buckley CD, Gilroy DW, Haslett C, O'Neill LA, Perretti M, Rossi AG, Wallace JL: Resolution of inflammation: state of the art, definitions and terms. FASEB J 2007; 21: 325-332.

[90] Lawrence T, Gilroy DW: Chronic inflammation: a failure of resolution? Int J Exp Path 2007; 88: 85-94.

[91] Agarwal AK, Auchus RJ: Minireview: Cellular redox state regulates hydroxysteroid dehydrogenase activity and intracellular hormone potency. Endocrinology 2005; 146: 2531-2538.

[92] Ghosh S. Hayden MS: New regulators of NF-κB in inflammation. Nature Rev 2008; 8: 837-849

[93] Pasini E, Aquilani R, Dioguardi FS, D'Antona G, Gheorghiade M, Taegtmeyer H: Hypercatabolic syndrome: Molecular basis and effects of nutritional supplements with aminoacids. Am J Cardiol 2008; 101(Suppl 1): 11E-15E.

[94] Hasenboehler E, Williams A,Leinhase I, Morgan SJ, Smith WR, Moore EE, Stahel PF: Metabolic changes after polytrauma: an imperative for early nutritional support.World J Emerg Surg 2006; 1:29

[95] Rajakariar R, Lawrence T, Bystrom J, Hilliard M, Colville-Nash P, Bellingan G, Fitzgerald D, Yaqoob MM, Gilroy DW: Novel biphasic role for lymphocytes revealed during resolving inflammation. Blood 2008; 111: 4184-4192.

[96] Sauer S, Bruno L, Hertweck A, Finlay D, Leleu M, Spivakov M, Knight ZA, Cobb BS, Cantrell D, O'Connor E, Shokat KM, Fisher AG, Merkenschlager M: T cell receptor signaling controls Foxp3 expression *via* PI3K, Akt, and mTOR. Proc Natl Acad Sci U S A 2008; 105: 7797-7802.

[97] Mäkinen T, Norrmen C, Petrova TV: Molecular mechanisms of lymphatic vascular development. Cell Mol Life Sci 2007; 64: 1-15.

[98] Ohtani O, Ohtani Y: Organization and developmental aspects of lymphatic vessels. Arch Histol Cytol 2008; 71:1-22.

[99] Alberts B, Bray D, Lewis J, Raff M, Roberts K, Walter P: Small molecules, energy and biosynthesis. In: Molecular biology of the cell. Vol. 2. Garland Publishing Inc, New York: 1983: 43-89.
[100] Acquisti C, Kieffe J, Collins S: Oxygen content of transmembrane protein over macroevolutionary time scales. Nature 2007; 445: 47-52.
[101] Nakamura H, Hase A: Cellular differentiation in the process of generation of the eukaryotic cell. Orig Life Evol Biosph 1991; 20: 499-514.
[102] Raymond J, Segre D: The effect of oxygen on biochemical networks and the evolution of complex life. Science 2006; 311: 1764-1767.
[103] Baudin-Cornu P, Thomas D: Oxygen at life's boundaries. Nature 2007; 445: 35-36.
[104] Aller MA, Arias JI, Alonso-Poza A, Arias J. A Review of metabolic staging in severely injured patients. Scand J Trauma Resusc Emerg Med 2010; 18: 27.

Send Orders for Reprints to reprints@benthamscience.net

Surgical Inflammation, 2013, 180-213

CHAPTER 7

Inflammation Related with Surgical Infections

Maria-Angeles Aller[1], Manuel Giner[2], Gregorio Rodriguez–Boto[3], Manuel Losada[4], Alfredo Alonso-Poza[4], Jose- Ignacio Arias[5] and Jaime Arias[1,*]

[1]Surgery Department, School of Medicine, Complutense University of Madrid, Madrid, Spain; [2]General and Digestive Surgery Unit, Clinico San Carlos Hospital, Surgery Department, School of Medicine, Complutense University of Madrid, Madrid, Spain; [3]Neurosurgery Unit, Clinico San Carlos Hospital, Surgery Department, School of Medicine, Complutense University of Madrid, Madrid, Spain; [4]General and Digestive Surgery Unit, Sudeste Hospital, Arganda del Rey, Madrid, Spain and [5]General and Digestive Surgery Unit, Monte Naranco Hospital, Oviedo, Asturias, Spain

Abstract: The inflammatory response related to surgery is a systemic reaction considered as the expression of three overlapping trophic phases during which the oxygen consumption progressively increases. However, surgical inflammation could induce old functions in which life on the Earth has based on the expression of two hypothetical extraembryonic trophic axes *i.e.* coelomic-amniotic and trophoblastic-yolk sac related, when integrated in the interstitium of the injured tissues and organs to induce a gastrulation-related phenotype. This later phenotype would repair the tissues by fibrosis and/or regeneration. A coupling of this recapitulated extraembryonic axis would cause hyperacute or acute–on-chronic inflammation or sepsis. The mechanisms of this systemic inflammatory response could be reminiscences of some phylogenetic mechanisms that ultimately would favor a metabolic cross-talk between the eukaryotic cell and gut microbiome. These ontogenic and phylogenic hypotheses of the surgical inflammatory and septic responses could open new research pathways about the ancient co-evolution of humans with their microbiota.

Keywords: Eukaryotes, surgical infections, gut microbiome, fibrosis, regeneration, sepsis, intestinal bacterial translocation, multiorgan dysfunction syndrome, compensatory anti-inflammatory response syndrome, multiple organ failure, cholesterol, glucocorticoids, mineralocorticoids, postcapillary venules, biofilms, *quorum* sensing.

***Address correspondence to Jaime Arias:** Cátedra de Cirugía, Facultad de Medicina, Universidad Complutense, Pza. de Ramón y Cajal s.n., 28040 MADRID, Spain; Tel: +34 91 394 1389; Fax: +34 91 3947115; E-mail: jariasp@med.ucm.es

INTRODUCTION

The human microbiome project requires researchers to go beyond comparative genomics to an integrated "systems metagenomics" approach that accounts for microbial community structure (the microbiota), gene content (the microbiome), gene expression (the "meta-transcriptome" and "meta-proteome") and metabolism (the "meta-metabolome") [1].

Although microbial communities reside on all human body surfaces, including the skin, and respiratory, gastrointestinal and genitourinary tracts, our largest collection of microbes resides in the gut, where an estimated 10-100 trillions of organisms reside (the "gut microbiota") [2]. The human gut microbiota consists of bacteria and archaea and is composed of approximately 1,100 prevalent species, with approximately 160 such species per individual. In its entirety, the intestinal microflora contains approximately 150-fold more genes than our own host genomes [3, 4].

The intestinal microbiome is therefore more than just a simple organ of the human body. It could be considered as an associated organism and consequently an "exosymbiosis" phenomenon would be established in which different genera cooperate to their joint advantage, namely, humans with gut bacteria [5]. The principle of symbiogenesis is considered an evolutionary process, according to which the complex eukaryotic cells are produced *via* the fusion of archaic microbes and the subsequent cooperation of the partners [6]. Lynn Margulis, a brilliant scientist, (who is recently diseased) proposed the "serial endosymbiosis hypothesis of the origin of eukaryotic cells" based on Mereschowsky's insights and those of other cytologists [7-9]. Today the principle of symbiogenesis explains the evolutionary origin of eukaryotes, *i.e.* protists, fungi, plants and animals [6, 10].

Endosymbiosis could therefore constitute the ancestral way that favors eukaryogenesis [9] while exosymbiosis is essential to maintain our organism homeostasis [1]. This narrow relationship of our evolutionary development with microbes could explain how our survival has a mutual beneficial partnership with bacteria, starting with our unicellular origin to our present multi-specialized pluricellular condition [5, 6, 8-10].

Gut microbiota plays a central role in homeostasis, given its defensive capacity against incoming pathogens, in the development of mucosal immunity or in nutrient metabolism [11]. However, communications between the host and its gut microbiota are altered in pathophysiological processes, especially if associated with inflammation [11-13].

Diseases mediated by the inflammatory response could induce a change in our relationship with gut microbiota, whose intimate meaning is unknown [12]. Inflammatory conditions, not only alter the gut microbiota composition, but also cause epithelial and endothelial permeability to increase the intestinal bacteria and bacterial products, such as toxins [11]. In particular, bacterial translocation related to injury or infection could lead to bacterial overgrowth and disruption of gut homeostasis. This results in a "leaky gut" syndrome, with translocation of gut bacteria or bacterial products to systemic sites, that finally results in systemic complications [11, 12, 14]. This systemic microbial infiltration associated with the inflammatory response could be similar to our ancestral endosymbiotic origin [8, 10].

The term "metaorganism" refers to organisms which are between two levels of metabolic organization [15]. Nowadays, this term is used to name the multicellular organism derived from co-evolution with microbiota, including humans as a result of their close relationship with the intestinal microbiota [1, 15, 16]. However, inflammation of the human metaorganism could induce a strong modulation in its microbial counterpart [16]. The resulting inflamed human metaorganism could be functionally based on different mechanisms that control the cross-talk between the healthy body and its intestinal microbiota [11]. In particular the microbiome could acquire a complementary (or specific) metabolic phenotype or "metabotype" [1] to the human inflammatory metabolism itself.

THE SURGICAL INFLAMMATORY AND SEPTIC RESPONSES

The surgery, either elective or accidental/trauma-related induces an inflammatory response that could be considered a surgical inflammation [17]. Surgical inflammation usually triggered by psychophysiological stimuli takes place with pathophysiological changes associated with the stress response [18]. The considerable progress that has been made in discerning the cellular and molecular mechanisms of the stress-response [19-22] and the inflammatory response [17, 23-26] enables to establish close links between both types of reactions [18, 27-31]. This is the reason why the stress response could have evolved from and is intricately linked to the surgical inflammatory response [18].

The surgical inflammatory response is a systemic reaction of the body with variable intensity depending on the severity of the injury suffered. The pathophysiological characteristics of this systemic reaction are obvious in the cases of severe injury (*i.e.* polytraumatized patients) [32-37]. On the contrary, in the cases of mild injury (*i.e.* skin wound healing), the systemic response is imperceptible or subtle [18].

The surgical inflammatory response could be described as a succession of three phases during which the tissues use progressively oxygen for their metabolism [25, 38, 39]. Each one of these phases emphasizes the trophic role of the mechanisms developed in the damaged tissues. Hence nutrition by diffusion predominates in the first phase; trophism could be mediated by inflammatory cells in the second phase and finally, blood circulation and oxidative metabolism play the most significant nutritive role in the third phase [25, 36, 39] (Fig. **1**) (Table **1**).

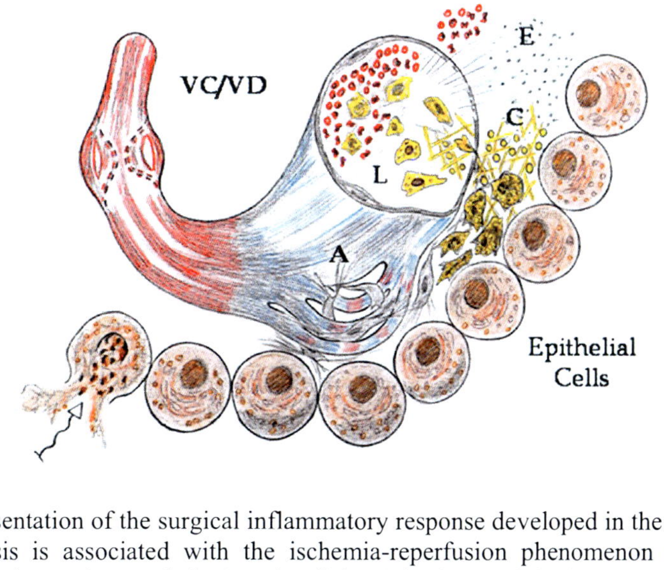

Figure 1: Representation of the surgical inflammatory response developed in the microcirculation. Epithelial necrosis is associated with the ischemia-reperfusion phenomenon that occurs with molecular (exudation and coagulation) and cellular (platelets and leukocytes) infiltration of the interstitium, angiogenesis and tissue repair at the same time.

Table 1: Surgical inflammatory response could be described as a succession of three overlapping phases of metabolic progressive complexity for using oxygen.

First or Immediate Phase	Second or Intermediate Phase	Third or Late Phase
- Vasomotor response - Ischemia-reperfusion - Oxidative and nitrosative stress - Interstitial edema - Up-regulated lymphatic circulation	- Interstitial infiltration by leukocytes and bacteria. - Enzymatic stress - Lymphocyte activation	- Angiogenesis - Blood circulation - Antioxidant and antienzymatic functions. - Resolution - Tissue repair - Remodeling

In the first or immediate phase of the inflammatory response, interstitial hydroelectrolytic alterations appear. The vasomotor response is responsible for the ischemia-reperfusion phenomenon with oxidative and nitrosative stress. In this phase, during the progression of interstitial edema, the lymphatic circulation is simultaneously activated [25].

In the following intermediate phase of the surgical inflammatory response, the tissues are infiltrated by inflammatory blood-borne cells, particularly leukocytes. Symbiosis of the leukocytes and bacteria for extracellular digestion by enzyme release and for intracellular digestion by phagocytosis produces enzymatic stress. Furthermore, macrophages, dendritic cells and bacteria take advantage of the lymphatic circulation activation and migrate through it until reaching the lymph nodes where they activate lymphocytes [25, 39].

During the third phase of the surgical inflammatory reaction, angiogenesis permits numerous substances, including hormones, to be transported by the blood circulation. Although the final objective of angiogenesis is to form new mature vessels for oxygen, substrates, and blood cell transport, other functions could be carried out before the new mature vessels are formed. Thus angiogenesis could have antioxidant and antienzymatic properties, favoring therefore the resolution of the inflammation, as well as tissue and organ repair by regeneration and/or scarring. Consequently, in this phase the new formed tissue is structured, specialized, and matured by remodeling [25, 38, 39] (Fig. **1**).

The sequence in the expression of progressively more elaborate and complex nutritional systems could hypothetically be considered the essence of the evolution of the surgical inflammatory response. Thus the incidence of harmful influences during its evolution could involve regression to the most primitive trophic stages, where nutrition by diffusion, which is simpler but also less costly, facilitates temporary survival until a more favorable environment makes it possible to initiate more complex nutritional methods [25, 36, 40, 41].

The initial trauma, the so-called “first hit”, causes a systemic inflammatory response with damage of external and internal barriers *i.e.* skin and gut mucosa, that facilitates invasion and translocation of microorganisms [32, 35]. In the case of an additional insult or “second hit”, such as extensive surgical procedures, anesthesiological interventions or additional stress *i.e.* hypoxia, hypothermia or microbiological invasion, the inflammatory response could get worse [35]. The “two-hit” hypothesis of post-traumatic multiple organ dysfunction syndrome (MODS) suggests that severe trauma and associated tissue hypoperfusion prime leukocytes (“first hit”), so that a subsequent, apparently minor insult (“second hit”) can generate an excessive inflammatory response leading to MODS [32, 35, 42, 43].

Since a primed cell has the ability to respond to a second stimulus in an altered way, which in turn can be an adaptive (constructive) response or a maladaptive (destructive) response [44], the response to a second stimulus could act in two ways. It could either favor the progression of the inflammatory response, *i.e.* beneficial through a tissue and organic differentiation process, or on the contrary, make it difficult, due to interruption and consequent regression to its initial stages, *i.e.* harmful through a tissue and organic dedifferentiation process [40, 41] (Fig. **2**).

The failed evolution of the inflammatory response to repair is based on the change in the phenotype of the damaged tissue, with regression or dedifferentiation of its metabolism to stages characterized by a deficient use of oxygen; this would explain the important role acquired by hypoxia inducible factors in the first phases of acute inflammation or when the inflammatory process begins [36, 45]. In particular the persistent activity of cell mechanisms for adapting to hypoxia, such as the prolyl-hydroxylase (PHD)-hypoxia-inducible transcription factor (HIF) system [46], would keep the tissue and the inflammatory cells (mast cells, neutrophils, macrophages and lymphocytes) active at the expense of an ancestral and limited metabolic capacity based on anaerobic glycolysis [36, 41, 43, 45]. In this situation, a link could be established between two diverse and significant settings such as hypoxia and inflammation [46, 47].

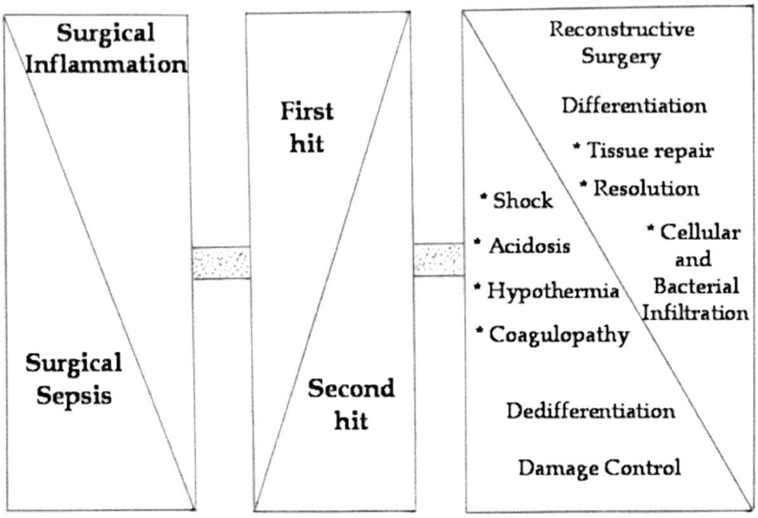

Figure 2: Surgical inflammation and surgical sepsis take place after two successive insults (first and second hits) that induce the dedifferentiation of tissues and organs with regression to the simplest and least costly trophic mechanisms (nutrition by diffusion) and therefore impair the evolution of a constructive or reparative response through dedifferentiation or specialization.

Post-traumatic hibernation during ischemia could therefore be a situation of dedifferentiation, with an intention of adapting to the imposed noxious changes [36]. This is the case with patients after trauma if they have uncontrolled hemorrhage. Uncontrolled bleeding injuries are thought to induce a "lethal triad of trauma", consisting of hypothermia, acidosis and coagulopathy [36, 48]. The implementation of "damage control" principles during resuscitation and surgery has enabled better control of these effects of trauma previously associated with high mortality rates [48-50]. In addition, it has been shown that blood loss induces a suppression of the immune system with impairment of NK-cell activity and reduction of major histocompatibility complex 2 (MHC II) expressions on monocytes [51, 52]. Therefore, it is generally agreed that reconstructive surgery should be postponed until pH, temperature, coagulopathy and immunosuppression are normalized [36, 43, 48-51] (Fig. **2**).

In addition to ischemia/reperfusion-induced mechanisms, *i.e.* hemorrhagic shock and resuscitation, trauma *i.e.* fractures, has been shown to independently contribute to the inflammatory response following major injury [53]. Several animal models have been used to investigate the mechanisms of postoperative and post-traumatic immunosuppression, the most simple model includes surgical induced immune dysfunction in mice through laparotomy by manipulating the small intestine in the antegrade direction [54]. The immunological changes in the postoperative period generally include inhibition of macrophage activity, lymphocytopenia and increased serum IL-10 concentrations [52, 54]. In particular, the degree of lymphocyte suppression correlates with the complexity of surgery or severity of injury [52].

This post-traumatic failure of immune defense systems is considered the primary mechanism for containing bacterial contamination and preventing colonization, infection and sepsis [37]. A number of animal models have been proposed and developed to investigate the post-traumatic septic response. Among them, the most prevalent is cecal ligation and puncture (CLP) in rodents [55, 56]. In brief, the experiment involves midline laparotomy, exteriorization of the caecum, ligation of the caecum distal to the ileocecal valve, and punctures of the ligated cecum [55, 57]. Mortality in sepsis is significantly lower if sepsis is acquired spontaneously, *i.e.* perforated diverticulitis compared to postoperative septic complications [54]. In the case of CLP in the rat, injuries, such as surgery, trauma and infection, are noticed. These injuries induce the activation of a pro-inflammatory response characterized by the enhanced synthesis of acute-phase proteins, increased metabolic rate and oxidative stress induced damage. The presence of more severe signs of oxidative stress and cellular damage in CLP, compared with rats with surgery without infection, is consistent with the stronger, more sustained up-regulation of pro-inflammatory mediators in septic traumas with respect to aseptic (surgery) injury [56]. A model of early and late MODS that depends on the initial degree of injury severity has been described [58]. An initial massive traumatic insult can create an early intensive pro-inflammatory response with severe systemic inflammatory response syndrome free of infection, resulting in early MODS. At the same time, in relation with the "two-hit" hypothesis, initially less severely-injured patients eventually develop late MODS as a result of the inflammatory response caused by ischemia/reperfusion injury or bacterial infection [43, 52, 58]. Depending on the severity of injury and the post-traumatic course, anti-inflammatory mediators are also produced. An overwhelming anti-inflammatory response, also called compensatory anti-inflammatory response syndrome (CARS) seems to be responsible for post-traumatic immunosuppression, with a high susceptibility to infections and septic complications [32, 52, 59].

Surgical sepsis requires surgical intervention for its source control [60, 61] and is considered different from medical sepsis for several reasons. First, surgical trauma and anesthetic agents used during surgery alter host local and systemic immune function [62]. Additionally, patients who have surgical sepsis often require source control in the form of urgent surgical intervention [62]. It has been suggested that infection and sepsis are a manifestation of organ system dysfunction rather than its cause [14]. If so, gastrointestinal dysfunction and associated microbiome dysfunction may cause intestinal bacterial translocation to colonize the inflamed interstitium in the sickest patients with immunoparalysis [14, 36].

RECAPITULATED EXTRAEMBRYONIC FUNCTIONS RELATED TO SURGICAL INFLAMMATION AND SURGICAL SEPSIS

Surgical inflammation could recapitulate ontogeny through the re-expression of two hypothetical extraembryonic trophic axes that is, coelomic-amniotic and trophoblastic-yolk sac-related, in the interstitial space of the injured tissues [18, 63]. If so, surgical inflammation could mean the use of the same biochemical mechanisms that cause the embryonic development in mammals. The re-expression of these ancient mechanisms with a prenatal solvent path is perhaps hard to recognize since they are anachronistic during postnatal life and because they are established in a different environmental medium [18, 63].

Embryogenesis starts after fertilization with the zygote, which undergoes cleavage by mitosis. When the morula stage is reached, the embryo establishes polarity. The cells bind tightly to each other, forming a compact sphere with two different cell layers. The outermost layer becomes the trophoblast and the inner cells become the inner cell mass or embryoblast [64]. The extraembryonic *coeloum* or exocoelomic cavity surrounds the blastocyst which is composed of two structures, the amnion and the primary yolk sac. At the end of the fourth week of gestation, the developing exocoelomic cavity splits the extraembryonic mesoderm into two layers, the somatic mesoderm, lining the trophoblast, and the splanchnic mesoderm covering the secondary yolk sac and the embryo [65]. Coelomic fluid results from an ultrafiltration of maternal serum with the addition of specific placental and secondary yolk-sac products [65, 66] (Fig. **3**).

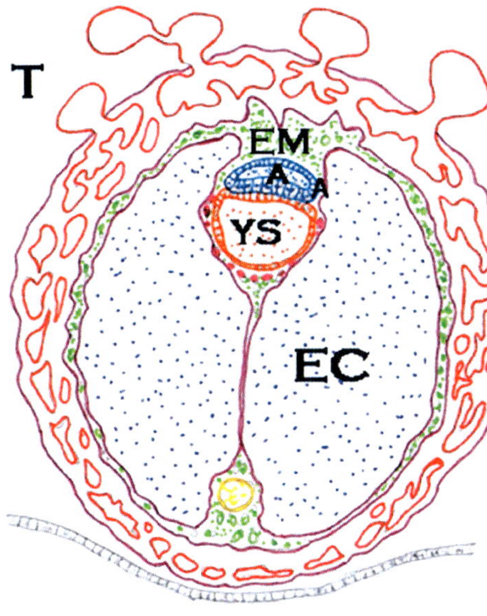

Figure 3: Representative drawing of the early mammalian embryo. The developing exocoelomic cavity (EC) splits the extraembryonic mesoderm (EM) into two layers, the somatic mesoderm, lining the trophoblast (T), and the splanchnic mesoderm covering the secondary yolk sac (YS) and the amnion (A).

The hypothetical recapitulation of these initial phases of embryonic development during the early surgical inflammatory response would imply the expression of functions similar to the extraembryonic *coelum* that surrounds the blastocyst. If so, this phenotype could be adopted by the inflamed interstitium that subsequently induces the accumulation of fluid with characteristics resembling the coelomic fluid in an environment with low pH and oxygen [65, 67]. In essence, this would mean interstitial edema with high levels of proteins, in particular albumin, as well as electrolytes, metals, amino-acids, antioxidants and cytokines [67-71]. This initial interstitial pro-inflammatory edema secondary to ischemia-reperfusion would play the leading role in injured tissue trophism [18]. The biological data and the anatomical location of the exocoelomic cavity also suggest that it is as an essential nutritional pathway for the embryo and early fetus before the placental circulation is fully established [66] (Table **2**).

Table 2: Hypothetical recapitulated extraembryonic functions during the surgical inflammatory response

Exocoelomic-Amniotic-Related Functional Axis	Trophoblastic-Yolk Sac-Related Functional Axis
- Low pH - Hypoxia - Albumin - Aminoacids - Electrolytes - Metals - Antioxidant - Neural potential - Amnion-derived cellular cytokine solution - Pluripotent stem cells - Bacteriostatic - Anti-inflammatory	- Trophoblast-related phagocytic activity - Trophoblast inflammatory mediators production • Immunomodulation • Invasiveness - Blood islands • Hematopoiesis • Angiogenesis - Endocytosis/digestion - Acute phase proteins - *Vitellum* (carbohydrate, protein and lipid storage for embryo nutrition)

The amnion complements this extraembryonic functional axis, with its strong neural potential [72] and since it secretes a unique combination of cytokines and growth factors, known as the "amnion-derived cellular cytokine-solution", which establishes a communication network between mesenchymal and epithelial cells during embryo development [73]. The amniotic fluid that surrounds the fetus may therefore be considered an extension of the extracellular space of the fetal tissues [74]. Furthermore, pluripotent stem cells can be isolated from amniotic fluid, which suggests that the amniotic fluid represents a new and very promising source for stem cell research [75, 76]. The adoption of an amniotic-like phenotype for the inflamed interstitium could offer stem cells a hypoxic and hydrated environment [74], with cytokines and growth factors [73] favoring not only nutrition by diffusion, but also transport, excretion and bacteriostatic and anti-inflammatory protection [74, 76] (Table **2**).

In turn, the re-expression of the trophoblastic-yolk sac-related functional axis in the injured tissues provides molecular and cellular mediators that complement the development of the inflammatory response when in particular it is not sterile. The wall of the secondary yolk sac in mammals is formed by an external mesothelial layer facing the exocoelomic cavity, a vascular mesenchyme and an endodermal layer facing the yolk sac cavity [75] (Fig. **2**).

"Blood islands" develop in the mesenchymal layer of the yolk-sac supporting hematopoiesis and angiogenesis [77]. The endothelial and blood progenitors of blood islands arise independently from the epiblast before they migrate to the extraembryonic yolk-sac. Then, hemangioblasts in the blood islands could generate blood cells through specialized intermediate progenitors known as the hemogenic endothelium [78]. By the sixth week of gestation, the secondary yolk-sac starts appearing as a cystic structure covered by numerous superficial small vessels [65]. The mesothelial and endodermal layers have absorptive functions and are active in endocytosis/digestion [77, 79]. The endodermal layer is also the source of several proteins including acute phase proteins such as pre-albumin, albumin, transferring and α_1- antitrypsin [75] (Table **2**).

A major function of the yolk sac is carbohydrate, protein and lipid accumulation for embryo nutrition and, for this reason it is also called the "*vitellum*" [80]. Therefore, the yolk sac plays a vital role in providing lipids and lipid-soluble nutrients to embryos during the early phase of development [80]. However, during the 10th week of gestation, the yolk sac starts to degenerate and rapidly ceases to function [65]. During the inflammatory response, the re-expression of the yolk sac-related phenotype could favor the regulation of lipid metabolism genes [81], the hematopoietic-cell derived control with recruitment of immune cells, in particular leukocytes and the induction of an angiogenic switch [78] to permit new tissue immunological tolerance. In addition, through the synthesis and release of acute phase proteins, this extraembryonic phenotype reduces the oxidative, nitrosative and enzymatic stress, activates the complement-coagulation system, regulates the lipid metabolism, and favors phagocytosis [82, 83] a specific form of endocytosis primarily associated with nutrition in unicellular organisms, *i.e.* phagotrophic nutrition and to innate and adaptative immunity in mammals [84]. In particular during trophoblast differentiation, trophoblast cells also exhibit intense phagocytic activity leading to events as diverse as engulfment and destruction of extracellular material and the production of inflammatory mediators that may modulate both the immune response [84] and trophoblast invasiveness [85, 86]. These functions expressed by the trophoblast cells recall those of the leukocytes themselves in the inflammatory response, especially when septic [32, 34-36, 54] (Table **2**).

The major alterations in lipid metabolism during the systemic inflammatory response syndrome include increased lipolysis and fatty acid recycling, hyper-triglyceridemia and hepatic steatosis [43]. In fact, lipid metabolism predominance with cholesterol accumulation in the inflamed tissue could be attributed to its role as a precursor molecule of many hormones, like aldosterone, corticoids, progesterone, androgens and estrogen [87] and even vitamin D [88].

The molecular and cellular contribution made by the above-mentioned extraembryonic membranes, *i.e.* exocoelomic cavity, amnion, yolk sac and trophoblast to the intra-embryonic mesoderm, could be essential for embryo development and organogenesis [63]. Moreover, it has been proposed that the functions of these primitive extraembryonic structures are internalized by the embryo at early developmental stages [89]. Consequently, the hypothesized re-expression of these extraembryonic functions after injury during postnatal life could be a key process need to repair the injured organism [18, 63]. However, the exaggerated re-expression of these extraembryonic functions could produce a diverse pathology according to the different predominating functions derived from the coelomic-amniotic axis or the trophoblastic-yolk sac axis.

PATHOLOGICAL INFLAMMATORY AND SEPTIC AXES RELATED TO RECAPITULATED EXTRAEMBRYONIC FUNCTIONS

The systemic surgical inflammatory response is a complex process involving systemic alterations related to a stress response. In this review, we have been trying to establish certain similarities between the complex pathophysiological mechanisms developed in surgical inflammation and surgical sepsis and the pluripotent extraembryonic pathways during embryo development.

Interestingly enough, during the evolution of the surgical inflammatory response, the re-expressed extraembryonic functions focus on the injured tissues and this fact would condition the evolution of the repair response. In this way, the systemic recapitulation of the extraembryonic coelomic and amniotic functions could be represented by the initial activation of the systemic neurogenic axis, while the latter recapitulation of the trophoblast and yolk sac functions would be performed by the activation of a systemic bone-marrow-related axis [18, 63] (Fig. **4**).

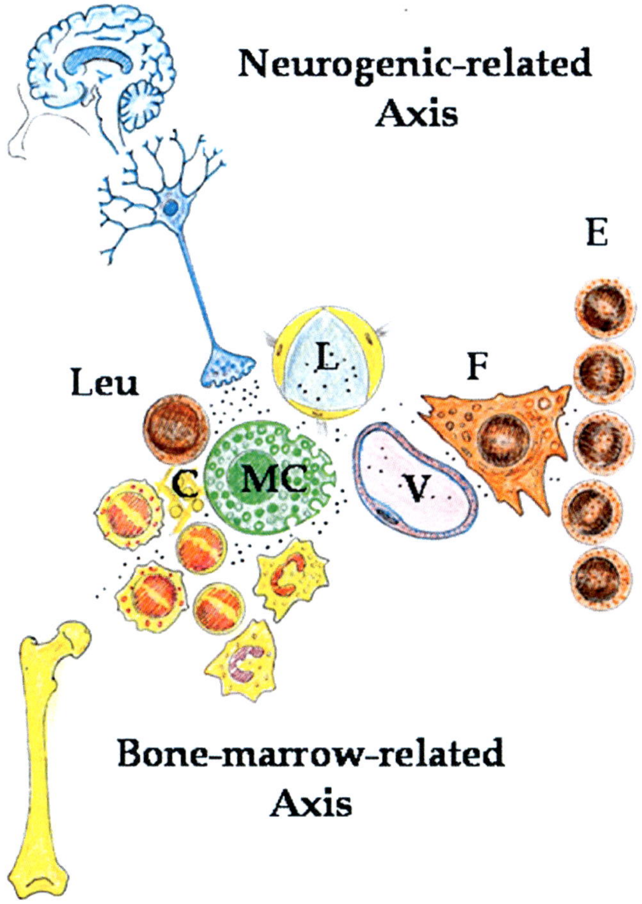

Figure 4: Surgical inflammatory and septic response. Surgical inflammation could be the result of the activation of two pathological systemic axes: the neurogenic axis and the bone-marrow-related

axis, which produce molecular and cellular infiltration, including bacteria, in the interstitium of the injured tissues and organs. Coupling of both axes in the interstitial space could enable the recapitulation of a gastrulation-like phenotype, with tissue and organ repair by fibrosis and/or regeneration. On the contrary, the excessive activation of these systemic axes would induce an interstitial uncoupling, as in hyperacute or acute-on-chronic inflammation, wasting the embryo-like process that enables curing. MC: mast cell; L: lymphatic capillary; V: post-capillary venule; F: fibroblast; E: epithelial cells; Leu: leukocytes; C: coagulation.

The activation of these pathological systemic axes, neurogenic and bone-marrow related could be produced in two steps. The upregulated coelomic-amniotic phenotype would be responsible for a sudden and early neurogenic response with sensory changes (stress, inflammatory pain, analgesia), and motor alterations (light-to-flight and withdrawal reflexes, tachycardia and vasoconstriction and vasodilation) which causes in turn systemic cardiovascular, hemodynamic and hydroelectrolytic alterations [25, 36]. In this early response, those cells that produce substances for export, first synthesize and then store large amounts of molecules in secretory vesicles that are ready for rapid release [90] *i.e.* biogenic amines, which play the leading role [18]. In this early response, mast cells would also participate by the rapid and instant release of preformed mediators including histamine, proteoglycans, neutral proteases and certain cytokines in particular tumor necrosis factor-alpha (TNF-α) [91, 92]. Mast cells play an important role in the systemic response to severe trauma (Fig. **4**). Mast cell deficiency resulted in a damped systemic inflammatory response, greatly attenuated multiple organ failure and more stable hemodynamics in the experimental hemorrhagic shock/trauma inflammatory response [93]. Since mast cells are located in high density in tissues that form large host barriers such as gastrointestinal tract [94], sensitization of enteric neurons as well as extrinsic visceral afferent neurons by mast cell mediators, in particular histamine and proteases may be operative in the gut of poly-traumatized patients [95]. In particular in the human intestine histamine influences a variety of gut functions including fluid and ion transport, which is partly nerve mediated [95]. Mast cell mediators could therefore be involved in the increased permeability of the intestinal mucosal barrier as well in the microvascular intestinal changes which explain the "two-hit" theory of multiple organ failure (MOF) [96]. In this way, gastrointestinal distress caused by microcirculatory dysfunction and associated mitochondrial depression underlies the condition in shock and sepsis [97] (Fig. **4**) (Table **3**).

Table 3: Pathological systemic axes activated during the surgical inflammatory and septic responses.

Neurogenic Axis (Coelomic-Amniotic-Related Phenotype)	**Bone-Marrow-Related Axis (Trophoblastic-Yolk Sac-Related Phenotype**
- Sensory changes (stress, inflammatory pain, analgesia) - Motor alterations: - light-to-flight reflex - Withdrawal reflex - Vasoconstriction/vasodilatation - Cardiovascular and hemodynamic alterations. - Hydroelectrolytic alterations - Release of preformed mediators(suprarenal medulla, mast cell) - Vasoactive mediators - Increase gut permeability (gut lymph hypothesis)	- Stimulation of hematppoietic stem cells - Stimulation of mesenchymal stem cells - Acute phase response - Steroidogenic response (cholesterol derived hormones) - Peripheral neuroendocrine autonomy - Intestinal bacterial translocation - Gut-derived sepsis

In this early neurogenic stress response the activation of the hypothalamo-pituitary-adrenocortical, sympathetic-adrenal medullary and renin-angiotensin-aldosterone axes occur with the release of catecholamines, glucocorticoids and mineralocorticoids [18]. Consequently, selective accumulation of these substances in the interstitial space of tissues suffering from ischemia-reperfusion, including the injured tissues and the gastrointestinal tract, is produced because endothelial permeability is increased, especially in post-capillary venules [25, 36, 41, 63].

In turn, the upregulated systemic trophoblastic-yolk sac-related phenotype could mediate the inflammatory bone marrow response with a lipid and protein metabolic switch linked to steroid and acute phase response protein synthesis, respectively [18] (Table **3**). Therefore, this slower response would be developed first by steroidogenic cells that store very little steroid hormones, so that a rapid steroidogenic response would require rapid synthesis of new steroids, *i.e.* cholesterol-derived hormones [90]. The increase of the acute-phase protein synthesis *i.e.* innate immunity, by the hepatocytes is linked with the acute phase response and follows the upregulation of pro-inflammatory cytokines and chemokines [82, 83]. In this sense, human intestinal mast cells are a potent source of chemokines [98].

Nowadays, the inflammatory bone marrow-related response induced by wounds is considered both a key and complementary arm of the stress response [18]. The inflammatory activation of the bone marrow stem cell niche indicates the stimulation of hematopoietic stem cells and mesenchymal stem cells, both multipotent stem cells [99-101]. Hematppoietic stem cells are the progenitors of all blood and immune cells [102]. Inflammatory signaling molecules appear to stimulate hematopoietic stem cell proliferation in response to surgical inflammation and surgical sepsis [32-35, 103]. Neutrophils and macrophages generated from hematopoietic stem cells are the dominant phagocytes at inflammatory locations [38, 39]. Although macrophages are required for the initiation and maintenance of the inflammatory response, they are also involved in its suppression, resolution and reversal [104].

The collection of cells that infiltrate the interstitium in the inflamed tissues and organs acquires in turn metabolic characteristics that transform them into tissues with great functional autonomy. Monocytes, macrophages and lymphoid cells express β- and α_1-adrenoceptors and synthesize catecholamines [105-107]. Furthermore, the pro-opiomelanocortin (POMC)-peptides found in leukocytes share the same structure of those present in the pituitary [108, 109]. POMC-derived peptides have a very ancient origin and an extremely high level of conservation [110]. They also play a critical role in regulating energy balance [111]. These might be the reasons why the stress response axis can be retrieved by the immunocytes participating in the inflamed interstitium of tissues and organs, where the corticotrophin-releasing hormone (CRH) adrenocorticotrophin (ACTH)-like and biogenic amines are present [109] (Table **3**).

Mast cells are thought to use the same basic migration mechanisms as other granule-containing inflammatory cells. Chemoattractant molecules generated in the inflamed tissues recruit mast cells by acting on surface receptors causing adhesion on the venular endothelium [112]. Stem cell factor (SCF) also known as stell factor or c-Kit-ligand, is a hematopoietic growth factor that promotes survival, proliferation and differentiation of hematopoietic cells [113]. SCF is crucially important for mast cell function. Mice deficient in SCF, or its receptor, c-Kit, lack tissue mast cells [93-112]. Mature mast cells in the gastrointestinal tract of surgical patients could be extremely plastic and could adapt synthesis and release of their mediators to tissue conditions [95]. In particular, mast cells in a late inflammatory response could synthesize cytokines, chemokines, lipid mediators, and growth factors [91, 92] which, at the same time, could influence the gut microbiota [11, 13, 114] and gut permeability [94, 95]. In this phase of the systemic inflammatory response (SIRS), the acute phase response, to which diverse pathophysiological changes such as pyrexia, leukocytosis and dramatic changes in the plasmatic concentrations of acute phase proteins are attributed, becomes more prominent [82].

Therefore, the early onset of the systemic inflammatory surgical response could be due to pro-inflammatory factors released from the stressed gut that reach the systemic circulation through the mesenteric lymphatics. This pathophysiological mechanism of the SIRS syndrome and MODS syndrome ("gut-lymph hypothesis") [115] would represent one of the pathological consequences of the upregulated coelomic-amniotic phenotype (Table **3**). In turn, in a later phase, intestinal bacterial translocation and gut-derived sepsis would be produced, secondary to the upregulated trophoblastic-yolk sac phenotype. These patient populations are generally critically ill and the bacterial overgrowth of aerobic and anaerobic germs in the small and large intestine could induce marked hemodynamic, metabolic and immunological alterations, with associated multiple organ failure and finally septic shock secondary to an acute-on-chronic SIRS (Fig. **2**).

On the contrary, if the above-mentioned systemic extraembryonic phenotypes are focused on and coupled in the interstitium of the injured tissues and organs including the gastrointestinal tract, they could finally induce a gastrulation-like process with repair by regeneration and/or fibrosis [18]. The gastrulation-like process with neo-formation of a reparative tissue could be based on the integration of both extraembryonic–related phenotypes, namely coelomic-amniotic and trophoblast-vitelline, by the multipotent mesenchymal stem/stromal cells [101, 102]. Therefore, the coupled interaction of the extraembryonic-related functional axes *i.e.* neurogenic and bone-marrow-related responses, in the interstitium of the damage tissues and organs, allows them to recapitulate the mechanisms characteristic of gastrulation and subsequently forms a mesenchyma similar to that present in the early development phases [63] (Fig. **5**).

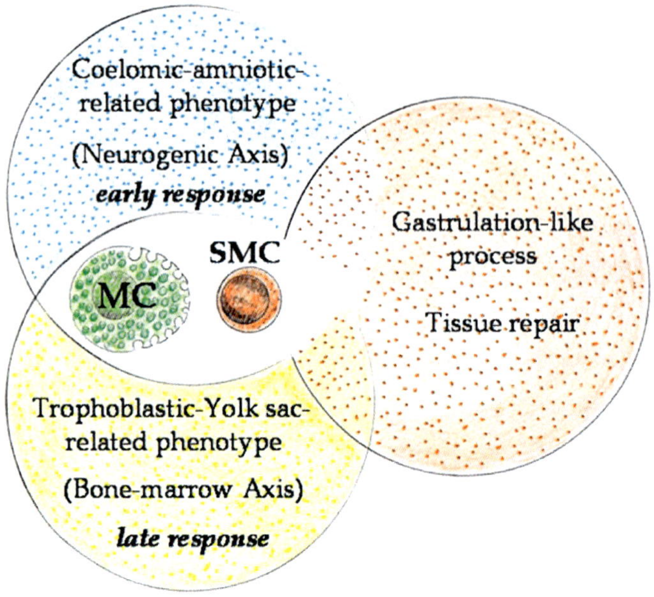

Figure 5: Coupling of the recapitulated extraembryonic functions, *i.e.* coelomic-amniotic- related and trophoblastic yolk sac-related in the injured tissue and organs could induce a gastrulation-like phenotype, need for repair by fibrosis and/or regeneration. MC: mast cell; SMC: stem mesenchymal cell.

Mesodermal derived cells, in particular fibrocytes [116] or alternatively epiblast-derived pluripotent stem cells, survive beyond embryonic development in adult tissues [117]. There is substantial information available supporting the hypothesis that fibrocytes are derived from the bone marrow [118]. Human fibrocytes may represent an intermediate stage of differentiation of a monocyte subset into mature fibroblast and myofibroblasts in tissues [119]. In addition, fibrocytes have ambivalent repair functions, so they can accelerate tissue and organ healing by stimulating cell proliferation, reepithelization and angiogenesis [120], but on the contrary, they can also be involved in inflammatory fibrotic processes [118, 121-123] (Fig. **5**).

Inflammatory chemokines trigger the interstitial recruitment of fibrocytes [118], and also serve as a signal for the homing of endothelial progenitor cells from the bone marrow to the sites of angiogenesis [124]. During vasculogenesis or neovascularization, precursor cells from adult bone marrow are mobilized into circulation in response to various signals, including chemokines and their receptors, and are homed to the source where they differentiate into mature endothelial cells [125]. However, mesodermal derived cells, in particular fibrocytes, can accelerate the recovery of homeostasis by the injured organism through stimulating proliferation and vessel remodeling. Specifically, the recruitment of mural mesenchymal derived cells *i.e.* pericytes and vascular smooth muscle cells, to nascent blood vessels, plays an essential role in stabilizing and maturing new vascular networks [126, 127]. Nutrition mediated by mature blood capillaries is established through the expression of this angiogenic and/or vasculogenic phenotype, which makes tissue and organ regeneration possible or, by default, their repair by fibrosis [118, 119].

Since the above-mentioned extra-embryonic phenotypes become autonomous when they are expressed in the peripheral inflamed tissues and organs [63] during the last gastrulation-like phenotype expression, the body progressively recovers control of the neuro-endocrine and immune functions. This progressive centralization of the neuroendocrine functions could be related with wound repair during the convalescence phase [18, 36]. On the contrary, the failure in this right centralization of the neuroendocrine and immune functions, secondary to the uncoupling of the recapitulated extraembryonic-like phenotypes, maintains the neuroendocrine, immunological and peripheral functional autonomy and therefore prevents patient recovery.

PHYLOGENY DICTATES THE RULES IN SURGICAL INFLAMMATORY AND SEPTIC STATES

During the surgical inflammatory and septic responses, extraembryonic aces, *i.e.* coelomic-amniotic and trophoblastic-yolk sac-related, could be systemically re-expressed and converge into the interstitium of injured tissues and organs. Therefore, it seems appropriate to propose that the final aim of this process could also be collaborating in some type of development similar to embryonic development during the postnatal life [18].

If so, the repair process after injury could have properties comparable to an embryo. One of the main objectives of above-mentioned upregulated extraembryonic axes could be collaborating during the early phase of the acute inflammatory response to establish an open circulation in the injured tissues and organs. An open circulatory system could facilitate the interstitial fluid diffusion and concomitantly tissue nutrition when the blood circulation loses its prominent role [18, 128].

Animals adapted changes in their circulatory system during evolution. Vertebrates have a closed circulatory system and a heart that drives blood through closed blood vessels [129], whereas in invertebrates, like insects, the body fluid called hemolymph is pumped by a dorsal heart through the tissues without closed vessels [130]. The closed circulatory system in the inflamed tissues and organs suffers a switch to acquire some of the characteristics of the open circulatory system and perhaps of the hemolymph [128]. In this way, the inflammatory exudates bath the cells of the injured tissues and organs, thanks to the quick infiltration of the extracellular matrix [25, 32, 36]. Consequently, through the activation of the post-capillary venules, the endothelium and the high endothelial venules, extravasation of plasma and blood cells is produced during the inflammatory response [18]. In turn, by means of the associated simultaneous activation of the lymphatic circulation, an open anaerobic pathway in the inflamed tissues and organs would be established [18, 128]. Thanks to this new open microcirculatory system, in which venous hemo-lymphatic circulation becomes predominant, the tissues and organs are provided with molecules and cells coming from the up-regulated extraembryonic coelomic-amniotic (*i.e.* neurogenic-related axis) and the trophoblast-yolk sac (*i.e.* bone marrow-related axis) axes [18]. So perhaps through the up-regulation of ancestral phylogenetic mechanisms, the plasma, the interstitial fluid and lymph compartments are closely linked during inflammation, thus favoring the continuous flow of fluid and cells from one compartment to the next in an environment predominated by anaerobiosis [18, 128]. Thus, the venous endothelium acquires trophoblastic properties since it becomes an intermediary between the stressed host and the inflamed interstitium to play the leading role in the host trophism [84, 85]. The inflamed venous endothelium phenotype recognizes cell damage or pathogen invasion with surface-expressed or intracellular pattern recognition receptors (PRPs). These receptors detect, either directly or indirectly, damage-associated molecular patterns (DAMPs) released from injured cells such as DNA, adenosine triphosphate (ATP), uric acid, histones and DNA-binding nuclear protein high-mobility group box-1 (HMGB1) or pathogen-associated molecular patterns (PAMPs), such as microbial nucleic acids, lipoproteins and carbohydrates [131-133]. Specific-interactions between DAMPs and PAMPs with PPRs activate the specific signals that promote production of pro-inflammatory mediators and increase the vascular permeability [131] favoring the transport *via* the plasma-interstititum-lymphatic pathway of microorganisms and their substances. In surgical patients, the post-traumatic open circulatory phenotype would therefore worsen if sepsis develops during its evolution since the endogenous (DAMPs) and exogenous (PAMPs) danger signals would increase, which in turn increase the endothelial barrier permeability of the post-capillary venules causing severe sepsis and finally septic shock [134].

Based on the "two-hit" hypothesis of post-traumatic MODS, the "first-hit" could induce the expression of a low grade open circulatory phenotype that facilitates intestinal translocation of microorganisms [32, 35]. However, an additional insult or "second-hit" generates the induction of a high grade open circulatory phenotype (acute-on-chronic response) that leads to an excessive increase in the endothelial barrier permeability of the post-capillary venules, which not only aggravates intestinal bacterial translocation but also favors the loss of intravascular volume in the interstitial space, resulting in greater risk of shock [36, 42, 43]. In addition, the intense interstitial edema would induce an anaerobic environment which would be extremely favorable for the translocated human gut microbiota proliferation. In fact, the impossibility of recovery of more than 20-30% of the total gastrointestinal tract bacterial richness by the traditional microbiology is attributed to insufficient anaerobic cultivation technologies [135] (Fig. **6**).

Vertebrate cells contain cholesterol and although different tissues have characteristic patterns of cholesterol metabolism, the basic pattern is similar in all cells [136]. During inflammation, cholesterol esters may be transferred from high density lipoproteins (HDL) to apolipoprotein E and apolipoprotein B (apo B)-containing particles, such as low-density lipoproteins (LDL) and very low density lipoproteins (VLDL). Trapping of this apolipoproteins, particularly apo B containing particles, is an essential initiating event for the development of vascular inflammation [137]. It is now therefore accepted that inflammation and the concomitant acute phase response induce marked changes in the lipoprotein profile [12, 138] and cholesterol metabolism [139] (Fig. **6**). In this way, the characteristics of the inflammatory acute phase response and the associated cholesterol traffic have been compared with those playing the lead role in the accumulation of yolk materials into oocytes during oogenesis and their mobilization during embryogenesis (vitellogenic phenotype) [128].

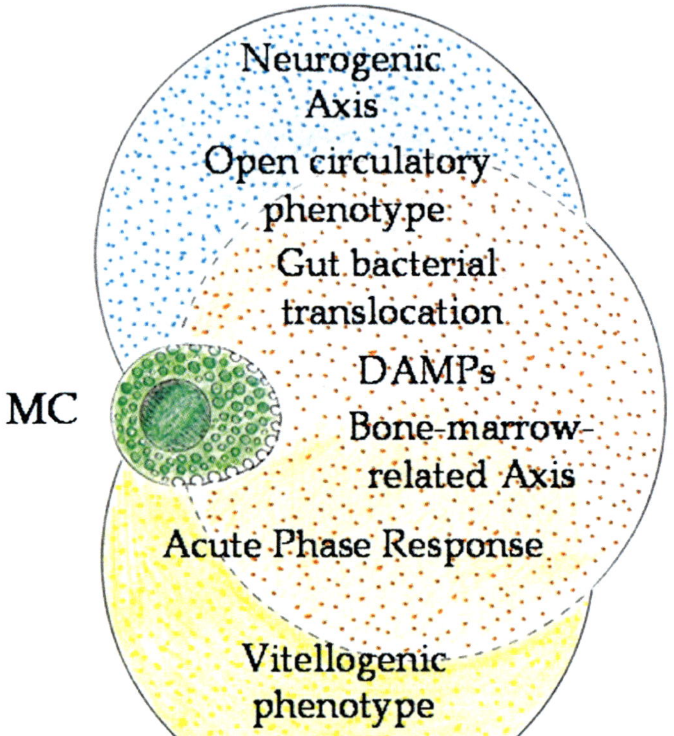

Figure 6: The surgical inflammatory and septic responses could also be viewed as a recapitulation in the injured body of ancestral phylogenetic functions. The neurogenic axis activation could therefore favor the re-expression of an open circulatory pathway used by molecules, cells and bacteria to reach the interstitial space of the injured tissues and organs. Meanwhile, through the activation of the bone-marrow related axis, the cells and substrates would be provided for the said interstitium, allowing to achieve peripheral autonomy of the immune and neuro-endocrine functions.

An isoform of apolipoprotein B and apolipoprotein B 48 particles are chylomicrons, which transport dietary cholesterol and triglycerides from the intestine to the site of storage for use within the body, such as the adipose tissue, skeletal and cardiac muscle and the liver [137]. This is one of the reasons why considering digestion as a physiologic inflammatory state is allowed. In particular, dietary fat is thought to increase intestinal transcellular and/or paracellular permeability by the transient activation of mucosal mast cells [140]. Also short chain fatty acids, which are the major metabolic products of anaerobic bacteria fermentation in the gastrointestinal tract, could modulate the production of pro- or anti-inflammatory mediators by leukocytes and may predispose to or prevent regional and systemic inflammatory responses [141].

Both cholesterol acquisition and leukocyte infiltration by the inflamed tissue collaborate to establish its new neuro-endocrine autonomy. Cholesterol is used locally to synthesize glucocorticoids and mineralocorticoids that could regulate microcirculatory functions and activate immune cells [87]. A growing body of evidence demonstrated the novo synthesis of glucocorticoids and mineralocorticoids in primary lymphoid organs, skin, brain and intestine [142]. Perhaps this ability of local corticosteroid synthesis is upregulated in the inflamed tissue, due to the new metabolic and functional needs. The pro-inflammatory and anti-inflammatory functions of androgens and estrogens and progesterone, respectively suggest that endogenous sex steroids may influence immune functions [143, 144]. In addition, leukocytes in the inflamed interstitium could develop neuroendocrine functions [107-111] (Fig. **6**). Lastly, it is widely known that bile acids are steroid acids that are produced in the liver from cholesterol and are biotransformed extensively through degradation by intestinal anaerobic bacteria of the genera *Bacteroides, Eubacterium* and *Clostridium* [13]. At the same time, the gut microbiota could, through effects on bile acid metabolism in the gut lumen, influence signaling pathways involved in energy and lipid metabolism [13]. It could therefore be concluded that the predominance of the lipid metabolism, and particularly of cholesterol, is a fundamental regulating factor of the inflammatory response.

It has been suggested that lipid metabolism inflammatory alterations are phylogenetically influenced [128]. In particular, the ability to transport fat in the form of lipoprotein through the circulatory system by eukaryotes is one of their most significant functions right from the beginning of existence [145]. Over the past several years, it has become increasingly evident that lipids and lipid modifying enzymes play important roles in the autophagy process [146] and *vice versa,* in eukaryotes, autophagy regulates lipid content [147]. Autophagy is a cellular process mobilizing intracellular nutrient resources and plays an important role in contributing to survival during unfavorable conditions [148]. Autophagy could be induced by cellular stress and nutrient starvation [148] two processes frequently associated to the surgical patient with systemic inflammation or sepsis [33, 35, 37, 43]. Among the numerous components involved in the regulation of autophagy TOR (target of rapamycin) is a key component in mammalian cells and also in yeast, involving stress responses, nutrient sensing pathways and growth factor signaling [146, 148]. Because autophagy prevents the accumulation of random molecular damage and provides a means to reallocate cellular resources from one biochemical pathway to another [149] it would be very interesting to understand its implication in the hypothetical process of dedifferentiation suffered by the injured body through the inflammatory response (Fig. **6**).

Increasing evidence implicates mast cells in the systemic inflammatory response to severe injury [93]. In particular, mast cell deficient mice subjected to hemorrhagic shock and fractures (exhibited) resulted in a damped systemic inflammatory response [93]. Mast cells produce serine proteases that could activate metalloproteinases leading to extracellular matrix remodeling. The tissue distribution of mast cells containing serine proteases varies across animal species and the large number of functions described to these enzymes clearly indicates their importance in mast cell biology. In fact, serine proteases appear to be a major link between innate immunity and tissue remodeling. This is one of the reasons why it has been proposed that the mast cell phylogenetic progenitor evolved from a phylogenetic progenitor that evolved from a primitive local innate immunity cell into a tissue regulatory and remodeling cell [150]. Thus, mast cells would play an integrating role orchestrating the surgical inflammatory and septic responses. Particularly important would be their ability for up-regulating the neurogenic and bone-marrow-related axes and therefore, for re-expressing ancestral phenotypes in cases of severe trauma and sepsis (Fig. **6**).

Intestinal microorganisms communicate and cooperate to perform a wide range of multicellular behaviors, such as dispersal, nutrient acquisition, biofilm formation and *quorum* sensing [151-155]. Therefore, they can recognize and respond to almost all the human body changes and especially to the inflammatory changes imposed by trauma [11, 12]. Since we have suggested that the surgical inflammatory response could represent the re-expression of ancestral phylogenetic mechanisms, colonic microbiota could also adopt an old behavior in their relationship with eukaryotic cells. So through the use of the recapitulated phylogenetic mechanisms in the surgical inflamed body, colonic microbiota could restore old metabolic interrelations with the eukaryotic cells that would increase their resistance to aggression and favor survival.

The establishment in the severe traumatized human body of an anaerobic pathway from the intestinal lumen through the lymphatics and post-capillary venules until reaching the interstitial edematous interstitium of inflamed tissues and organs could favor the invasion of certain microbial populations in the body. In addition, the selective interstitial accumulation of substrates and pro- and anti-inflammatory mediators could constitute the factors that would establish the metabolic cross-talk between bacteria and eukaryotic cells in an anaerobic environment. This new metabolic anaerobic microenvironment might recall old but successful symbiotic relations. In this sense, surgical sepsis ultimately represents the final and desperate attempt of intestinal microbiota to rescue its old travelling companion, the eukaryotic cell, from death.

ACKNOWLEDGEMENTS

We would like to thank Maria Elena Vicente for preparing the manuscript, Elizabeth Mascola for translating it into English and librarians of Complutense University Medical School, particularly the Director, Francisco Javier Jorge García-Reyes, and Manuela Crego and María José Valdemoro and B. Braun Surgical S.A. for their technical assistance.

This study was carried out in part with grants from Mutua Madrileña Research Foundation (Ref. nº PA 3077/2008 and AP5966/2009), MICINN PSI2010-19348 and with the special collaboration of the INEUROPA (Instituto de Neurociencias del Principado de Asturias)

CONFLICT OF INTEREST

The author(s) confirm that this chapter content has no conflict of interest.

REFERENCES

[1] Turnbaugh PJ, Ley RE, Hamady M, Fraser-Liggett CM, Knight R, Gordon JI. The human microbiome project. Nature 2007; 449: 804-810.

[2] Turnbaugh PJ, Gordon JI. The core gut microbiomes, energy balance and obesity. J Physiol 2009; 587: 4153-4158.

[3] Qin J, Li, R.; Raes, J.; Arumugam, M.; Burgdorf, K.S.; Manichanh, C.; Nielsen, T.; Pons, N.; Levenez, F.; Yamada, T.; Mende, D.R.; Li, J.; Xu, J.; Li, S.; Li, D.; Cao, J.; Wang, B.; Liang, H.; Zheng, H.; Xie, Y.; Tap, J.; Lepage, P.; Bertalan, M.; Batto, J.M.; Hansen, T.; Le Paslier, D.; Linneberg, A.; Nielsen, H.B.; Pelletier, E.; Renault, P.; Sicheritz-Ponten, T.; Turner, K.; Zhu, H.; Yu, C.; Li, S.; Jian, M.; Zhou, Y.; Li, Y.; Zhang, X.; Li, S.; Qin, N.; Yang, H.; Wang, J.; Brunak, S.; Doré, J.; Guarner, F.; Kristiansen, K.; Pedersen, O.; Parkhill, J.; Weissenbach, J.; MetaHIT Consortium; Bork, P.; Ehrlich, S.D.; Wang, J. A human gut microbial gene catalogue established by metagenomic sequencing. Nature 2010; 464: 59-65.

[4] Tilg H, Kaser A. Gut microbiome, obesity and metabolic dysfunction. J Clin Invest 2011; 121: 2126-2132.

[5] Fox R. Symbiogenesis. J R Soc Med 2004; 97: 559.

[6] Kutschera U. From the scala naturae to the symbiogenetic and dynamic tree of life. Biol Direct 2011; 6: 33.

[7] Margulis L. The conscious cell. Ann N Y Acad Sci 2001; 929: 55-70.

[8] Dolan MF, Melnitsky H, Margulis L, Kolnicki R. Motiligy proteins and the origin of the nucleus. Anat Rec 2002; 268: 290-301.

[9] Margulis L, Chapman M, Guerrero R, Hall J. the last eukaryotic common ancestor (LECA): Acquisition of cytoskeletal motility from aerotolerant spirochetes in the Proterozoic Era. Proc Natl Acad Sci USA 2006; 103: 13080-13085.

[10] Kutschera U. Symbiogenesis, natural selection and the dynamic Earth. Theory Biosci 2009; 128: 191-203.

[11] Sekirov I, Russell S, Antunes RE, Finlay BB. Gut microbiota in health and disease. Physiol Rev 2010; 90: 859-904.

[12] Hakansso A, Molin G. Gut microbiota and inflammation. Nutrients 2011; 3: 637-682.

[13] Nicholson JK, Holmes E, Kinross J, Burcelin R, Gibson G, Jia W, Pettersson S. Host-gut microbiota metabolic interactions. Science 2012; 336: 1262-1267.

[14] Marshall JC, Christou NV, Meakins JL. The gastrointestinal tract. The "undrained abscess" of multiple organ failure. Ann Surg 1993; 218: 111-119.

[15] Bosch TCG, McFall-Ngai MJ. Metaorganisms as the new frontier. Zoology (Jena) 2011; 114: 185-190.

[16] Biagi E, Candela M, Fairweather-Tait S, Franceschi C, Brigidi P. Ageing of the human metaorganism: the microbial counterpart. Age (Dordr) 2012; 34: 247-267.

[17] Kohl BA, Deutschman CS. The inflammatory response to surgery and trauma. Curr Opin Crit Care 2006; 12: 325-332.

[18] Aller MA, Blanco-Rivero J, Arias JI, Balfagon G, Arias J. The wound healing response and the upregulated systemic extraembryonic phenotypes: brothers-in-arms forever. Exp Dermatol 2012; 21: 497-503.
[19] Laborit H. The major mechanisms of stress. In: Stress revisited. 2. Systemic effects of stress. G. Jasmine, Proschek, L. Eds. Pp.1-26. Methods and Achivements in Experimental Pathology. Vol. 15. JASMIN J. Ed. Krager. Basel Switzerland. 1991.
[20] Pruett SB. Stress and the immune system. Pathophysiology 2003; 9: 133-153.
[21] Baumann N, Turpin J-C. Neurochemistry of stress. An overview. Neurochem Res 2010; 35: 1875-1879.
[22] Nadal E, Ammerer G, Posas F. Controlling gene expression in response to stress. Nat Rev Genet 2011; 12: 833-845.
[23] Cone JB. Inflammation. Am J Surg 2001; 182: 558-562.
[24] Nathan C. points of control in inflammation. Nature 2002; 420: 846-852.
[25] Aller MA, Arias JL, Nava MP, Arias J. Post-traumatic inflammation is a complex response based on the pathological expression of the nervous, immune and endocrine functional systems. Exp Biol Med (Maywood) 2004; 229: 170-181.
[26] Hotamisligil GS. Inflammation and metabolic disorders. Nature 2006; 444: 860-867.
[27] Selye H. Stress and inflammation. In: The Stress of Life. Revised edition. New York. Mc Graw-Hill Book Co. chapter 6, 1978, 129-143.
[28] Black PH, Garbutt LD. Stress, inflammation and cardiovascular disease. J Psychosom Res 2002; 52: 1-23.
[29] Rosmond DR. Role of stress in the pathogenesis of the metabolic syndrome. Psychoneuroendocrinology 2005; 30: 1-10.
[30] Arch PC, Slominski A, Theoharides TC, Peters EM, Paus R. Neuroimmunology of stress: Skin takes center stage. J Invest Dermatol 2006; 126: 1697-1704.
[31] Hänsel A, Hong S, Camara RJA, Von Känel R. Inflammation as a psychophysiological biomarker in chronic psychosocial stress. Neurosci Biobehav Reviews 2010; 35: 115-121.
[32] Keel M, Trentz O. Pathophysiology of polytrauma. Injury 2005; 36: 691-709.
[33] Lenz A, Franklin GA, Cheadle WG. Systemic inflammation after trauma. Injury 2007; 38: 1336-1345.
[34] Stahel PF, Smith WR, Moore EE. Role of biological modifiers regulating the immune response after trauma. Injury 2007; 38: 1409-1422.
[35] Gebhard F, Huber-Lang M. Polytrauma-pathophysiology and management principles. Langenbecks Arch Surg 2008; 393: 825-31.
[36] Aller MA, Arias JL, Alonso-Poza A, Arias J. A review of metabolic staging in severely injured patients. Scand J Trauma Resusc Emerg Med. 2010; 18: 27
[37] Blackburn GL. Metabolic considerations in management of surgical patients. Surg Clin N Am 2011; 91: 467-480.
[38] Arias JI, Aller MA, Arias J. Surgical inflammation: a pathophysiological rainbow. J Transl Med 2009; 7: 19.
[39] Aller MA, Arias JI, Giner M, *et al.* Oxygen-related inflammatory wound phenotypes. In: Wound healing: Process, Phases and Promoting. J.E. Middelton Ed. Nova Sciences Publishers-Huntington N.Y. USA. Chapter 2, 2011; 1-26.
[40] Aller MA, Arias JL, Nava MP, Arias J. Evolutive trophic phases of the systemic acute inflammatory response, oxygen use mechanisms and metamorphosis. Psicothema 2004; 16: 369-372.

[41] Aller MA, Arias JL, Sanchez-Patan F, Arias J. The inflammatory response: An efficient way of life. Med Sci Monit 2006; 12: RA225-RA234.
[42] Meakins JL. Etiology of multiple organ failure. J Trauma 1990; 30: S165-S168.
[43] Mizock BA. The multiple organ dysfunction syndrome. Dis Mon 2009; 55: 476-523.
[44] Meldrum DR, Cleveland JC, Moore EE, *et al.* Adaptive and maladaptive mechanisms of cellular priming. Ann Surg 1997; 226: 587-598.
[45] Singer M, De Santis V, Vitale D, Jeffcoate W. Multiorgan failure is an adaptative, endocrine-mediated, metabolic response to overwhelming systemic inflammation. Lancet 2004; 364: 545-548.
[46] Eltzschig HK, Carmeliet P. Hypoxia and inflammation. N Engl J Med 2011; 364: 656-665.
[47] Nathan C. Oxygen and the inflammatory cell. Nature 2003; 422: 657-676.
[48] Thorsen K, Ringdal KG, Strand K, SØreide K. Clinical and cellular effects of hypothermia, acidosis and coagulopathy in major injury. Br J Surg 2011; 98: 894-907.
[49] Kouraklis G, Spirakos S, Glivanov A. Damage control surgery: an alternative approach for the management of critically injured patients. Surg Today 2002; 32: 195-202.
[50] Germanos S, Gourgliotis S, Villias C, Bertucci M, Dimopoulos N, Salemis N. Damage control surgery in the abdomen: An approach for the management of severe injured patients. Int J Surg 2008; 6: 246-252.
[51] BrØchner AC, Toft P. Pathophysiology of the systemic inflammatory response after major accidental trauma. Scand. J Trauma. Resusc Emerg Med 2009; 17: 43
[52] Kimura F, Shimizu H, Yoshidome H, Ohtsuka M, Miyazaki M. Immunosuppression following surgical and traumatic injury. Surg Today 2010; 40: 793-808.
[53] McGhan LJ, Jaroszewski DI. The role of toll-like receptor-4 in the development of multi-organ failure following traumatic haemorrhagic shock and resuscitation. Injury 2012; 43: 129-137.
[54] Menges P, Kessler W, Kloecker C, *et al.* Surgical trauma and postoperative immune dysfunction. Eur Surg Res 2012; 48: 180-186.
[55] Cuenca AG, Delano MJ, Kelly-Scumpia KM, Moldawer LL, Efron PA. Cecal ligation and puncture. Curr Protoc Immunol 2010; Chapter 19, Unit 19-13.
[56] Yang Q, Mattick JSA, Orman MA, Nguyen TT, Ierapetritou MG, Berthiaume F, Androulakis IP. Dynamics of hepatic gene expression profile in a rat cecal ligation and puncture model. J Surg Res 2012; 176: 583-600.
[57] Rittirsch D, Huber-Lang MS, Flierl MA, *et al* – Immunodesign of experimental sepsis by cecal ligation and puncture. Nat Protoc 2009; 4: 31-36.
[58] Moore FA, Moore EE. Evolving concepts in the pathogenesis of postinjury multiple organ failure. Surg Clin North Am 1995; 75: 257-277.
[59] Bone RC. Sir Isaac Newton, sepsis, SIRS and CARS. Crit Care Med 1996; 24: 1125-1128.
[60] Moore LJ, Moore FA, Todd SR, *et al.* Sepsis in general surgery: The 2005-2007 national surgical quality improvement program perspective. Arch Surg 2010; 145: 695-700.
[61] Bosma E, Veen EJ, De Jongh MAC, Roukema JA. Variable impact of complications in general surgery: a prospective cohort study. Can J Surg 2012; 5: 163-170.
[62] White LE, Chaudhary R, Moore LJ, Moore FA, Hassoun HT. Surgical sepsis and organ crosstalk: The role of the kidney. J Surg Res 2011; 167: 306-315.
[63] Aller MA, Arias JI, Arias J. Pathological axes of wound repair: Gastrulation revisited. Theor Biol Med Model 2010; 7: 37.

[64] De Miguel MP, Arnalich-Montiel P, Lopez-Iglesias A, *et al.* Epiblast-derived stem cells in embryonic and adult tissues. Int J Dev Biol 2009; 53: 1529-1540.
[65] Jauniaux E, Gulbis B. Fluid compartments of the embryonic environment. Hum Reprod Uptadate 2006; 6: 268-278.
[66] Jauniaux E, Gulbis B, Jurkovic D, Campbell S, Collins WP, Ooms HA. Relationship between protein concentrations in embryological fluids and maternal serum and yolk sac size during human pregnancy. Hum Reprod 1884; 9: 161-166.
[67] Burton GJ, Hempstock J, Jauniaux E. Nutrition of the human fetus during the first trimester – A review. Placenta 2001; 22: S70-S77.
[68] Jauniaux E, Sherwood RA, Jurkovic D, Boa FG, Campbell S. Amino acid concentrations in human embryological fluids. Hum Reprod 1994; 9: 1175-1179.
[69] Wathen NC, Delves HT, Campbell DJ, Chard T. The coelomic cavity – A reservoir for metals. Am J Obstet Gynecol 1995; 173: 1884-1888.
[70] Jauniaux E, Hempstock J, Teng C, Battaglia FC, Burton GJ. Polyol concentrations in the fluid compartments of the human conceptus during the first trimester of pregnancy: maintenance of redox potential in a low oxygen environment. J Clin Endocrinol Metab 2005; 90: 1171-1175.
[71] Calleja-Agius J, Jauniaux E, Muttukrishna S. Inflammatory cytokines in maternal circulation and placenta of chromosomally abnormal first trimester miscarriages. Clin Dev Immunol 2012; 2012: 175041.
[72] Chang YJ, Hwang SM, Tseng CP, *et al.* Isolation of mesenchymal stem cells with neurogenic potentials from the mesoderm of the amniotic membrane. Cell Tissues Organs 2010; 192: 93-105.
[73] Ubertu MG, Pierpont YN, Ko F, *et al.* Amnion-derived cellular cytokine solution (ACCS) promotes migration of Keratinocytes and fibroblasts. Ann Plast Surg 2010; 64: 632-635.
[74] Bellini C, Boccardo F, Bonioli E, *et al.* Lymphodynamics in the fetos and newborn. Lymphology 2006; 39: 110-117.
[75] Siegel N, Rosner M, Hanneder M, *et al.* Human amniotic fluid stem cells: a new perspective. Aminoacids 2008; 35: 291-293.
[76] Shaw SW, David AL, De Coppi P. Clinical applications of prenatal and postnatal therapy using stem cells retrieved from amniotic fluid. Curr Opin Obstet Gyencol 2011; 23: 109-116.
[77] Fraser ST, Baron MH. Embryonic fates for extraembryonic lineages: new perspectives. J Cell Biochem 2009; 107: 586-591.
[78] Ueno H, Weissman IL. The origin and fate of yolk sac hematopoiesis: application of chimera analyses to developmental studies. Int J Dev Biol 2010; 54: 1019-1031.
[79] Gulbis B, Jauniaux E, Cotton F, Stordeur P. Protein and enzyme patterns in the fluid cavities of the first trimester gestational sac: relevance to the absorption role of secondary yolk sac. Mol Hum Reprod 1998; 4: 857-862.
[80] Yoshida S, Wada Y. Transfer of maternal cholesterol to embryo and fetus in pregnant mice. J Lipid Res 2005; 46: 2168-2174.
[81] Nakazawa F, Alev C, Jakt LM, *et al.* Yolk sac endoderm is the major source for serum proteins and lipids and is involved in the regulation of vascular integrity in early chick development. Dev Dyn 2011; 240: 2002-2010.
[82] Gabay C, Kushner I. Acute-phase proteins and other systemic responses to inflammation. N Engl J Med 1999; 340: 448-454.

[83] Jain S, Gautam V, Naseem S. Acute-phase proteins: As diagnostic tool. J Pharm Bioallied Sci 2011; 3: 118-127.

[84] Bevilacqua E, Hoshida M-S, Amarante-Paffaro A, Albieri-Borges A, Gomes SZ. Trophoblast phagocytic program: roles in different placental systems. Int J Dev Biol 2010; 54: 495-505.

[85] Knöfler M. Critical growth factors and signaling pathways controlling human trophoblast invasion. Int J Dev Biol 2010; 54: 269-280.

[86] Knöfler M, Pollheimer J. IFPA Award in Placentology Lecture: Molecular regulation of human trophoblast. Placenta 2012; 33: S55-S62.

[87] Miller WL, Bose HS. Early steps in steroidogenesis: intracellular cholesterol trafficking. J Lipid Res 2011; 52: 2111-2135.

[88] Chagas CEA, Borges MC, Martini LA, Rogero MM. Focus on Vitamin D, inflammation and type 2 diabetes. Nutrients 2012; 4: 52-67.

[89] Rohen JW, Lütjen-Drecoll E. Introduction. Fundamental concepts. In: Funktionell Embryology. Schattauer. Sttutgart. Germany. Chapter 1, 2006; 1-37.

[90] Crivellato E, Nico B, Ribatti D. The chromaffin vesicle: Advances in understanding the composition of a versatile, multifunctional secretory organelle. Anat Rec (Hoboken) 2008; 291, 1587-1602.

[91] Galli SJ, Kalesnikoff J, Grimbaldeston MA, Piliponsky AM, Williams CMM, Tsai M. Mast cells as "tunable" effector and immunoregulatory cells: recent advances. Ann Rev Immunol 2005; 23: 749-786.

[92] Gri G, Frossi B, D'Inca F, Danelli L, Betto E, Mion F, Sibilano R, Pucillo C. Mast cell: an emergin partner in immune interaction. Front Immunol 2012; 3: 1-11.

[93] Cai C, Cao Z, Loughran PA, Kim S, Darwiche S, Korff S, Billiar TR. Mast cells play a critical role in the systemic inflammatory response and end-organ injury resulting from trauma. J Am Coll Surg 2011; 213: 604-615.

[94] Bischoff SC, Wedemeyer A, Hermann PN, Meier C, Trautwein C, Cetin H, Maschek M, Stolte M, Gebel M, Manns MP. Quantitative assessment of intestinal eosinophils and mast cells in inflammatory bowel disease. Histopathology 1996; 28: 1-13.

[95] Buhner S, Schemann M. Mast cell-nerve axis with a focus on the human gut. Biochim Biophys Acta 2012; 1822: 85-92.

[96] Garrison RN, Spain DA, Wilson MA, Keelen PA, Harris PD. Microvascular changes explain the "two-hit" theory of multiple organ failure. Ann Surg 1998; 227: 851-860.

[97] Ince C. The microcirculation is the motor of sepsis. Crit Care 2005; 9: S13-S19.

[98] Feuser K, Thon K-P, Bischoff SC, Lorentz A. Human intestinal mast cells are a potent source of multiple chemokines. Cytokine 2012; 1822: 85-92.

[99] Hocking AM, Gibran NS. Mesenchymal stem cells: Paracrine signaling and differentiation during cutaneous wound repair. Exp Cell Res 2010; 316: 2213-2219.

[100] Dazzi F, Krampera M. Mesenchymal stem cells and autoimmune diseases. Best Pract Res Clin Haematol 2011; 24: 49-57.

[101] Otto WR, Wright NA. Mesenchymal stem cells: from experiment to clinic. Fibrogenesis Tissue Repair 2011; 4: 20.

[102] Ehninger A, Trumpp A. The bone marrow stem cell niche grows up: mesenchymal stem cells and macrophages move in. J Exp Med 2011; 208: 421-428.

[103] Balbridge MT, King KY, Goodell MA. Inflammatory signals regulate hematopoietic stem cells. Trends Immunol 2011; 32: 57-64.

[104] Serhan CN, Brain SD, Buckley CD, *et al.* Resolution of inflammation: State of the art, definitions and terms. FASEB J 2007; 21: 325-332.
[105] Flierl MA, Rittirsch D, Huber-Lang M, Sarma JV, Ward PA. Catecholamines-crafty weapons in the inflammatory arsenal of immune/inflammatory cells or Opening Pandora's box? Mol Med 2008; 14: 195-204.
[106] Grisanti LA, Evanson J, Marchus E, *et al.* Pro-inflamatory responses in human monocytes are β_1-adrenergic receptor subtype dependent. Mol Immunol 2010; 47: 1244-1254.
[107] Sarkar C, Basu B, Chakroborty D, *et al.* The immunoregulatory role of dopamine: an update. Brain Behav Immun 2010; 24: 525-528.
[108] Smith EM, Galin FS, Le Boeuf RD, Coppenhauer DH, Harbour DV, Blalock JE. Nucleotide and amino acid sequence of lymphocyte-derived corticotrophin: endotoxin induction of a truncated peptide. Proc Natl Acad Sci USA 1990; 87: 1057-1060.
[109] Smith EM. Neuropeptides as signal molecules in common with leukocytes and the hypothalamic-pituitary-adrenal axis. Brain Behav Immunol 2008; 22: 3-14.
[110] Malagoli D, Accorsi A, Ottaviani E. The evolution of pro-opiomelanocortin: looking for the invertebrate finger prints. Peptides 2011; 32: 2137-2140.
[111] Wardlan SL. Hypothalamic proopiomelanocortin processing and the regulation of energy balance. Eur J Pharmacol 2011; 660: 213-219.
[112] Collington SJ, Williams TJ, Weller CL. Mechanisms underlying the localization of mast cells in tissues. Trends Immunol 2011; 32: 478-485.
[113] Halova I, Draberova L, Draver P. Mast cell chemotaxis-chemoattractants and signaling pathways. Front Immunol 2012; 3: 1-17.
[114] Greenham S, Clarke G, Cryan JF, Dinan TG. Brain-gut-microbiome communication in health and disease. Front Physiol 2011; 2: 1-15.
[115] Deitch EA. Gut-origin sepsis: Evolution of concept. Surgeon. **2012** Apr 23. pii: S1479-666X(12)00033-9. doi: 10.1016/j.surge.**2012**.03.003 [Epub ahead of print]
[116] Kao H-K, Chen B, Murphy G, *et al.* Peripheral blood fibrocytes: Enhancement of wound healing by cell proliferation, re-epithelialization, contraction and angiogenesis. Ann Surg 2011; 254: 1066-1074.
[117] Ratajczak MZ, Liu R, Ratajczak J, *et al.* The role of pluripotent embryonic-like stem cells residing in adult tissues in regeneration and longevity. Differentiation 2011; 81: 153-161.
[118] Kelley EC, Mehrad B, Strieter RM. Fibrocytes: Bringing new insights into mechanisms of inflammation and fibrosis. Int J Biochem Cell Biol 2010; 42: 535-542.
[119] Bellini A, Mattolli S. The role of the fibrocyte, a bone marrow-derived mesenchymal progenitor, in reactive and reparative fibroses. Lab Invest 2007; 87: 858-870.
[120] Jones CP, Rankin SM. Bone marrow-derived stem cells and respiratory disease. Chest 2011; 140: 205-211.
[121] Wasmuth HE, Tacke F, Trautwein C. Chemokines in liver inflammation and fibrosis. Semin Liver Dis 2010; 30: 215-225.
[122] Meran S, Steadman R. Fibroblasts and myofibroblasts in renal fibrosis. Int J Exp Pathol 2011; 92: 158-167.
[123] Bucala R. Fibrocytes and fibrosis. Q J Med 2012; 105: 505-508.
[124] Raman D, Sobolik-Delmaire T, Richmond A. Chemokines in health and disease. Exp Cell Res 2011; 317: 575-589.
[125] Masuda H, Asahara T. Post-natal endothelial progenitor cells for neovascularization in tissue regeneration. Cardiovasc Res 2003; 58: 390-398.

[126] Herbert SP, Stainier DYR. Molecular control of endothelial cell behavior during blood vessel morphogenesis. Nat Rev Mol Cell Biol 2011; 12: 551-564.
[127] Potente M, Gerhardt H, Carmeliet P. Basic and therapeutic aspects of angiogenesis. Cell 2011; 146: 873-887.
[128] Aller MA, Arias N, Fuentes-Julian S, Blazquez-Martinez A, Argudo S, De Miguel MP, Arias JL, Arias J. Coupling inflammation with evo-devo. Med Hypotheses 2012; 78: 721-731.
[129] Aird WC. Discovery of the cardiovascular system: from Galen to William Harvey. J Thromb Haemost 2011; 9: 118-129.
[130] Eble JA, Nilands S. The extracellular matrix of blood vessels. Curr Pharm Des 2009; 15: 1385-1400.
[131] Arshad MI, Piquet-Pellorce C, Samson, M. IL-33 and HMGB1 alarmins: sensors of cellular death and their involvement in liver pathology. Liver Int 2012; 32:1200-1210.
[132] Denk S, Perl M, Huber-Lang M. Damage- and pathogen-associated molecular patterns and alarmins: Key to sepsis? Eur Surg Res 2012; 48: 171-179.
[133] Newton K, Dixit VM. Signaling in innate immunity and inflammation. Cold Spring Harb Perspect Biol 2012; 4: a006049.
[134] Puskaich MA. Emergency management of severe sepsis and septic shock. Curr Opin Crit Care 2012; 18:295-300.
[135] Maccaferri S, Biagi E, Brigidi P. Metagenomics: Key to human gut microbiota. Dig Dis 2011; 29: 525-530.
[136] Goedeke L, Fernandez-Hernando C. Regulation of cholesterol metabolism. Cell Mol Life Sci 2012; 69: 915-930.
[137] Sniderman A, Couture P. De Graaf, J. Diagnosis and treatment of apolipoprotein B dyslipoproteinemias. Nat Rev Endocrinol 2010; 6: 335-346.
[138] Jahangiri A. High-density lipoprotein and the acute phase response. Curr Opin Endocrinol Diabetes Obes 2010; 17: 156-160.
[139] Targher G, Day CP, Bonora E. Risk of cardiovascular disease in patients with nonalcoholic fatty liver disease. N Engl J Med 2010; 363: 1341-1350.
[140] Ji Y, Sakata Y, Tso P. Nutrient-induced inflammation in the intestine. Curr Opin Clin Nutr Metab Care 2011; 14: 315-321.
[141] Vinolo MAR, Rodrigues HG, Nachbar RT, Curi R. Regulation of inflammation by short chain fatty acids. Nutrients 2011; 3: 858-876.
[142] Taves MD, Gomez-Sanchez CE, Soma KK. Extra-adrenal glucocorticoids and mineralocorticoids: evidence for local synthesis, regulation and function. Am J Physiol Endocrinol Metab 2011; 301: E11-E24.
[143] Gilliver SC. Sex steroids as inflammatory regulators. J Steroid Biochem Mol Biol 2010; 120: 105-115.
[144] Cunningham M, Gilkeson G. Estrogen receptors in immunity and autoimmunity. Clin Rev Allergy Immunol 2011; 40: 66-73.
[145] Arukwe A, GoksØyr A. Eggshell and egg yolk proteins in fish: hepatic proteins for the next generation: oogenetic population and evolutionary implications of endocrine disruption. Comparative Hepatology 2003; 2: 4.
[146] Knaevelsrud H, Simonsen A. Lipids in autophagy: Constituents, signaling molecules and cargo with relevance to disease. Biochim Biophys Acta 2012; 1821: 1133-1145.
[147] Singh R, Kaushik S, Wang Y, Xiang Y, Novak I, Komatsu M, Tanaka K, Cuervo AM, Czja MJ. Autophagy regulates lipid metabolism. Nature 2009; 458: 1131-1135.

[148] Jung CH, Ro S-H, Cao J, Otto NM, Kim D-H. mTOR regulation of autophagy. FEBS letters 2010; 584: 1287-1295.

[149] Neufeld TF. Autophagy and cell growth- the yin and yang of nutrient responses. J Cell Sci 2012; 125: 2359-2368.

[150] Crivellato E, Ribati D. The mast cell: an evolutionary perspective. Boil Rev 2010; 85: 347-360.

[151] Costerton JW, Stewart PS, Greenberg EP. Bacterial biofilms: A common cause of persistent infections. Science 1999; 284: 1318-1322.

[152] Parsek MP, Greenberg EP. Sociomicrobiology: the connections between quorum sensing and biofilms. Trends Microbiol 2005; 13: 27-33.

[153] West SA, Griffin AS, Gardner A, Diggle SP. Social evolution theory for microorganisms. Nat Rev Microbiol 2006; 4: 597-607.

[154] Donelli G, Vuotto C, Cardines R, Mastrantonio P. Biofilm-growing intestinal anaerobic bacteria. FEMS Immunol Med Microbiol 2012; 65: 318-325.

[155] Stevens AM, Schuster M, Rumbaugh KP. Working together for the common good: Cell-cell communication in bacteria. J Bacteriol 2012; 194: 2131-2141.

Send Orders for Reprints to reprints@benthamscience.net

Surgical Inflammation, 2013, 214-249

CHAPTER 8

Cancer: Using the Inflammatory Way to Invade the Host

Jose-Ignacio Arias[1], Maria-Angeles Aller[2], Isabel Prieto[3], Ana Arias[4], Heping Yang[5] and Jaime Arias[2,*]

[1]General Surgery Unit, Monte Naranco Hospital, Oviedo, Asturias, Spain; [2]Surgery Department, School of Medicine, Complutense University of Madrid, Madrid, Spain; [3]Surgery Department, La Paz Hospital, Autonoma University of Madrid, Madrid, Spain; [4]Internal Medicine Department, Puerta de Hierro Hospital, Autonoma University of Madrid, Majadahonda, Madrid, Spain and [5]Division of Gastroenterology and Liver Diseases, USC Research Center for Liver Diseases, Keck School of Medicine USC, Los Angeles, California, USA

Abstract: Inflammation has been implicated in tumor development, invasion and metastasis. Hence, it has been suggested that common cellular and molecular mechanisms are activated in wound repair and in cancer development. In addition, it has been previously proposed that the inflammatory response, which is associated with the wound healing process, could recapitulate ontogeny through the re-expression of the extraembryonic, *i.e.* amniotic and vitelline, functions in the interstitial space of the injured tissue. If so, the use of inflammation by the cancer-initiating cell can also be supported in the ability to reacquire extraembryonic functional axes for tumor development, invasion and metastasis. Thus, the diverse components of the tumor microenvironment could represent the overlapped re-expression of amniotic and vitelline functions. These functions would favor a gastrulation-like process, that is, the creation of a reactive stroma in which fibrogenesis and angiogenesis appear.

Keywords: Cancer, tumor development, tumor invasion, metastasis, cancer-related inflammation, angiogenesis, wound healing, myofibroblast, epithelial-mesenchymal transition, mesenchymal-epithelial transition lymphangiogenesis, hypoxia, interstitial-lymphatic tumoral axis, Warburg effect, leukocytic cancer cell phenotype, immunotolerance.

INTRODUCTION

In the nineteenth century, Rudolf Virchow postulated a link between cancer and

***Address correspondence to Jaime Arias:** Cátedra de Cirugía, Facultad de Medicina, Universidad Complutense, Pza. de Ramón y Cajal s.n., 28040 MADRID, Spain; Tel: +34 91 394 1389; Fax: +34 91 3947115; E-mail: jariasp@med.ucm.es

Jaime Arias, Maria-Angeles Aller and Jose-Ignacio Arias (Eds)

inflammation on the basis of observations that tumors often arose at sites of chronic inflammation and the inflammatory cells were present in biopsied samples from tumors [1]. Twenty-five years ago, Dvorak recognized that the composition of tumor stroma is very similar to that of granulation tissue of healing skin wounds. He therefore suggested that "tumors are wounds that do not heal" [2]. Since that time, inflammation has been implicated in tumor development, invasion, and metastasis and in the development of clinical features as fever and cachexia [3]. These observations suggested that common cellular and molecular mechanisms are active in wounds and in cancer tissue [4].

WOUND REPAIR PHENOTYPES: GASTRULATION REVISITED

The inflammatory response that is induced in the injured skin could be described as a succession of three overlapped phases during which the phenotypes of metabolic progressive complexity in using oxygen are expressed. Each one of these phases emphasizes the trophic role of the mechanisms developed in the damaged tissue. Hence, nutrition by diffusion predominates in the first phase; trophism is mediated by inflammatory cells in the second phase; and finally blood circulation and oxidative metabolism play the most significant nutritive role in the third phase [5].

In the first or immediate phase of the inflammatory response, interstitial hydroelectrolytic alterations stand out. The vasomotor response, with vasoconstriction and vasodilation, is responsible for the ischemia-reperfusion phenomenon, which in turn causes oxidative and nitrosative stress in the injured tissue. In this phase, during the progression of the interstitial edema, the lymphatic circulation is simultaneously activated. In the following intermediate phase of the inflammatory response, the tissues are infiltrated by inflammatory blood-born cells, particularly leukocytes. Symbiosis of the leukocytes and bacteria for extracellular digestion by enzyme release, *i.e.* phagocytosis, produces enzymatic stress. Furthermore, macrophages and dendritic cells take advantage of the lymphatic circulation activation, and migrate through it until reaching the lymph nodes, where they activate lymphocytes [5, 6].

During the third phase of the inflammatory response, angiogenesis permits numerous substances, including hormones, to be transported by the blood circulation. Although the final objective of angiogenesis is to form new mature vessels for oxygen, substrates and blood cells transport, other functions could be carried out before the new mature vessels are formed. Thus, angiogenesis could have antioxidant and antienzymatic properties, favoring therefore the resolution of the inflammation, as well as wound repair by epithelial regeneration and scarring. Consequently, in this phase the new formed tissue is structured, specialized and matured by remodeling [5, 6,7] (Table **1**).

Table 1: Phenotypes expressed in the acute inflammatory wound healing response

- Ischemia-Reperfusion Phenotype
. Oxidative stress
. Nitrosative stress
. Interstitial hydroelectrolytic alterations
. Hemodynamic impairments
. Edema
. Increased lymphatic circulation (circulatory switch)
- Leukocytic Phenotype
.Infiltration by granulocytes, macrophages and lymphocytes
. Enzymatic stress
. Lymphangiogenesis
. Lymph node reaction
. Wound immunotolerance
. Resolution
- Angiogenic Phenotype
. Endothelial cell proliferation
. Energetic stress
. Fibrogenesis
. New vascular network
. Epithelial regeneration

It has been previously proposed that the inflammatory response associated with the wound healing process in the skin could recapitulate ontogeny through the re-expression of two hypothetical embryonic trophic axes, *i.e.*: amniotic and yolk sac or vitelline, in the interstitial space of the injured tissue. If so, inflammation could represent the debut during post-natal life of ancestral biochemical mechanisms that were used for normal embryonic development. The re-expression of these ancient mechanisms, with a prenatal solvent path, is perhaps inappropriate and hard to recognize since they are anachronistic during post-natal life and because they are established in a different environmental medium [8].

The molecular and cellular contribution made by the two extraembryonic tissues that surround the fetus, the amnion and yolk sac, to the interstitial space located between them, namely the mesoderm, is essential for organogenesis [9]. It could be assumed that both cavities are controlled by an array of inductive and inhibitory signals originating from the adjacent extraembryonic mesenchyma [8] (Fig. **1**).

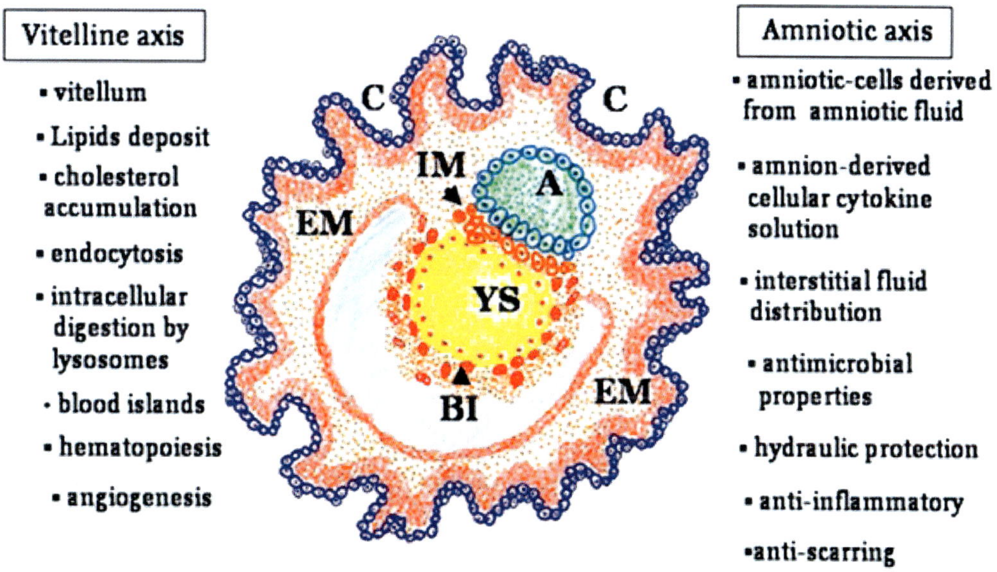

Figure 1: Representative drawing of the early mammalian embryo during gastrulation. The internalization of the extraembryonic mesoderm (EM) during gastrulation, allows the creation of the intraembryonic mesoderm (IM) that could thus join functional amniotic and vitelline properties from the amnion (A) and yolk sac (YS), respectively. BI: blood islands; C: chorionic vellosities.

The amniotic axis could play a leading role in primitive interstitial hydroelectrolytic changes. The early mammalian embryo already has the ability to manage fluids in the interstitial space. Body fluid is distributed among three major fluid spaces, *i.e.* intracellular fluid, interstitial fluid and plasma. Nevertheless, the fluid distribution in each of these compartments is dramatically different in the fetus compared to the adult. Particularly, the amniotic fluid that surrounds the fetus may be considered an extension of the extracellular space of the fetus. Thus the lymphatic system plays an essential role in the regulation of fluid distribution between the plasma and the interstitial fluid and, probably with the amniotic fluid [10]. In addition to the rich amino acid content, amniotic fluid contains abundant peptides, carbohydrates, lipids, hormones and electrolytes with water [11]. The amniotic fluid has antimicrobial properties, and this may be part of the innate immune system. A reduced volume of amniotic fluid may decrease the natural host defense conferred by this fluid and predispose it toward intrauterine infections [12]. Finally, it has been shown that amniotic fluid-derived stem cells are able to differentiate into neurogenic, mesodermal and endodermal lineages [13].

The vitelline axis, represented by the yolk sac, is the final destination of migrating visceral endoderm cells. The visceral yolk sac expands and blood islands, structures consisting of hematopoietic progenitors surrounded by a loose network of endothelial cells, appear [14]. Endothelial cell precursors associated with blood islands differentiate and coalesce to form a primitive circulation bed, which later connects to the embryo *via* the vitelline vessels [15]. Also a major function of the yolk sac is the accumulation of carbohydrates, proteins and lipids (vitellum) for the embryo nutrition [16, 17]. Particularly, the yolk sac plays a vital role in providing lipids and lipid-soluble nutrients to embryos during the early phases of development [16, 18]. The yolk sac uses high-density lipoproteins (HDL) and very low-density lipoproteins (VLDL) as carriers to incorporate cholesterol from the maternal circulation and to transfer it to the embryonic side [16]. In turn, the interstitial lipid accumulation of cholesterol, a precursor molecule of many hormones like aldosterone, corticoids, androgens, estrogens and progesterone, may favor fluid infiltration and cell migration, proliferation and differentiation during embryo development [19]. The ability to transport fat in the form of lipoprotein through the circulatory system by eukaryotes is one of their most significant functions right from the beginning of existence [20].

It could be accepted that these primitive functions are internalized during gastrulation to create the intraembryonic mesoderm. Thus, this germ layer would integrate the amnion- and yolk sac-related functions [8]. Fibroblasts are mesodermal derived cells and perhaps this embryonic origin could justify their great postnatal plasticity. The mesodermal cells of the embryo participate in the extraembryonary structures, including the corion, the amnion and the yolk sac [9]. In the human body, the fibroblasts form a heterogeneous collection of mesenchymal cells and they are the principal cellular constituents of connective tissues [21]. The major role of the mesodermal cells and their ability to differentiate from the first stages of embryonic development allow for considering them as the cell prototype that should be resorted to when the repair of any tissue in the body is needed [9]. And for this reason, perhaps the post-traumatic inflammatory response after wound skin has the same intention, namely, to use the embryonic mesodermal phenotype with a therapeutic objective [8].

Local fibroblasts residing in the skin are considered the most prominent source of myofibroblasts. However, a variety of other precursor cells contribute to the myofibroblast population, depending on the nature of the injured tissue and the particular microenvironment [22]. Activated myofibroblasts are generated from a variety of sources, including resident mesenchymal cells, epithelial and endothelial cells, *via* the epithelial/endothelial mesenchymal transition as well as from circulating fibroblast-like cells called fibrocytes, derived from bone-marrow stem cells [21, 23]. In addition, circulating monocytes have the capacity to differentiate into non-phagocytes, *i.e.* mesenchymal cells and endothelial cells [24].

The reason why the myofibroblasts are attractive to a broad scientific and clinical audience is due to the large panel of cells that can develop this phenotype upon activation. It appears that myofibroblasts can be recruited from any local cell type and they are suitable for rapidly repairing injured tissue [22]. Fibroblast can be induced to acquire the myofibroblast phenotype during wound repair. Several days after injury a subset of wound fibroblasts can differentiate into myofibroblasts, which are responsible for repopulating the wounded area in parallel to angiogenesis, thus forming the granulation tissue [6, 7]. Granulation tissue is then repopulated with fibroblasts to produce a more densely collagenous extracellular matrix which is more akin to the matrix found in interstitial stroma [25].

Tissue remodeling requires the removal of granulation tissue and maturation of collagen is oxygen dependent [6]. Indeed increasing wound oxygenation results in increased collagen deposition and tensile strength [26]. However, hypoxia benefits the expansion, differentiation, adhesion, growth factor secretion and regenerative potential of mesenchymal stem cells derived from subcutaneous adipose tissue [27]. Finally, the phenotypic changes suffered by the keratinocytes during re-epithelization suggest a partial epithelial-mesenchymal transition. Following the completion of wound-repair, keratinocytes revert from their mesenchymal-like phenotype to an epithelial phenotype [28, 29].

In the adult organism, many pathways that play an essential role during embryo development are inactivated later in life although some of them may be transiently expressed during adult repair [30]. That is why we have considered that wound repair would require the up-regulation of signaling pathways characteristic of the extraembryonic functions, *i.e.*: amniotic and vitelline, during the embryo development. If so, emulation by the wound tissue of these extraembryonic functions perhaps requires retracing the mechanisms that produce and distribute the extracellular fluid and substrates; activating the migration and invasion of stem or progenitor cells and hematopoietic-derived cells and inducing the establishment of a complex vascular network by lymphangiogenesis and angiogenesis- all of which are required to mediate normal new tissue growth and development [8]. The abovementioned extraembrionary mechanisms seem to be aimed at favoring the grafting of new repairing tissue. Thus, through the successive expression of functions related to natural immunity and later with the acquired immunity, the neoformed tissue is accepted by the host.

This transient recapitulation of embrionary mechanisms through the hypothetical succession of overlapped amniotic-like and vitelline-like functions would get the cellular and metabolic diversity necessary for repairing the injured adult tissue with a graft (Table **1**).

THE INFLAMMATORY CANCER CELL

Nowadays, the causal relationship between inflammation and cancer is widely accepted [1, 3, 4, 31-37]. Inflammation has long been thought to have contributed to the development of cancer [1, 35, 37]. Particularly, chronic inflammation is a major cause of cancer [32, 34, 36].

The understanding of the pathogenesis and progression of cancer requires the establishment of the altered genetic/metabolic factors that are essential to the development, growth and proliferation of malignant cells [38]. This new frontier of cancer research requires the appropriate marriage of genetic/proteomic studies or the geneticist approach to the biochemical/metabolic cellular studies or the biochemical approach [38].

With regards to the geneticist approach, in many cancers a stem cell tumor model probably takes place [39]. Although a stem cell may sustain the first oncogenic hit, subsequent alterations required for the genesis of a cancer stem cell can occur in descendent cells [40]. This mechanism could explain the marked tumoral heterogeneity, either interturmoral, *i.e.* variability between tumors arising in the same organ, as intratumoral, *i.e.* variability within individual tumors [40].

With regards to the biochemist approach, metabolic transformation of malignant cells is essential to the development and progression of all cancers [38, 41-43]. Cancer cells, similar to normal cells, live in niches and microenvironments that are heterogeneous. Specifically, intratumoral gradients of nutrients and oxygen could play a profound role in modulating tumor cell metabolism [42].

The comparison of tumors with wounds that do not heal [2] suggests that during the host invasion, the malignant tumor cells could express the previously proposed inflammatory phenotypes during wound repair [44]. Due to the plasticity of cancer stem cells it should be kept in mind that while a malignant tumor develops, it can express phenotypes that also share the inflammatory response such as: an ischemic phenotype (hypoxic) with edema and lymphangiogenesis (circulatory switch); the adoption of a leukocytic phenotype, with migration to the regional lymph nodes and development of cachexia, and an angiogenic phenotype with the supply of nutrients and oxygen and tumoral mass growth [44-46] (Fig. **2**).

It has already been proposed that these phenotypes represent the expression of trophic functional systems of increasing metabolic complexity in the wound inflammatory response [5, 6]. Their expression by cancer cells could have a similar significance [46]. In this hypothetical circumstance, malignant tumor cells could adopt an inflammatory-like phenotype that evolves in three hypothetical functional phases of increasing metabolic complexity and which would also have a trophic significance [44, 45, 46].

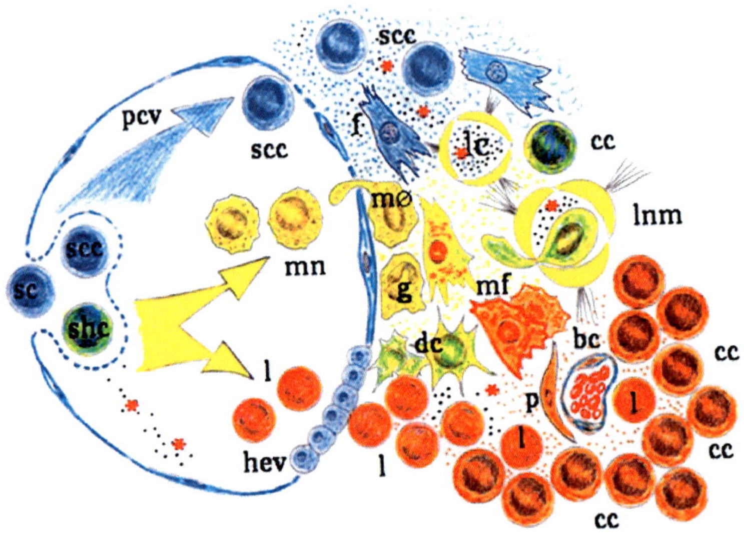

Figure 2: Evolutive phases of the inflammatory cancer cell. Cancer cells can adopt an inflammatory phenotype to invade neighboring tissues and survive in these ectopic sites. In the successive phases of tumorigenesis, the cancer cells invade the host by expressing natural and adaptive immune-related mechanisms. sc: stem cell; scc: stem cancer cell; shc: stem hematopoietic cell; f: fibroblast; mn: monocyte; mf: myofibroblast; g: granulocyte; mØ: macrophage; lc: lymphatic capillaries; cc: cancer cell; lnm: lymph node metastasis; hev: high endothelial venule; l: lymphocytes; pcv: post-capillary venule; bc: blood capillaries; p: pericyte; * tumoral antigen.

Moreover, acute wounds are initially hypoxic and chronic ischemic wounds are essentially hypoxic [47, 48]. However, in the wounded tissue molecular and functional heterogeneity could be related to the heterogeneous distribution of oxygen with hypothetical pockets of graded levels of hypoxia [48].

The hypothesized similarity of the inflammatory response in wounds and tumors, based on the molecular-related, *i.e.* genetic and metabolic, pathways is an interesting proposal because it could allow for translational inflammatory research between tissue repair and cancer. Moreover, the cancer cell also successively uses the natural and acquired immunity to be grafted into the host. The need to be recognized by the host, by both the cells that make the wound repair as by the cells that cause tumorigenesis to develop would indicate that in the adult organism the creation of a new tissue without a previous immunologic acceptation could not be possible. Regardless of whether the neoformed tissue is normal, like during embrionary development and wound repair, or pathological, like in cancer, the expression of extraembrionary functions would be essential for homing in the host. Therefore, the different inflammatory-related extraembryonic ways that converge in the embryo, in the wound repair process and in tumor growth may have the final aim of getting their immunological acceptation.

THE EVOLUTIVE PHASES OF THE INFLAMMATORY CANCER CELL

It has been proposed that the relation between inflammation and tumor development depends on whether the tumor is benign or malignant [44]. The benign tumor cells seem to be able to induce the inflammatory response in the host. Therefore, it is possible that the host participates in establishing the tumor through a process called desmoplasia, which consists of fibroblastic cells and the extracellular matrix, a leukocytic response represented by lymphocytes, macrophages and dendritic cells as well as lymphangiogenesis and angiogenesis [49]. Essentially, all the elements that constitute the inflammatory response participate in the "host reaction", which could, therefore, have a trophic purpose for the tumor cells [44, 46]. Consequently, this inflammatory response of the host would develop in the interstitial space of the tumor, which invades in order to be more efficient, trophically [46].

However, when tumor cells reach higher grades of malignancy their invasive capacity reflected in the classic metastatic cascade, *i.e.* primary tumor (T), lymph node invasion (N) and distant metastases (M), seems to be more a reflection of the new capacity to express the inflammatory response than to induce it in the host [45]. In this hypothetical circumstance the inflammatory phenotypes would be expressed by tumor cells to invade the host.

Therefore, it should be kept in mind that while a malignant tumor develops it can express phenotypes that are common to the inflammatory response, including a hypoxic phenotype with edema and lymphangiogenesis; a leukocytic phenotype with migration to the regional lymph nodes and distant metastasis; and an angiogenic phenotype with granulation tissue development and tumor and metastasis growth.

The Hypoxic Phenotype and the Interstitial-Lymphatic Tumoral Axis

Hypoxia and inflammation meet at several points in the setting of cancer [50]. During the initial avascular stages of tumor growth, which is when the tumor mass measures less than 0.5 cm [51], the cells seem to adopt an anoxic-hypoxic phenotype [52]. When tumor cells come into contact with oxygen, they could undergo a process of reoxygenation, with oxidative stress and edema [44].

The experimental evidence indicates that the cell mechanism for adapting to hypoxia is the prolyl-hydroxylases (PHDs)-hypoxia-inducible transcription factor (HIF) system [50]. The distribution of PHD-HIF system within the inflamed tumor is involved in both, its growth and vascularization [50]. In this way, cancer cells could adopt a hypoxic metabolism to survive. Most cancer cells rely on aerobic glycolysis, a phenomenon termed "the Warburg effect". Thus cancer cells can convert glucose and glutamine into biomass most efficiently and can proliferate faster [53]. In addition, glutamine metabolism has important "non anabolic" functions, including the regulation of oxidative stress, signal transduction and autophagy [43].

Cancer cells at this stage can over-express matrix metalloproteinases (MMPs). In many instances, therefore, the extensive alterations produced by MMPs in the stromal microenvironment could promote tumor progression [54, 55]. Thus, during the earlier phase of tumor progression, the metabolic autonomy and invasive capacity of the tumor cells would induce their premature migration to the peripheral tissue [56].

Metabolically active cancer cells could induce interstitial edema [57]. There is increasing evidence that conditions characterized by an intense inflammatory response are associated with alterations in cellular membrane potential, with subsequent depolarization and abnormal ion transport. Moreover, disturbances in ion transport are associated with intracellular as well as interstitial edema [58].

Interstitial fluid flow is elevated in tumors, favoring thus the diffusion of solutes and proteins and inducing a substantial influence on cancer cells [59, 60]. The tumor interstitial fluid is absorbed by lymphatic capillaries and drains through lymph nodes in the thoracic duct, where it reaches the blood *via* the large veins of the neck [60]. Tumor interstitial fluid is suggested to be a rich sample from which biomarker discovery can be conducted [61].

Compared with non-neoplastic tissue, the tumor stroma contains increased amounts of collagens, proteoglycans and glycosaminoglycans [61, 62]. Particularly, the accumulation of glycosaminoglycan fragments has been proposed as an important mechanism for edema formation because of its hydrophilic properties [63]. Glycosaminoglycans, *i.e.* hyaluronan, are long unbranched polysaccharide chains which tend to adopt highly extended random-coil conformations and occupy a huge volume for their mass [63]. They attract and entrap water and ions, thereby forming hydrated gels, while permitting the flow of cellular nutrients [63]. Thus, interstitial edema could favor nutrition by diffusion through the malignant tumor. Under inflammatory conditions, hyaluronan is more polydisperse with a preponderance of lower-molecular forms, and favors edematous infiltration of the tissues as well as the interstitial fluid flow and the tissue lymph pressure gradient [63-65].

Tumor interstitial fluid represents the early microenvironment of the tumor cells [57, 59]. One may therefore envisage that access to tumor interstitial fluid bathing the cancer cells is of considerable importance to understand how tumor develops and progresses [57, 59]. It could be suspected that during this early phase of the inflammatory cancer cell response, while edema progresses, the lymphatic circulation is simultaneously activated and this circulatory switch establishes an interstitial-lymphatic tumoral axis by which lymph can reach the systemic blood circulation [60]. In this way, lymphatic tumoral vessels are transformed in routes for trafficking through the body, exploited not only by immune cells but also by cancer cells [66]. Nevertheless, the interstitial tumoral fluid flow associated with edema can have important effects on tumoral tissue morphogenesis and function, cancer cell migration and differentiation and matrix remodeling, among other processes [67] (Fig. **3**).

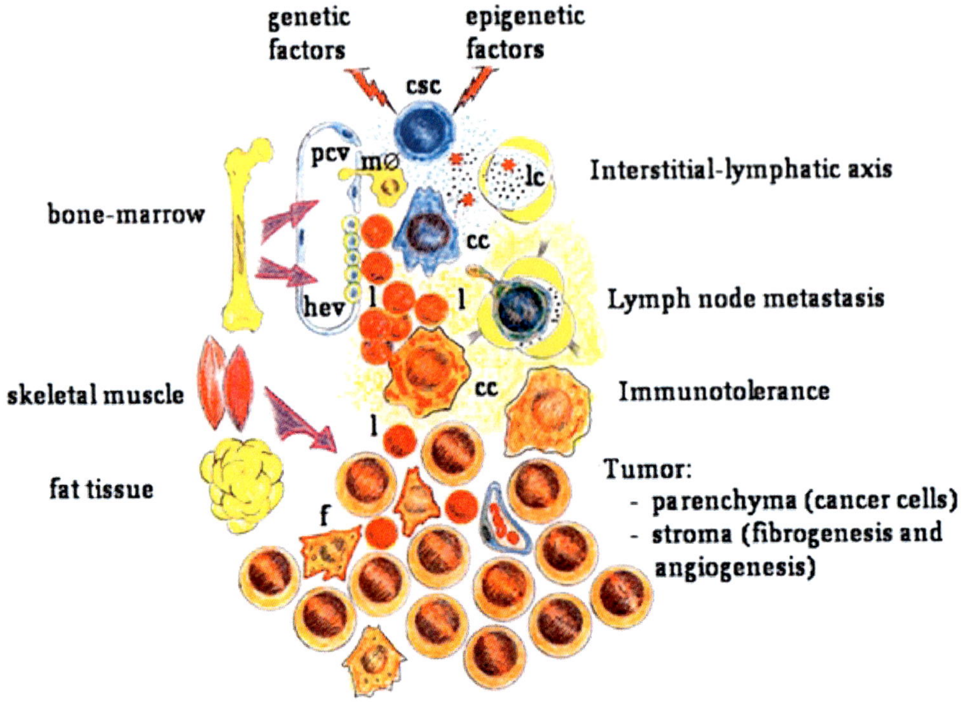

Figure 3: Successive and overlapped stages of tumorigenesis. Genetic and epigenetic factors stimulate the formation of a cancer stem cell that invades the interstitial space favored by the inflammatory interstitial-lymphatic axis, which steers the tissue circulation of fluid and the cellular migration. The tumor cell, by means of using the natural and adaptive immune mechanisms becomes immunotolerated, which favors the following phases of tumor development. Then the cancer cell induces the creation of a stroma formed by a special type of granulation tissue and this allows the creation of a tumoral parenchyma provided with functional heterogeneity. Finally, this heterogeneous tumor mass devastates the trophic stores of the host inducing cachexia.

A number of studies in animal tumor models have established the concept that tumors, rather than just accidentally invading pre-existing lymphatic vessels in their vicinity, can actively induce tumor-associated lymphangiogenesis by secreting appropriate growth factors such as vascular endothelial growth factor (VEGF)-C, VEGF-D or VEGF-A [66]. The formation of new lymphatic vessels, termed lymphangiogenesis, is often observed around or within the tumors [68]. With tumor progression, cancer cells secrete lymphangiogenic cytokines and growth factors which result in the formation of lymphatic vessels [69]. Tumor-associated lymphangiogenesis leads to a more extensive drainage network to capture the increased interstitial fluid flowing from the tumor cells and through the microenvironment [60]. Lymphatic vessels are also active modulators of immunity. Tumor association with the lymphatic system may not only affect the local microenvironment, but also the host immune response against the tumor [70]. Recent findings raise the possibility that the tumor-associated lymphatic vessel and draining lymph nodes may be important in tumor immunity which, in turn govern metastasis. Peritumoral lymphangiogenesis associated with increased drainage to the lymph nodes could activate and maintain tumor tolerance by the host [70]. Hence, targeting lymphangiogenesis by developing anti-lymphangiogenesis agents might constitute a novel way to prevent lymphatic progression in some tumors [71].

It has been shown that tumoral lymphatic vessels could display a retrograde draining pattern. At present, the mechanisms of tumoral lymphatic dysfunction are not entirely known [69]. It is hypothesized that the rapid growth of tumor results in tissue edema, which generates mechanical forces to compress the lymphatics, or tumor cells can destroy the intratumoral lymphatic structure [69]. However, the high colloid osmotic pressure and protein concentration of the tumoral interstitial fluid [59] associated with the tumoral lymphatic dysfunction could favor cancer cells trophism by diffusion, modulate their metabolic microenvironment and, therefore, play a key role in tumor growth and metastasis.

The Adoption of a Leukocytic Phenotype by Cancer Cells

The cancer cell could express a leukocytic phenotype with anaerobic glycolysis as the main source of energy, which permits lymphatic migration and invasion of the host [44-46].

Hypoxic tumor cells may suffer oxidative and nitrosative stress, like what occurs to leukocytes in the chronic inflammatory response by the generation of reactive oxygen and nitrogen species. Increased oxidative damage levels in malignant cells could result from more reactive species formation with unaltered antioxidant defenses; unaltered reactive species formation with decreases in antioxidant defenses; failure to repair oxidative damage, so that levels rise; or any combination of the above [72]. Overall, evidence supports the view that at least some malignant cells produce more reactive species for their own benefit and the antioxidant defense and repair activities may sometimes rise, but not enough to cope with the extra reactive species [72].

In most inflammatory responses, the actions of reactive species are mediated by IκB kinase/nuclear factor (NF)-κB (IKK/NF-κB) system, and in turn, this system can be regulated by hypoxia and/or reoxygenation [52, 73]. More specifically, the expression of inducible genes leading to the synthesis of cytokines, chemokines, chemokine receptors, adhesion molecules and autacoids relies on transcription factors; and among the primary transcription factors, NF-κB plays a main role in the regulation of inflammatory mediators [74]. In addition, reactive oxygen and nitrogen species generated by both oncogene-expressing cells and inflammatory cells could cause oxidative damage to host DNA resulting in activation of oncogenes and/or inactivation of tumor suppressor genes and various epigenetic changes that favor tumor progression [73].

The activated IKK/NF-κB pathway may play a tumor-promoting role by protecting tumor cells from death, *i.e.* antiapoptotic or enhancing their proliferation [73]. However, much attention regarding NF-κB has focused on inflammatory responses and tumor development, the current upsurge of interest in stem cell biology has led to studies of the function of NF-κB in stem cells of the bone marrow. NF-κB has been suggested to regulate secretion of growth factors and cytokines in adult and neonatal stem cells from the bone marrow environment [75].

Tumors in their development share an array of inflammatory activation mechanisms with leukocytes, including toll-like receptors (TLR) [32, 76], prostaglandin and leukotrienes metabolism [77], mitogen activated protein kinases (MAPKs), *i.e.* extracellular signal-regulated kinases (ERKs), c-Jun NH2-terminal kinases (JNKs) and p38 isoforms (p38s) [78], deregulation of phosphoinositide 3-kinase (CI3K)/Phosphatase and tensin homolog (PTEN)/AKT pathway [79], infiltrating tumor associated macrophages (TAMs) [31] and lymphocytes T and B [34] and microRNA expression [36].

The activation of a leukocytic phenotype by the tumor cells could imply their transition to a more elaborated inflammatory response. Hence tumor cells may usurp key mechanisms by which inflammation interfaces with cancer to further colonize the host [46].

The association between inflammation and cancer can be established by studying the influence of inflammatory cells in tumor progression, including neutrophils, eosinophils, macrophages, myeloid-derived suppressor cells, mast cells and lymphocytes [1, 31, 35]. However, opposing effects of inflammation on cancer have been described, and, at the risk of oversimplifying for the sake of clarity, it can be said that acute inflammation counteracts while chronic inflammation promotes cancer development [80, 81]. Nevertheless, such a link may not be as simple as the one currently portrayed because certain types of inflammatory processes in skin, such as psoriasis or atopic dermatitis, and possibly other tissues as well, may also serve as a tumor suppressor function [82].

Chronic inflammation is involved in shaping the tumor microenvironment and has been referred to as "host reaction", although it might be more appropriate to think of it as "tumor promoting" reaction [31]. In this way, cancer cell could reconvert the inflammatory host response to obtain an immunosuppressive inflammatory microenvironment and thus may escape from the host aggression [1, 31, 83]. An upregulation of immune tolerance by cancer cell could be induced using adaptive immunity [31, 34, 83, 84]. On the contrary, an inflammatory host response that switches the nature of the tumor-promoting an immunosuppressive microenvironment could kill tumor cells and produce cancer regression [31, 83, 85].

Independently of the action of host leukocytes and, owing the great plasticity of malignant cells, we could suspect that among the wide variety of phenotypes that they could express, it has been shown that tumor cells co-opt some of the signaling molecules of the host innate immune system, like chemokines, selectins and their receptors, for invasion, migration and metastasis [85]. Inflammation-associated products can also be secreted by the tumor cells themselves, giving rise to tumor microenvironment, which is overloaded and enriched with inflammatory factors with marked immunosuppressive abilities [81, 86]. In addition, immune cells in the tumor microenvironment not only fail to exercise antitumor effector functions, but they are co-opted to promote tumor growth and metastasis [31, 87] (Fig. **3**).

The hypothetical activation by chemokines of the leukocytic phenotype in the tumor cells could permit these cells to fulfill functions characteristic of activated inflammatory cells. For example, functions associated with neutrophils, for example the hyperproduction of extracellular proteases, including MMPs and other protease enzymes that carry out a true extracellular digestion of the basement membrane and the extracellular matrix, also aid invasiveness in the early stages of the disease [55, 88]. The extracellular matrix is a reservoir for many molecules, including growth factors and cytokines, which are only released upon their dissolution [89]. Also, cancer cells can present pseudopodia formation and directional migration [90]. Other functions seem to correspond to a monocyte-macrophage phenotype in the sense that tumor cells migrate to the regional lymph nodes through the lymphatic capillaries [70, 91]. Moreover, the so-called fusion theory explains that the acquisition of metastatic phenotype occurs when a healthy migratory leukocyte fuses with a primary tumor cell. Interestingly, the fusion of genetic and cytoplasmic material between cells of different origins is an important physiological process during development [92].

Cancer cells dissociated from the primary tumor could change their phenotype to become more autonomous, express specific adhesion molecules, produce lymphangiogenic factors and eventually evade the host defense [69]. The hypothetical adoption of a leukocytic phenotype by most tumor cells would also imply the acquisition of a similar metabolism. In this situation, like the activated leukocytes, their function would require glycolysis as the main source to obtain substrates and energy [93]. In this sense, the metabolic regulation of cancer metastatic cells could be closely related to a specific mutational activation of oncogenes and inactivation of tumor suppressor genes [94]. In contrast to normal cells, cancer cells tend to convert glucose into lactate even in the presence of sufficient oxygen, a term called "Warburg effect" or aerobic glycolysis [95]. Glutamine is also a major cancer cell energy and anabolic substrate [94]. The oncogenes Akt, Myc and Ras, MAP-kinase, PI3K and mammalian target of rapamycin (mTOR) pathways and HIF can stimulate the transcription of a number of genes that encode the proteins that mediate the glycolysis and glutaminolysis pathways [94, 95]. This metabolic characteristic of the tumor cell in this stage would explain why tumors grow, regardless of their angiogenic ability, in the lymph node [96]. In turn, nutrition of cancer cells during the expression of a leukocytic phenotype could also be based on extracellular, *i.e.* proteolytic enzymes, and intracellular, *i.e.* phagocytic functions including autophagy, digestion [44, 45].

During the adoption of a leukocytic phenotype, soluble factors could push tumor cells towards premature migration to peripheral tissue [45]. Considerable progress has been made in recent years regarding how tumor cells circulating in the blood and lymphatic system interact with and extravasate into secondary sites, and what determines whether these disseminated tumor cells survive, remain dormant or go on to form macrometastases [97]. Hence the leukocytic phenotype would favor the homing of metastatic tumor cells to specific organs, especially those where populations of resident macrophages are abundant, *i.e.* lung (alveolar macrophages), liver (Kupffer cells), brain (glia) and bone (osteoclasts) [44]. Particularly, specific chemokines in distant organs and chemokine receptors on the tumor cells dictate a metastasis pattern according to the cancer cells [98].

Tumor cell-derived factors, which also could partially be contributed by tumor-infiltrating macrophages [31], have been found to induce the expansion of the lymphatic network in the lymph nodes, even before the arrival of the metastatic cancer cells, as if to create a favorable environment for the future metastasis [99, 100]. Also, disseminated tumor cells in bone marrow can be detected in 20-40% of cancer patients without any clinical or histopathological signs of metastasis [101]. The particular bone marrow environment may induce these cells to survive and disseminate later into other distant organs. This "dormant stage" of disseminated tumor cells may explain why these cells are relatively resistant to chemotherapy [102].

The adoption of a leukocytic phenotype by cancerous cells could be associated with an increased degree of lymphangiogenesis. In animal models, a strong relationship between lymphangiogenesis and survival has been shown [68]. Lymphangiogenesis at the site of the primary tumor as well as in the draining lymph node actively contribute to metastatic cancer spread and its inhibition might be of interest for preventing tumor metastasis [68, 99, 103]. Lymphangiogenesis is not only crucial for cancer cells to metastasize, but also offer the tumor the possibility to disseminate inflammatory mediators in the host, which would produce a systemic inflammatory response syndrome (SIRS) [45, 104]. The SIRS, mediated in part by pro-inflammatory mediators including cytokines, plays a role in the genesis of cachexia associated with both critical illness and chronic inflammatory diseases [105]. The systemic inflammatory and immune response to the presence of a tumor is manifested in different ways, according to the type and extent of the tumor. Fever, night sweats, weight loss, fatigue, and malnutrition may all be attributable to tumor-induced inflammation [3]. Cancer cachexia is a continuum with three stages of clinical relevance: precachexia, cachexia and refractory cachexia, but not all patients traverse the entire spectrum [106]. Additionally, although an acute phase protein response is usually produced, the C-reactive protein in serum is the most widely accepted index of systemic inflammation, and cachexia can be present in the absence of overt systemic inflammation [106]. Thus, the host, as a yolk sac-like structure, becomes a vitellum supplier for the tumor growth.

The tumor cell, through the lymphatic system, can also modulate the host immunity, using its own antigen production. Tumoral antigens in the interstitial fluid are collected into open-ended lymphatic capillaries, which can form a mesh-like network by lymphangiogenesis, which could then be transported to the lymph nodes [107]. However, tumoral antigens in prenodal lymph, before entering the node and once inside, could be filtered by dendritic cells and nodal antigen-presenting cells, respectively [107]. Thus, lymph-carried tumoral antigens might have particular relevance for the induction and maintenance of peripheral tolerance to cancer cells.

The functional plasticity of dendritic cells allows for adapting the immune system to mount functionally distinct types of responses, including the immunologic tolerance that could contribute to tumor development [83]. In this way, it is accepted that dendritic cell vaccines will be offered to patients either with early- or late-stage disease to elicit a strong and long-lived antigen-specific T cell immunity [83].

Additionally, lymphatic vessel density can increase in the chronic inflamed tumoral tissue, although without reestablishing an efficient lymphatic connection with the draining lymph nodes [108]. This defective lymphatic drainage, associated with the enduring local tumoral antigen stimulation, could be a crucial trigger of the cascade of events leading to lymphoid neogenesis [109]. *De novo* lymphoid tissue formation or tertiary lymphoid organs occur during states of chronic inflammation [70]. Tertiary lymphoid organs may accumulate tumor antigens and tumor antigen presenting cells, bypassing the lymph node function and therefore bypassing relevant lymph node function and therefore circumventing their tolerance-maintaining function [70, 109]. In addition, myeloid-derived suppressor cells, a heterogenic population of immature myeloid cells that consists of myeloid progenitors and precursors of macrophages, granulocytes and dendritic cells, use a number of mechanisms to suppress various T cell functions as well as to the induction of regulatory T cells [110].

Granulation Tissue-Related Cancer Cells

Cancer cells, to grow inside the host, need to induce the formation of a stroma to change in an organ. Therefore, the comparison of tumors with wounds that do not heal includes, among other characteristics, the development of a stroma in which the formation of fibroblasts, through a process named fibroplasia, mainly takes place [6]. This phase of cutaneous wound healing, also called granulation phase is basically characterized by active fibroplasia and angiogenesis [111] (Fig. **3**).

The role of fibroblasts in wound healing has been extensively studied over the past years. Fibroblasts and myofibrolasts mainly produce the new extracellular matrix necessary for supporting cells and blood vessels, which provides nutrients and oxygen needed for cell growth and proliferation [111]. This new matrix consists of collagen, proteoglycans and fibronectins produced by the fibroblasts. Fibroblasts activity is predominantly regulated by platelet-derived growth factor (PDGF) and transforming growth factor β (TGFβ) [112]. Growth factors involved in fibrogenesis also include fibroblasts growth factor-2 (FGF-2) and hepatocyte growth factor (HGF), which are also chemotactic factors for mesenchymal stem cells. Complementary to this, it has been demonstrated that keloid-derived fibroblasts induce higher mesenchymal stem cell migration toward themselves than normal fibroblasts [113]. Also, it must be noted that keloids are locally aggressive scars that typically invade into healthy surrounding tissues [113].

Recent studies indicate that mesenchymal stem cells from the bone marrow contribute to provide "fibroblasts" to the skin in adults and are thought to enhance cutaneous repair/regeneration [33, 114].

In recent years the tumor stroma has become the focus of intense research. In particular, fibroblasts, a heterogeneous collection of mesenchymal cells, are among the most abundant cell types in the microenvironment of solid tumors [37]. Cancer-associated fibroblasts through the release of cytokines and growth factors could modulate the cancer stem cell phenotype and could also lead to enhanced angiogenesis [33, 37]. It has been suggested that cancer-associated fibroblasts may be derived from tumor cells that undergo epithelial-mesenchymal transition [115]. One characteristic of the cancer-associated fibroblasts is their heterogeneity, which is also expressed through the formation in solid tumors of a very different profile of extracellular matrix proteins [37]. Mesenchymal stromal cells also can suppress immune responses, favoring tumor cells to escape the host immune response [116].

Angiogenesis characterizes a phase of cancer evolution that permits numerous substances, including hormones, to be transported by the blood. Angiogenesis requires migration of endothelial cells into the interstitial space with the subsequent proliferation and differentiation into capillaries [44]. Tumors induce angiogenesis by activating tumor stromal cells, by releasing angiogenic factors from the extracellular matrix to which they bind by the emergence new epitopes in the extracellular matrix that promotes angiogenesis, and *via* the switching of neoplastic cells to an angiogenic phenotype [117]. However, tumor-angiogenesis produces a tumor-associated vasculature that is chaotic, both in structure and function. Although angiogenesis supplies a growing tumor with nutrients and oxygen, the neo-vasculature is poorly formed often with leaky blood vessels that do not link the arterial to the venous circulation but are rather dead-end [42, 118]. This characteristic impairs tumor blood flow and delivering of oxygen [119], but they favor its growth since without angiogenesis tumors rarely grow larger than 2 to 3mm [120]. However, the tumor during its growth seems to prioritize the venous-lymphatic circulation in detriment of the arterio-venous circulation, which is characteristic of the specialized tissues. This circulatory switch perhaps could offer some metabolic advantages to the tumor biology, for instance, it would favor an environment poor in oxygen, strengthening therefore an efficient anaerobic metabolism that forms biomass; to the blood endothelium with an inflammatory phenotype, it would give more permeability to molecules and cells and it would also enrich the composition of the interstitial space. In essence, a "reactive stroma" would be created [59, 121]. The normal stroma in most organs contains a minimal number of fibroblasts, whereas a reactive tumor stroma could be associated with an increased number of cells, including fibroblasts, enhanced vessel density and protein deposition [59].

Cancer cells are also associated with high endothelial venule development. Lymphocytes get into lymph nodes from the blood through high endothelial venules. T and B cells subsequently move into the T zone and B-cell follicles, respectively and then migrate in a stromal guided random walk [122]. In contrast to the flat endothelial cells that line other types of blood vessels, high endothelial venule endothelial cells are almost cuboidal, and they selectively express certain tissue specific adhesion molecules and chemokines [123]. High endothelial venules are mainly found in the paracortical and interfollicular areas of the lymph node and are surrounded by an intricate stromal network consisting of fibroblastic reticular cells but also high-endothelial venule-like structures are associated with tertiary lymphoid organs, which represent highly organized lymphoid tissues induced by inflammation [123]. In addition, recruitment of lymphocytes and dendritic cells to inflamed lymph nodes by *trans*-high-endothelial venule migration involves the mediation of heparan sulfate [124].

Tumors build their blood vessels by mechanisms that involve endothelial cell response, including circulating endothelial precursors and circulating endothelial cells, to tumor signaling [98]. Recent works provide evidence indicating that the state of endothelial cell activation in the tumoral niche, rather than angiogenesis itself may dictate tumor dormancy or escape. In essence, the cross-talk between tumor cells and stromal cells, including endothelial cells within the tumor microenvironment, mediates tumor evolution [98, 125].

Within the factors that play a role in initiating tumoral neovascularization, the "classical", *i.e.* VEGF, fibroblast growth factor-2 (FGF-2), also termed basic fibroblast growth factor (bFGF), platelet-derived growth factor (PDGF), transforming growth factors (TGFs) and angiopoietins (Angs); and the "non-classical" mediators of angiogenesis, *i.e.* erythropoietin, angiotensin II, endothelins and thyroid hormones, stand out [126].

However, as it has been previously explained, tumor vasculature is typically aberrant [118] with a reduced pericyte coverage which, in turn destabilizes vascular integrity and function [127]. Additionally, vascular heterogeneity could be associated with subpopulations of cancer cells that differ in their energy-generating pathways macromolecular biosynthesis and redox control [42, 43, 127, 128]. These populations may function symbiotically since the cells proximal to a better-oxygenated tumoral tissue consume oxygen with glucose and glutamine, serving as substrates and secreting lactate that can be used by another subpopulation of hypoxic cancer cells as their main energy source [42, 127]. In a similar compensatory way, the activation of HIF in the hypoxic cancer cell subpopulation or in stromal cells within the tumor could augment their vascularization and oxygenation. This change could be associated in turn, with tumoral blood flow redistribution, rendering ischemic other areas of the tumor, and therefore with a hypoxic metabolism that induces an increase in tumor invasiveness and risk of metastasis [50]. In this way, it can be suspected that the metabolic and functional heterogeneity of the tumors, which is imposed by their stroma, *i.e.* granulation tissue-like, is dynamic. This tumoral dynamic heterogeneity could constitute a favoring factor of chronicity.

CANCER CELL MEETS AMNIOTIC AND VITELLINE FUNCTIONAL AXES

The concept that cancer and embryonic cells have much in common is an old idea. The morphological resemblance between cancer cells and the cells of fetal tissues has been repeatedly discussed in current biomedical literature [129]. During the mid-19th century, upon observing cancer tissue under the microscope, the forefathers in pathology noticed the similarities between embryonic tissue and cancer, and suggested that tumors arise from embryo-like cells [130]. More recently, it became clear that neoplastic cells possess a more embryonic phenotype than their tissue of origin and that this involves the expression (or re-expression) of embryonic genes [131]. Both, embryos and tumors, display similar antigens, elaborate angiogenic growth factors and subvert apoptotic cell death. Furthermore, they may both escape immune destruction by similar mechanisms [131].

Epithelial to mesenchymal transitions (EMT) are transdifferentiation programs that are also required for tissue morphogenesis both during embryonic and cancer development [132, 133]. The conversion of epithelial cells to mesenchymal cells is fundamental for embryonic development and involves profound phenotypic changes, including the loss of cell-cell adhesion and the acquisition of migratory and invasive properties [115, 132]. Recent evidence suggests that normal stem cells and cancer stem cells share a mesenchymal phenotype that enhances their ability to preserve stemness, to retain migratory properties and to respond to different stimuli during expansion and differentiation [132]. Thus, EMT induction in cancer cells results in the acquisition of invasive and metastatic properties [132, 133]. Interestingly these invasive cells with both a stem cell-like and mesenchymal phenotype can generate an epithelial-like structure by mesenchymal to epithelial transition (MET) and therefore, could be involved in the formation of macrometastasis [132]. Furthermore, nowadays it is accepted that metastasis progression should be considered as an independent and parallel process in tumorigenesis governed by the EMT that occurs among tumor cells [92, 115, 133]. In addition, although the majority of tumors are epithelial, they also exert mesenchymal characteristics [92, 132, 133].

An EMT process also occurs in the mammalian embryos during gastrulation [115]. Gastrulation is a developmental phase that delineates the three embryogenic germ layers, named ectoderm, endoderm and mesoderm. Haeckel coined the term gastrulation derived from the Greek word *"gaste"*, meaning stomach or gut, that transforms the rather unstructured early embryo into a gastrula with several specific characteristics: the three primary germ layers are formed; the basic body plan is established, including the construction of the rudimentary body axes; and the cells assume new positions, allowing them to interact with cells that were initially not close to them [134]. The nascent mesoderm generated during gastrulation could involve an internalization process of extraembryonic phenotypes [115]. In essence, gastrulation could be represented as the creation of an interstitial space in which extraembryonic, *i.e.* amniotic and vitelline, functions are expressed using mesenchymal cells. If so, the mesoderm would represent the vehicle or the mediator for the internalization of the extraembryonic functions into the embryos [8] (Fig. **1**).

The vast arrangement of the mesenchyma around and between the developing amniotic and yolk sac cavities suggests an important role of the mesenchyma in orchestrating embryo development. Mesenchyma isolated specifically from the amniotic membrane could differentiate into neuronal-like cells which are identified to secrete dopamine [135]. Cells derived from amniotic fluid also have a neuronal, dopaminergic phenotype [136]. These results allow for considering the amnion as an embrionary functional axis with strong neural potential [135, 136]. In addition, experimental and clinical studies have demonstrated that amniotic membrane transplantation has important biological properties, including anti-inflammatory, anti-microbial, anti-fibrosis and anti-scarring, as well as low immunogenicity [137, 138]. Amnion-derived multipotent progenitor cells secrete a unique combination of cytokines and growth factors, known as "amnion-derived cellular cytokine solution", which establish a communication network between mesenchymal and epithelial cells during embryo development. That is why using the amnion to accelerate wound healing through its functions has been proposed, which regulates migration, proliferation and differentiation of fibroblasts as well as of keratinocytes [139].

In turn, the extraembryonic visceral yolk sac in mammals is composed of two layers, *i.e.* the visceral endoderm, which is active in endocytosis/digestion and has large lysosomes, and the underlying mesoderm layer [140]. In the embryonic mesoderm layer "blood islands" develop supporting hematopoiesis and angiogenesis [141]. While formation of the various primitive hematopoietic populations is restricted to the yolk sac, progenitors of definitive hematopoietic cells that arise in the yolk sac may contribute to hematopoiesis in the embryo proper [141]. Also a major function of the yolk sac is associated with the accumulation of carbohydrates, proteins and lipids for embryo nutrition (vitellum) [142]. Particularly, the yolk sac plays a vital role in providing lipids and lipid-soluble nutrients to embryos during the early phases of development [142]. Interstitial lipid accumulation of cholesterol, a precursor molecule of many hormones, like aldosterone, corticoids, androgens, strogens and progesterone, may favor fluid infiltration and cell migration, proliferation and differentiation during embryo development [143].

Dissecting out the possible contribution of extraembryonic lineages to the embryo has been difficult, in large part because of the inaccessibility of the mammalian embryo within the uterus [141]. In addition, the term "extraembryonic" is somewhat a misnomer, as there is no clear anatomical or molecular demarcation to separate the embryonic from the extraembryonic tissues during the early steps of the development, and at later stages both are integral components of the developing embryo [144]. However, recent studies suggest that extraembryonically-derived functions and cells make an increasingly significant and possibly exclusive contribution to the embryonic development [141, 44]. Thus, the molecular and cellular contribution made by both extraembryonic structures, *i.e.* the amnion and the yolk sac, to the interstitial space located between them, namely the mesoderm, is essential for organogenesis. Particularly, both in the amnion axis as in the yolk sac axis, the extraembryonic mesenchyma plays an important role [9].

The internalization of extraembryonic functions, *i.e.* amniotic-like and vitelline-like, by mesenchymal cells not only could be a key process of the embryonic development, but it could be also used by the postnatal organism when it suffers an injury and, therefore it needs to be repaired. Thus, an acute or chronic injury could induce a dedifferentiation process with the expression of different and overlapped inflammatory phenotypes that resemble similar phenotypes expressed during embryo development. Particularly, molecular and cellular amniotic and vitelline mechanisms involved in gastrulation would return [8].

Moreover, the relationship between inflammation and cancer also could be based on the orchestration of extraembryonic functions. If so, tumorigenic cancer cells could successively induce the expression of overlapped amniotic and vitelline-like phenotypes that promote the invasion, control and remodeling of interstitium. The amniotic-like phenotype could offer the cancer cells an interstitial-lymphatic axis [59], favoring transport, nutrition by diffusion, excretion, and bacteriostatic and anti-inflammatory protection [139]. In turn, the vitelline phenotype could favor

Table 2: Hypothesized cancer cell extraembryonic (amniotic and vitelline) and embryonic (gastrulation) phenotypes.

- ***Amniotic-Like Phenotype***
. Abnormal ion transport
. Extracellular matrix degradation and permeability increase
. Diffusion
. Increased interstitial fluid (cytokines-substrates)
. Interstitial-lymphatic axis
. Circulatory switch
. Stem cancer cell recruitment and activation
- ***Vitelline-Like Phenotype***
. Fat transport – lipoproteins
- cholesterol
. Hematopoiesis – bone marrow control
- platelets
- neutrophils
- mast cells
- tumor associated macrophages
- lymphocytes
- dendritic cells
. Lymphatic metastasis
. Immunotolerance
. Angiogenic switch
. Cachexia – Using the host as vitellum
- ***Gastrulation–Like Phenotype***
. Tumoral stroma
- Epithelial-mesenchymal transition
- Granulation tissue
- Fibrosis
. Tumoral parenchyma
- Mesenchymal epithelial transition
- Epithelial proliferation
. Tumoral organ – Tumoral tissue growth and heterogeneity

the regulation of lipid metabolism genes, including cholesterol and eicosanoids homeostasis [145], the hematopoietic/bone marrow control [114] and the induction of an "angiogenic switch" [118, 127] to permit tumor and metastatic growth. The integration of both extraembryonic phenotypes by the cancer cell would render them the functional and metabolic heterogeneity that they need to successively modulate their microenvironment during their development in the host (Table **2**).

The new point of view proposed in the current review would be based on considering the extra-embrionary mechanisms like the expression of an ancient type of inflammatory response. Ancestral mechanisms of natural and acquired immunity immersed into the amniotic and vitelline axes would allow the acceptation of new and foreign tissues by the host. Therefore, the neoformed tissues, either physiological, *i.e.* embryo and repair tissue, or pathological, *i.e.* cancer, both of them being alien to the host organism, would need to use similar extra-embrionary mechanisms to be grafted successfully.

The involvement of these extraembryonic mechanisms, which are individualized in each patient in tumorigenesis, would be a key inducing factor of the vast heterogeneity of cancer [146, 147]. Moreover, cancer cells could be modified through epigenetic modifications that alter gene-expression patterns. Like all the cells that constitute the human body, a cancer cell is a direct descendent of the fertilized egg from which the cancer patient is developed. Compared with the fertilized egg, the cancer genome will also have acquired epigenetic changes with an altered chromatin structure and gene expression [148].

It could be concluded that cancer cells acquire the ability to invade the host organism through the recapitulation of extraembryonic, amniotic and vitelline functions. In this way, through the hypothesized overlapped expression of these two extraembrionary functional axes, cancer cells would adopt the different phenotypes that they need to develop. Maybe this is the reason why the pluripotent cancer-initiating cells would acquire the nature of embryonic cells. Thus the cancer-initiating cells would have the amazing ability of inducing, in their own benefit, the expression in the host of functional mechanisms of extraembrionary nature.

The immunological properties of the extraembrionary functions would have the aim of inducing the acceptance of the embryo by the maternal immune system. In addition, the adoption during the post-natal life of the above mentioned extraembrionary functions for developing new tissues during wound repair and tumorigenesis could have the same objective. Therefore, an appropriate immunological and trophic microenvironment would be created to live together with the host.

Since tumor tissue is what induces the expression of extraembryonic functions in the host that favor its development, it would become an autonomous organism that progressively takes over of its nutritional stores. This behavior could be compared with that which the cuckoo adapts for reproduction. This bird uses foreign nests to lay its eggs, which are incubated by other birds. After hatching, the newborn cuckoos throw out the nest all their potential competitors and thus monopolize the nutritional support of the deceived parents. In the same way, tumor cells adopt a selfish behavior, against the altruistic behavior characteristic of the normal cells of the host. Hence, in cancer, new immunotolerant tissues monopolize the nutritional resources of the host. This behavior could represent a last attempt to survive of this indomitable eukaryotic cell even at the expense of "murdering" its supporter.

ACKNOWLEDGEMENTS

We would like to thank Maria Elena Vicente for preparing the manuscript, Elizabeth Mascola for translating it into English and librarians of Complutense University Medical School, particularly the Director, Francisco Javier Jorge García-Reyes, and Manuela Crego and María José Valdemoro and B. Braun Surgical S.A. for their technical assistance.

This study was carried out in part with grants from Mutua Madrileña Research Foundation (Ref. nº PA 3077/2008 and AP5966/2009), MICINN PSI2010-19348 and with the special collaboration of the INEUROPA (Instituto de Neurociencias del Principado de Asturias).

CONFLICT OF INTEREST

The author(s) confirm that this chapter content has no conflict of interest.

REFERENCES

[1] Mantovani A, Allavena P, Sica A, Balkwill F. Cancer-related inflammation. Nature 2008; 454: 436-44.

[2] Dvorak HF. Tumors: wounds that do not heal. Similarities between tumor stroma generation and wound healing. N Engl J Med 1986; 315: 1650-9.

[3] Moore MM, Chua W, Charles KA, Clarke SJ. Inflammation and cancer: causes and consequences. Clin Pharmacol Ther 2010; 87: 504-8.

[4] Schâfer M, Werner S. Cancer as an overhealing wound: an old hypothesis revisited". Nature Mol Cell Biol 2008; 9: 628-38,.

[5] Aller MA, Arias JL, Nava MP, Arias J. Post-traumatic inflammation is a complex response base don the pathological expresión of the nervous, immune and endocrine functional systems. Exp Biol Med (Maywood) 2004; 229: 170-81.

[6] Aller MA, Arias JI, Giner M, Losada M, Cruz A, Alonso-Poza A, Arias J. Oxygen-related inflammatory wound phenotypes, In: Wound healing: Process, phases and promoting. Ed. Middleton, J.E., Nova Science Publishers, Inc. 2011; Chapter 2, pp. 1-26.

[7] Aller MA, Arias JL, Sanchez-Patan F, Arias J. The inflammatory response: An efficient way of life. Med Sci Monit 2006; 2: RA225-RA234.

[8] Aller MA, Arias JI, Arias J. Pathological axes of wound repair: Gastrulation revisited. Theor Biol Med Model 2010; 7: 1-32.

[9] De Miguel MP, Arnalich-Montiel F, Lopez-Iglesias P, Blázquez-Martinez A, Nistal M. Epiblast-derived ítem cells in embryonic and adult tissues. Int J Dev Biol 2009; 54: 1529-40.

[10] Bellini C, Boccardo F, Bonioli E, Campisi C. Lymphodynamic in the fetus and newborn. Lymphology, 2006; 39: 110-7.

[11] Underwood MA, Gilbert WM, Sherman MP. Amniotic fluid: not just fetal urine anymore. J Perinatol 2005; 25: 341-8.

[12] Kim BJ, Romero R, Lee SM, Park C-W, Park JS, Jun JK, Yoon BH. Clinical significance of oligohydramnios in patients with preterm labor and intact membranes. J Perinat Med 2011; 39: 131-6.

[13] Parolini O, Soncini M, Evangelista M, Schmidt D. Amniotic membrane and amniotic fluid-derived cells: potential tools for regenerative medicine. Regen Med 2009; 4: 275-91.

[14] Bielinska M, Narita N, Wilson DB. Distinct roles for visceral endoderm during embryonic mouse development. Int J Dev Biol 1999; 43: 183-205.

[15] Collardeau-Franchon S, Scoazec JY. Vascular development and differentiation during human liver organogenesis. Anat Rec (Hoboken) 2008, 291: 614-27.

[16] Yoshid S, Wada Y. Transfer of maternal cholesterol to embryo and fetus in pregnant mice. J Lipid Res 2005.; 46: 2168-74.

[17] Koike S, Keino-Masu K, Ohto T, Sugiyama E, Takahash S, Masu M. Autotaxin/lysophospholipase D-mediated lysophosphatidic acid signaling is required to form/distinctive large lysosomes in the visceral endoderm cells of the mouse yolk sac. J Biol Chem 2009; 284: 33561-70.

[18] Terasawa Y, Cases SJ, Wong JS, Jamil H, Jothl S, Traber MG, Packer L, Gordon DA, Hamilton RL, Farese RV. A poliprotein B-related gene expression and ultrastructural characteristics of lipoprotein secretion in mouse yolk sac during embryonic development. J Lipid Res 1999; 40: 1967-77.

[19] Rantakaki P, Lagerbohm H, Kalmairen M, Suomela JP, Strauss L, Sainio K, Pakarinen., Poutanen M. Hydroxysteroid (17β) dehydrogenase-12 is essential for mouse organogenesis and embryonic survival. Endocrinology 2010; 151: 1893-1901.

[20] Arukwe A, GoksØyr A. Eggshell and egg yolk proteins in fish: hepatic proteins for the next generation: oogenetic, population, and evolutionary implications of endocrine disruption. Comp Hepatol 2003; 2: 4.

[21] Sorrel JM, Caplan AI. Fibroblast-a diverse population at the center of it all. Int Rev Cell Mol Biol 2009; 276: 161-214.

[22] Hinz B. The myofibroblast: Paradigm for a mechanically active cell. J Biomechanics 2010; 43: 146-55.

[23] Pilling D, Fan T, Huang D, Kaul B, Gomer RH. Identification of markers that distinguish monocyte-derived fibrocytes from monocytes, macrophages and fibroblasts. PLoS One 2009; 4: e7475.

[24] Seta N, Kuwana M. Human circulating monocytes as multipotential progenitors. Keio J Med 2007; 56: 41-7.

[25] Eckers B, Nischt R, Krieg T. Cell-matrix interactions in dermal repair and scarring. Fibrogenesis Tissue Repair 2010; 3: 4.

[26] Sen CK. Wound healing essentials: let there be oxygen. Wound Rep Reg 2009; 17: 1-18.

[27] Chung HM, Wan CH, Sung JH. Responses of adipose-derived stem cells during hypoxia: enhanced skin-regenerative potential. Expert Opin Biol Ther 2009;9: 1499-508.

[28] Gurtner GC, Werner S, Barrandon Y, Longaker MT. Wound repair and regeneration. Nature 2008; 453: 314-21.

[29] Kalluri R, Weinberg RA. The basics of epithelial-mesenchymal transition. J Clin Invest 2009; 119: 1420-28.

[30] Selman M, Pardo A, Kaminski N. Idiopathic pulmonary fibrosis: Aberrant recapitulation of development programs? PLoS Med 2008; 5: e62.

[31] Whiteside TL. The tumor microenvironment and its role in promoting tumor growth. Oncogene 2008; 27: 5904-12.

[32] Kluwe J, Mencin A, Schwab RF. Toll-like receptors, wound healing, and carcinogenesis. J Mol Med 2009; 87: 125-38.

[33] Patel SA, Heinrich AC, Reddy BY, Rameshwar P. Inflammatory mediators: Parallels between cancer biology and stem cell therapy. J Inflamm Res 2009; 1: 13-9.

[34] Grivennikov SI, Greten FR, Karin M. Immunity, inflammation and cancer". Cell 2010; 140: 883-99.

[35] Rodriguez-Vita J, Lawrence T. The resolution of inflammation and cancer. Cytokine Growth Factor Rev 2010; 21: 61-5.

[36] Schetter AJ, Heegaard N H-H, Harris CC. Inflammation and cancer: interweaving microRNA, free radical, cytokine and p53 pathways. Carcinogenesis 2010; 31: 37-49.

[37] Allen M, Louise Jones J. Jekyll and Hyde: the role of the microenvironment on the progression of cancer. J Pathol 2011; 223: 162-76.

[38] Costello LC, Franklin RB. Tumor cell metabolism: the marriage of molecular genetics and proteomics with cellular intermediary metabolism; proceed with caution! Mol Cancer 2006; 5: 59.

[39] Dalerba P, Cho RW, Clark MF. Cancer stem cells: Models and concepts. Annu Rev Med 2007; 48: 267-84.

[40] Visvader J.E. Cells of origin in cancer. Nature, 2011; 469: 314-22.

[41] De Berardinis RJ, Lum JJ, Hatzivassiliou G, Thompson C.B. The biology of cancer: Metabolic reprogramming fuels cell growth and proliferation. Cell Metab 2008; 7: 11-20.
[42] Dang CV, Hamaker M, Sun P, Lee A, Gao P. Therapeutic targeting of cancer cell metabolism. J Mol Med 2011; 89: 205-12.
[43] Shanware NP, Mullen PR, De Berardinis RJ, Abraham RT. Glutamine: pleiotropic roles in tumor growth and stress resistance. J Mol Med 2011; 89: 229-36.
[44] Arias JI, Aller MA, Arias J. The use of inflammation by tumor cells. Cancer 2005; 104: 223-28,.
[45] Arias JI, Aller MA, Sanchez-Patan F, Arias J. Inflammation and cancer: Is trophism the link? Surg Oncol 2006; 15: 235-42.
[46] Arias JI, Aller MA, Arias J. Cancer cell: using inflammation to invade the host. Mol Cancer 2007; 6: 29.
[47] Bishop A. Role of oxygen in wound healing. J Wound Care 2008; 17: 399-402.
[48] Schreml S, Szeimies RM, Prantl L, Karrer S, Landthaler M, Babilas P. Oxygen in acute and chronic wound healing. Br J Dermatol 2010; 163: 257-68.
[49] Marcel M, Leroy A. Clinical, cellular, and molecular aspects of cancer invasion. Physiol Rev 2003; 83: 337-76.
[50] Eltzschig HK, Carmeliet P. Hypoxia and inflammation. N Engl J Med 2011; 264: 656-65.
[51] Bamias A, Dimopoulos MA. Angiogenesis in human cancer: implications in cancer therapy. Eur J Intern Med 2003; 14: 459-69.
[52] Denko NC, Fontana LA, Hudson KM, Sutphin PD, Raychaudhuri S, Altman R, Giaccia AJ. Investigating hypoxic tumor physiology through gene expression patterns. Oncogene 2003; 22: 5907-14.
[53] Van der Heiden MG, Cantley LC, Thompson CB. Understanding the Warburg effect: The metabolic requirements of cell proliferation. Science 2009: 324: 1029-33.
[54] Hornebeck W, Emonard H, Monbolsse JC, Bellon G. Matrix-directed regulation of pericellular proteolysis and tumor progression. Semin Cancer Biol 2002; 12: 231-41.
[55] Gialeli C, Theocharis AD, Karamanos NK. Roles of matrix metalloproteinases in cancer progression and their pharmacological targeting. FEBS J 2011; 278: 16-27.
[56] Schmidt-Kittler O, Ragg T, Daskalakis A. From latent disseminated cells to overt metastasis: genetic analysis of systemic breast cancer progression. Proc Natl Acad Sci USA 2003; 100: 7737-42.
[57] Freitas I, Baronzio GF, Bono B, Griffini P, Bertone V, Sonzini N, Magrassi GR, Bonandrini L, Gerzeli G.Tumor interstitial fluid: Misconsidered component of the internal milieu of a solid tumor. Anticancer Res 1997; 17: 165-72.
[58] Eisenhut M, Wallace H. Ion channels in inflammation. Pflugers Arch Eur J Physiol 2011; 461: 401-21.
[59] Wiig H, Tenstad O, Iversen PO, Kalluri R, Bjerkvig R. Interstitial fluid: the overlooked component of the tumor microenvironment? Fibrogenesis andTissue Repair 2010; 3: 12.
[60] Shieh AC, Swartz M.A. Regulation of tumor invasion by interstitial fluid flow. Phys Biol 2011; 8: 1-8.
[61] Teng P-N, Hood BL, Sun M, Dhir R, Conrads TP. Differential proteomic analysis of renal cell carcinoma tissue interstitial fluid. J Proteome Res 2011; 10: 1333-42.
[62] Rønnov-Jessen L, Petersen OW, Bissell M.J. Cellular changes involved in conversion of normal to malignant breast: importance of the stromal reaction. Physiol Rev 1996; 76: 69-125.

[63] Jiang D. Liang J, Noble PW. Hyaluronan in tissue injury and repair. Annu Rev Cell Dev Biol 2007; 23: 435-61.
[64] Aukland K, Reed R.K. Interstitial-lymphatic mechanisms in the control of extracellular fluid volume. Physiol Rev 1993; 73: 1-78.
[65] Chen B, Fu B. A model for charged molecule transport in the interstitial space. Conf Proc IEEE Eng Med Biol Soc 2008; 1: 55-8.
[66] Cueni LN, Detmar M. The lymphatic system in health and disease. Lymphat Res Biol 2008; 6: 109-22.
[67] Rutkowski JM, Swartz MA. A driving force for change: interstitial flow as a morphoregulator. Trends Cell Biol 2006; 17: 44-50.
[68] Nagahashi M, Ramachandran S, Rashid OM, Takabe K. Lymphangio-genesis: A new player in cancer progression. World J Gastroenterol 2010; 16: 4003-12.
[69] Zhang Z, Helman JI, Li L-J. Lymphangiogenesis, lymphatic endothelial cells and lymphatic metastasis in head and neck cancer. A review of mechanisms. Int J Oral Sci 2010; 2: 5-14.
[70] Lund AW, Swartz MA. Role of lymphatic vessels in tumor immunity: Pasive conduits or active participients? J Mammary Gland Biol Neoplasia 2010; 15: 341-352.
[71] Al-Rawi MA, Jiang WG. Lymphangiogenesis and cancer metastasis. Front Biosci 2011; 16.: 723-39.
[72] Halliwell B. Oxidative stress and cancer: have we moved forward?, Biochem J 2007; 401: 1-11.
[73] He G, Karin M. NF-κB and STAT3-key players in liver inflammation and cancer. Cell Research 2011; 21: 159-68.
[74] Hanada T, Yoshimura A. Regulation of cytokine signaling and inflammation. Cytokine Growth Factor Rev 2002; 13: 413-21.
[75] Patel SA, Heinrich AC, Reddy BY, Rameshwar P. Inflammatory mediators: Parallels between cancer biology and stem cell therapy. J Inflamm Res 2009; 2: 13-19.
[76] Rakoff-Nahoum S, Medzhitov R. Toll-like receptors and cancer. Nat Rev Cancer 2009; 9: 57-63.
[77] Wang D, Dubois RN. Eicosanoids and cancer. Nature Rev Cancer 2010; 10: 181-92.
[78] Huang P, Han J, Hui L. MAPK signaling in inflammation-associated cancer development. Protein Cell 2010; 1: 218-28.
[79] Peyrou M, Bourgoin L, Foti M. PTEN in liver diseases and cancer. World J Gastroenterol 2010; 16: 4627-32.
[80] Philip M, Rowley DA, Schreiber H. Inflammation as a tumor promoter in cancer induction. Semin Cancer Biol 2004; 14: 433-9.
[81] Ben-Baruch A. Inflammation-associated immunesuppression in cancer: the roles played by cytokines, chemokines and additional mediators. Semin Cancer Biol 2006; 16: 38-52.
[82] Nickoloff BJ, Ben-Neriah Y, Pikarsky E. Inflammation and cancer: is the link as simple as we think?, J Invest Dermatol 2005; 124: 10-14.
[83] Palucka K, Ueno H, Fay J, Banchereau J. Dendritic cells and immunity against cancer. J Intern Med 2011; 269: 64-73.
[84] Mantovani A, Sica A. Macrophages innate immunity and cancer: balance, tolerance and diversity. Curr Opin Immunol 2010; 22: 231-37.
[85] Balkwill F, Mantovani A. Cancer and inflammation: implications for pharmacology and therapeutics. Clin Pharmacol Therap 2010; 87: 401-.

[86] Mishra P, Banerjee D, Ben-Baruch A. Chemokines at the crossroads of tumor-fibroblast interactions that promote malignancy. J Leukoc Biol 2011; 89: 31-9.
[87] Sica A. Role of tumour-associated macrophages in cancerrelated inflammation. Exp Oncol 2010; 32: 153-8.
[88] Hornebeck W, Emonard H, Monboisse JC, Bellon G. Matrix-directed regulation of pericellular proteolysis and tumor progression. Semin Cancer Biol 2002; 12: 231-41.
[89] Engbring JA, Kleinman H.K. The basement membrane matrix in malignancy. J Pathol 2003; 200: 465-70.
[90] Muller A, Homey B, Soto H, Ge N, Catron D, Buchanan MT. Involvement of chemokine receptors in breast cancer metastasis. Nature 2001; 410: 50-6.
[91] Al-Rawi MAA, Mansel RE, Jiang W.G. Lymphangiogenesis and its role in cancer. Histol Histopathol 2005; 20: 283-98.
[92] Pavelic SK, Sedic M, Bosnojak H, Spaventi S, Pavelic K. Metastasis: new perspectives on an old problem. Mol Cancer 2011; 10: 22.
[93] Sitkovsky MV, Lukashev D, Apasov S, Kojima H, Koshiba M, Caldwell C, Ohta A, Thiel M. Physiological control of immune response and inflammatory tissue damage by hypoxia-inducible factors and adenosine A2A receptors. Annu Rev Immunol 2004; 22: 657-82.
[94] Levine AJ, Puzio-Kuter A.M. The control of the metabolic switch in cancers by oncogenes and tumor suppressor genes. Science 2010; 330: 1340-44.
[95] Mentis A-FA, Kararizou E. Metabolism and cancer: An up-to-date review of a mutual connection. Asian Pac J Cancer Prev 2010; 11: 1437-44.
[96] Naresh KN, Nerurkar AY, Borges AM. Angiogenesis is a redundant for tumor growth in lymph node metastases. Histopathology 2001; 38: 466-70.
[97] Sleeman JP, Nazarenko I, Thiele W. Do all roads lead to Rome? Routes to metastasis development. Int J Cancer 2011; 128: 2511-26.
[98] Chouaib S, Kieda C, Benlalam H, Noman MZ, Mami-Chouaib F, Rüegg C. Endotelial cells as key keterminants of the tumor microenvironment: Interaction with tumor cells, extracellular matrix and immune killer cells. Critical Rev Immunol 2010; 30: 529-45.
[99] Cueni LN, Detmar M.The lymphatic system in health and disease. Lymphat Res Biol 2008; 6: 109-22.
[100] Ji RC. Lymph node lymphangiogenesis: a new concept for modulating tumor metastasis and inflammatory process. Histol Histopathol 2009; 24: 377-84.
[101] Pantel K, Woelfle U. "Detection and molecular characterisation of disseminated tumor cells: Implications for anticancer therapy", Biochim Biophys Acta 2005; 1756: 53-64.
[102] Braun S, Kentenich C, Janni W, Hepp F, De Waal J, Willgeroth F, Sommer H, Pantel K. Lack of effect of adjuvant chemotherapy on the elimination of single dormant tumor cells in bone marrow of high-risk breast cancer patients. J Clin Oncol 2000; 18: 80-86.
[103] Tammela T, Saaristo A, Holopainen T, Ylä-herttuala S, Anderson LC, Virolainen S, Immonen I, Alitalo K. Photodynamic ablation of lymphatic vessels and intralymphatic cancer cells prevents metastasis. Sci Transl Med 2011; 3: 69ra11.
[104] Deans C, Wigmore SJ. Systemic inflammation, cachexia and prognosis in patients with cancer. Curr Opin Clin Nutr Metab Care 2005; 8: 265-269.
[105] Delano MJ, Moldawer LL.The origin of cachexia in acute and chronic inflammatory diseases. Nutr Clin Pract 2006; 21: 68-81.
[106] Fearon K, Strasser F, Anker SD, Bosaeus I, Bruera E, Fainsinger RL, Jaoi A, Loprinzi C, MacDonald N, Mantovani G, Davis M, Muscaritoli M, Ottery F, Radbruch L, Ravaso P,

Walsh D, Wilcock A, Kaasa S, Baracos VE. Definition and classification of cancer cachexia: an international consensus. Lancet Oncol 2011; 12: 489-95.
[107] Clement CC, Rotzsche O, Santambrogio L.The lymph as a pool of self-antigens. Trends Immunol 2011; 32: 6-11.
[108] Bruyere F, Noël A. Lymphangiogenesis: *in vitro* and *in vivo* models. FASEB J 2010; 24: 8-21.
[109] Thaunat O, Kerjaschki D, Nicoletti A. Is defective lymphatic drainage a trigger for lymphoid neogenesis? Trends Immunol 2006; 27: 441-5.
[110] Condamine T, Gabrilovich DI. Molecular mechanisms regulating myeloid-derived suppressor cell differentiation and function. Trends Immunol 2010; 32: 19-25.
[111] Mahdavian Delavary B, Van der Veer WM, Van Egmond M, Niessen FB, Beelen RHJ. Macrophages in skin injury and repair. Immunobiology 2011; 216: 753-62.
[112] Goldberg SR, Diegelmann R.F. Wound healing primer. Surg Clin N Am 2010; 90: 1133-46.
[113] Shih B, Garside E, McGrouther DA, Bayat A. Molecular dissection of abnormal wound healing processes resulting in keloid disease. Wound Repair Regeneration 2009; 18: 139-53.
[114] Wu Y, Zhao RCH, Terdget EE. Concise Review: Bone marrow-derived stem/progenitor cells in cutaneous repair and regeneration. Stem Cells 2010; 28: 905-15.
[115] Acloque H, Adams MS, Fishwick K, Bronner-Fraser M, Nieto A. Epithelial-mesenchymal transitions: the importace of changing cell state in development and disease. J Clin Invest 2009; 119: 1438-49.
[116] Sioud M. New insights into mesenchymal stromal cell-mediated T-cell suppression through galectins. Scand J Immunol 2011; 73: 79-84.
[117] Norrby K. *In vivo* models of angiogenesis. J Cell Mol Med 2006; 10: 588-612.
[118] Fukumura D, Duda DG, Munn LL, Jain RK. Tumor microvasculature and microenvironment: novel insights through intravital imaging in pre-clinical models. Microcirculation 2010; 17: 206-25.
[119] Van Horssen R, Ten Hagen TLM, Eggermont AMM. TNF-α in cancer treatment: Molecular insights, antitumor effects, and clinical utility. Oncologist 2006; 11: 397-408.
[120] Byrne AM, Boucher-Hayes DJ, Harmey JH. Angiogenic and cell survival functions of vascular endothelial growth factor (VEGF). J Cell Mol Med 2005; 9: 777-94.
[121] Kalluri R, Zeisberg M. Fibroblasts in cancer. Nat Rev Cancer 2006; 6: 392-401.
[122] Grigorova IL, Panteleev M, Cyster JG. Lymph node cortical sinus organization and relationship to lymphocytes egress dynamics and antigen exposure. PNAS 2010; 107: 20447-52.
[123] Hayasaka H, Taniguchi K, Fukai S, Miyasaka M. Neogenesis and development of the high endotelial venules that mediate lymphocyte trafficking. Cancer Sci 2010; 101: 2302-8.
[124] Bad X, Moseman EA, Saito H, Petryanik B, Thiriot A, Hatakeyama S, Ito Y, Kawashima H, Yamaguchi Y, Lowe JB, Von Andrian UH, Fukuda M. Endothelial heparan sulfate controls chemokine presentation in recruitment of lymphocytes and dendritic cells to lymph nodes. Immunity 2010; 33: 817-29.
[125] Favaro E, Amadori A, Indraccolo S. Cellular interactions in the vascular niche: implications in the regulation of tumor dormancy. APMIS 2008; 116: 648-59.
[126] Pinto M, Soares P, Ribatti D. Thyroid hormone as a regulator of tumor induced angiogenesis. Cancer Lett 2011; 301: 119-26.

[127] Hanahan D, Weinberg RA. Hallmarks of cancer: the next generation. Cell 2011; 144: 646-74.
[128] Cairns RA, Harris IS, Mak TW. Regulation of cancer cell metabolism. Nat Rev Cancer 2011; 11: 85-95.
[129] Adinolfi A, Adinolfi M, Lessof MH. Alpha-feto-protein during development and in disease. J Med Genet 1975; 12: 138-51.
[130] Sell S, Pierce GB. Maturation arrest of stem cell differentiation is a common pathway for the cellular origin of teratocarcinomas and epithelial cancers. Lab Invest 1994; 70: 6-22.
[131] Brewer BG, Mitchell RA, Harandi A, Eaton JW. Embryonic vaccines against cancer: An early history. Exp Mol Pathol 2009; 86: 192-7.
[132] Thiery JP, Acloque H, Huang RYJ, Nieto A. Epithelial-mesenchymal transitions in development and disease. Cell 2009; 139: 871-86.
[133] Singh A, Settleman J. EMT, cancer stem cells and drug resistance: an emerging axis of evil in the war on cancer. Oncogene 2010; 29: 4741-51.
[134] Wang Y, Steinbeisser H. Molecular basis of morphogenesis during vertebrates gastrulation. Cell Mol Life 2009; 66: 2263-73.
[135] Chang YJ, Hwang SM, Tseng CP, Cheng FC, Huang SH, Hsu LW, Tsai MS. Isolation of mesenchymal stem cells with neurogenic potentials from the mesoderm of the amniotic membrane. Cell Tissues Organs 2010; 192: 93-105.
[136] Pfeiffer S, McLaughlin D. *In vitro* differentiation of human amniotic fluid derived cells: augmentation towards a neuronal, dopaminergic phenotype. Cell Biol Int 2010; 34: 959-67.
[137] Niknejad H, Peirov H, Jorjani M, Ahmadiani A, Ghanavi J, Seifalina M. Properties of the amniotic membrane for potential use in tissue engineering. Eur Cell Mater 2008; 15: 88-99.
[138] Yu SJ, Soncini M, Kaneko Y, Hess DC, Parolini O, Borlongan CV. Amnion: A potent graft for cell therapy in stroke. Cell Transplant 2009; 18: 111-8.
[139] Uberti MG, Pierpont YN, Ko F, Wright TE, Smith CA, Cruse CW, Robson M, Pay WG. Amnion-derived cellular cytokine solution (ACCS) promotes migration of keratinocytes and fibroblasts. Ann Plast Surg 2010; 64: 632-5.
[140] Koike S, Keino-Masu K, Ohto T, Suglyama E, Takahashi S, Masu M. Autotaxin/lysophospholipase D-mediated lysophosphatidic acid signaling is required to form distinctive large lysosomes in the visceral endoderm cells of the mouse yolk sac. J Biol Chem 2009; 284: 33561-70.
[141] Fraser ST, Baron MH. Embryonic fates for extraembryonic lineages: new perspectives. J Cell Biochem 2009; 107: 586-91.
[142] Yoshid S, Wada Y. Transfer of maternal cholesterol to embryo and fetus in pregnant mice. J Lipid Res 2005; 46: 2168-74.
[143] Rantakari P, Lagerbohm H, Kalmairen M, Soumela JP, Strauss L, Sainio K, Pakarinen P, Poutanen M. Hydroxysteroid (17β) dehydrogenase 12 is essential for mouse organogenesis and embryonic survival. Endocrinology 2010; 151: 1884-92.
[144] Sheng G. Primitive and definitive erythropoiesis in the yolk sac: a bird's eye view. Int J Dev Biol 2010; 54: 1033-43.
[145] Wang D, Dubois R.N. Eicosanoids and cancer. Nature Rev 2010; 10: 181-92.
[146] Lander ES. Initial impact of the sequencing of the human genome. Nature 2011; 470: 187-97.
[147] Perez-Losada J, Castellanos-Martin A, Mao J-H. Cancer evolution and individual susceptibility. Integr Biol (Camb) 2011; 3: 316-28.
[148] Stratton MR, Campbell PJ, Futreal PA. The cancer genome. Nature 2009; 458: 719-24.

Send Orders for Reprints to reprints@benthamscience.net

Surgical Inflammation, 2013, 250-276

CHAPTER 9

Mesenchymal Stem Cells: Advances and Surgical Applications

Maria-Angeles Aller[1], Maria-Paz de Miguel[2], Carlos Jiménez[3], Sherezade Fuentes-Julián[2], Alejandro Manrique[3], Alejandro Blázquez-Martínez[2], Jorge Calvo[3], Cristina Pascual[4], Francisco Arnalich-Montiel[5] and Jaime Arias[1,*]

[1]Surgery Department, School of Medicine, Complutense University of Madrid, Madrid Spain; [2]Cell Engineering Laboratory, IdiPaz, La Paz Hospital Research Institute, Madrid, Spain; [3]Abdominal Organ Transplantation and General and Digestive Surgery Department, 12 de Octubre University Hospital, Madrid, Spain; [4]Allergology Department, Infanta Sofia Hospital, Madrid, Spain and [5]Ophthalmology Department, Ramon y Cajal Hospital, Madrid, Spain

Abstract: Mesenchymal stem cells (MSCs) are used in regenerative medicine mainly based on their capacity to differentiate into specific cell types and also as bioreactors of soluble factors that will promote tissue regeneration from the damaged tissue cellular progenitors. Moreover, MSCs can stop a variety of immune cell functions: cytokine secretion and cytotoxicity of T and NK cells; B cell maturation and antibody secretion; DC maturation and activation; as well as antigen presentation. In this scenario, an inflammatory environment seems to be necessary to promote their effect. Preclinical studies have been conducted in rodents, rabbits and baboon monkeys among others for bone marrow, skin, heart, and corneal transplantation, graft-*vs.*-host disease, hepatic and renal failure, lung injury, multiple sclerosis, rheumatoid arthritis, and diabetes and lupus diseases. Preliminary results from some of these studies have led to human clinical trials; prevention of allograft rejection and enhancement of the survival of bone marrow and kidney grafts.

Keywords: Mesenchymal stem cells, regenerative medicine, immunosuppression, anti-inflammation, autoimmune diseases, inflammatory diseases, organ transplant-tation, graft *vs.* host disease, liver fibrosis, experimental microsurgical cholestasis.

MESENCHYMAL STEM CELLS: MECHANISM OF ACTION

Mesenchymal stem cells (MSCs) are considered some of the most promising cell

***Address correspondence to Jaime Arias:** Cátedra de Cirugía, Facultad de Medicina, Universidad Complutense, Pza. de Ramón y Cajal s.n., 28040 MADRID, Spain; Tel: +34 91 394 1389; Fax: +34 91 3947115; E-mail: jariasp@med.ucm.es

Jaime Arias, Maria-Angeles Aller and Jose-Ignacio Arias (Eds)

types for therapeutic applications. MSCs were first successfully isolated from the bone marrow over 20 years ago [1], and have subsequently been isolated from a variety of tissues, such as spleen and heart [2], skeletal muscle [3], synovium [4], amniotic fluid [5], dental pulp [6], bone [7], umbilical cord [8], adipose tissue [9] and from virtually all postnatal connective organs. They have also become a powerful tool in regenerative medicine for two reasons. Firstly, they can be expanded in culture while maintaining their multipontency [10] and secondly, they are capable of differentiating (or trans-differentiating) into different cell types, such as osteoblasts, chondrocytes, adipocytes, myocytes, cardiomyocytes, hepatocytes, epithelial cells, endothelial cells and neurons. However, a specific MSC-defining antibody is not available. Of note here is that MSCs are not considered a homogeneous group of cells and their heterogeneity makes them difficult to characterize [11]. Investigators use different methods of isolation and expansion, as well as varying differentiation protocols, making it difficult to compare and contrast study outcomes. The International Society for Cellular Therapy (ISCT) sets the minimal criteria for defining MSCs [12]. Firstly, MSCs must be plastic-adherent in standard culture conditions. Secondly, they must express CD105, CD73 and CD90, and lack expression of CD45, CD34, CD14 or CD11b, CD79α and CDA19 and the Major Histocompatibility Complex (MHC) class II cell surface receptor HLA-DR. And finally, they must be able to differentiate into osteoblasts, adipocytes and chondroblasts *in vitro*.

In addition to their capacity to serve as structural cells, when differentiating into the appropriate cell type of the damaged tissue, MSCs have been shown to modulate endogenous tissue by secreting a large spectrum of bioactive molecules (reviewed by [13]) that will promote progenitors. The expression of these factors by MSCs induces multiple responses: the survival and proliferation of endogenous cells [14]; induced angiogenesis [15]; inhibited inflammatory and immune responses; reduced apoptosis [16]; and even the transfer of mitochondria [17]. It is also known that MSCs are immune privileged due to their low expression of class II major histocompatibility complex (MHC-II) and co-stimulatory molecules in their cell surface, making them invisible to the immune system. Additionally, MSCs have an immunoregulatory capacity and elicit immunosuppressive effects in various settings. Such immense plasticity coupled with their ability to modulate the activity of immune cells makes them extremely valuable for stem cell-based therapy in the treatment of a wide array of illnesses.

IMMUNOSUPPRESSIVE PROPERTIES OF MSCs: *IN VITRO* ADVANCES

There is evidence to suggest that MSCs have immunosuppressive properties. In the year 2000, two groups proved that intraperitoneally injected human bone marrow-derived mesenchymal stem cells (hBM-MSCs) were able to survive for more than a year without being rejected in fetal sheep after the development of immunological competence [18, 19]. Even more outstanding were the unexpected *in vitro* and *in vivo* immunosuppressive effects that these MSCs showed in the mouse, baboon and human, even in an MHC-independent manner, regardless of differences in species [20-23]. Furthermore, after systemic infusion, MSCs distribute to almost every organ [24], but preferentially to injured places, sites of inflammation, and lymphoid organs [25-27]. All these properties led to the consideration of MSC therapy for immunomodulatory purposes.

Since then, a lot of information has been obtained about the different means in which MSCs exert their immunosuppressive properties. They can be classified by the different types of immune response, and the variety of immune cells and molecules implicated [28].

MSCs AND TUMOR DEVELOPMENT PROMOTION

Tumor induction is of major interest in MSC therapy research. There is great controversy over this issue, ranging from authors that completely rule out the possibility of malignant transformation of human MSCs *in vitro* [29] to those that report spontaneous transformation of these cells [30]. This transformation is attributed to chromosome instability, loss of contact inhibition and aberrant expression of *c-myc*. Moreover, some authors reported that when MSCs from a high passage are injected subcutaneously or intravenously intro immune-compromised mice, fibrosarcomas arise at different locations [30].

Apart from direct generation, MSCs can promote the development of non-MSC-derived tumors since they have immunosuppressive properties. MSCs have been demonstrated to selectively migrate and engraft in tumor sites when systemically infused [31-33]. B16 myeloma cells remain unrejected and induce tumor formation in mice only when MSCs are co-injected [23]. Similarly, adipose tissue-derived MSCs (AT-MSCs) co-injected with melanoma cells support the engraftment and tumor growth even when systemic delivery of MSCs is performed after melanoma injection [34]. Last but not least, Indoleamine,2, 3-dioxigenase (IDO) has been found to be over-expressed both in tumor-draining lymph nodes and in the tumor microenvironment itself, which helps suppression of the first immune response. Likewise, tumor cells transfected with IDO become resistant to rejection [35]. Human AT-MSCs isolated from breast adipose tissue from breast cancer patients have been demonstrated to express high levels of anti-inflammatory cytokines such as IL-10 and TGF-β [36]. In light of these findings, it is reasonable to suppose that MSCs physiologically favor tumor growth and that this property has to be taken into account when MSC therapy is performed [37].

IN VIVO ADVANCES: PRECLINICAL STUDIES

In vivo studies have shown many discrepancies regarding the immunomodulatory properties of MSCs. Mainstream analysis of the benefits of transplanting MSCs has been focused along two different lines: the suppression of the immune response in autoimmune and inflammatory diseases, and their capacity to prevent or treat allograft rejection [38, 39].

Cell and Solid Organ Transplants

Skin Grafts

The *in vivo* administration of donor MSC to MHC-mismatched recipient with transplanted allogenic skin grafts in baboons showed prolonged survival of donor and third-party skin grafts [20]. In contrast, some reports showed that MSC administration resulted in the acceleration of graft rejection in skin transplantation in rat and mouse models [39, 40], while the use of MSC and Cyclosporine A (CsA) as an adjunct immunosuppressor agent resulted in longer survival of the skin transplant in the same rat model [39].

Pancreatic Islets Transplant

Allogenic pancreatic islets transplanted beneath the kidney capsule in an immune-compromised experimental diabetic mouse were not rejected when introduced in concomitance with syngenic MSCs, as demonstrated by long-term normoglycemia [41]. In addition, on a diabetic rat model of allogenic islet transplantation, a sub-therapeutic dose of CsA in combination with autologous MSCs was successfully used [42].

Heart Transplant

Infusion of donor MSCs delayed graft rejection in a mice immunocompetent semiallogenic heart transplantation model [43]. However, in a mouse allogenic heart transplantation model, MSC infusion led to rejection, but when combined with rapamycin [26] or mycophenolate mofetil [44], it yielded a synergic effect and induced tolerance for up to 100 days post-transplantation [26].

Kidney Transplant

Donor MSCs greatly increased the survival of life-supporting allogenic kidney transplantation in mice [45]. Of note, both heart and kidney transplants required MSCs to be injected several days before organ transplant, suggesting that an induction of tolerance prior to engraftment is necessary.

Graft *vs.* Host Disease (GvHD)

GvHD is produced experimentally by injection of donor HSCs together with donor splenocytes into previously irradiated mice. BM-MSCs [46-49] and AT-MSCs [50] have been found to prevent or ameliorate experimental GvHD. Some authors did not corroborate this beneficial effect of MSCs [51, 52]; however the same MSCs, transduced to overexpress IL-10, ameliorated GvHD [51].

In all these autoimmune, inflammatory and transplantation studies, MSCs did not differentiate into cells of the injured tissue [53, 54] but were able to induce T-cell anergy and tolerance [25, 53, 54, 56], showing an impairment of Th1 response [26, 42, 43, 45]. MSCs were frequently found to engraft in the damaged tissue as well as in secondary lymphoid organs, confirming the early interaction between T cells and MSCs that leads to a tolerogenic effect [25, 26, 38, 42, 53, 57]. Furthermore, most transplantation models showed specific tolerance, as they were not able to support a secondary third-day skin graft. Human MSC therapy in rodent disease models has also been reported to bypass species differences even in immunocompetent models [38, 44, 57-59]

All these data support the usefulness of MSC therapy alone or in combination with sub-therapeutic doses of immunosuppressive drugs in the treatment of autoimmune and inflammatory diseases, as well as transplant rejection.

CURRENT AND FUTURE CLINICAL APPLICATIONS

A number of clinical studies have tested MSC therapy and autoimmune disorders, graft enhancement and rejection and graft-*vs.*-host diseases.

Prevention of Graft Rejection and Graft Enhancement

MSCs may delay graft rejection through multiple immunomodulatory mechanisms, including the generation of regulatory mediators, such as Regulatory T cells (Tregs) and tolerogenic Dendritic cells (DCs), in addition to the prevention of T-cell activation (in response to alloantigen presentation) [60].

Preclinical data suggests that combined therapy with immunosuppressive drugs and MSCs would probably improve graft survival and long-term function more than either therapy alone. Immunosuppressive drugs given after transplantation would allow MSC survival and would create an environment suitable for MSC activation. Conversely, MSCs could reduce the required dose of immunosuppressive drug therapy, thereby reducing the potential side effects of said drugs.

In humans, clinical trials using MSCs to prevent graft rejection for solid organ transplantation are at early stages with no results yet published, and mainly focus on kidney transplantation. Similarly, MSC therapy is also being tested in hematological malignancies following bone marrow allotransplantation to promote engraftment and prevent graft rejection (see www.clinicaltrials.gov/keywords: mesenchymal stem cells and grafts).

Graft *vs.* Host Disease

The most commonly explored therapeutic application for MSC is GvHD, a severe condition that develops after allogenic hematopoietic stem cell transplantation. After transplantation, donor T cells present in the graft mount an immune response to the antigenically foreign tissues of the recipient – mainly the liver, skin, mucosa and gastrointestinal tract. This reaction can be acute and potentially lethal or chronic.

Based on the fact that MSCs suppress inflammation by inhibiting T-cell proliferation, Le Blanc *et al.* first described this novel treatment in a 9-year-old boy with severe refractory stage IV GvHD of the gut and liver who was infused with MSCs in 2004 [61]. The boy's disease improved dramatically rapidly following 2 infusions and no significant side effects were noticed.

Since then, several small sample case-reports have been published, reporting successful outcomes in the treatment of steroid resistant acute GvHD (aGvHD) using MSCs [62, 63], such as MSCs derived from adipose tissue [64]. A multicenter phase II study by the European Group for Blood and Marrow Transplantation found that 70% of the GvHD patients treated with MSCs achieved complete resolution of the disease [65]. In this study, efficiency of the MSC treatment was independent from whether or not there was human leukocyte antigen (HLA)-match between donor and host. The results were even better in pediatric patients. Osiris Pharmaceutics Inc. conducted a phase III double blind, placebo-controlled study for the treatment of aGvHD that recruited 260 patients. MSCs were administered twice a week for 4 weeks at 2 $\times 10^6$ cells/kg per infusion. The primary endpoint for the trial was durable complete response, defined as complete resolution of GvHD for a period of at least 28 days. Preliminary results found no significant difference between placebo and MSC treatment regarding primary endpoint, but MSC therapy achieved a greater rate of complete remission than the control group (40% *vs.* 28% respectively). Treatment significantly improved response rates to liver and gut GvHD (29% and 88% respectively).

Mesenchymal Stem Cells Treatment in Experimental Extrahepatic Cholestasis

The bile duct-ligated rat is an experimental model used to study both portal hypertension and extrahepatic cholestasis [66, 67]. Regarding its use for studying extrahepatic cholestasis, an array of alterations in this experimental model can be studied that can be classified in hepatic and extra-hepatic alterations. The hepatic alterations due to microsurgical extrahepatic cholestasis in the rat are multiple, a slight portal inflammation associated to severe fibrosis and intense biliary duct proliferation stand out when long-term studies (6 to 9 weeks) are performed [68].

The hepatic fibrosis post-bile duct ligation or extra-hepatic bile route resection in rodents is the consequence of an inflammatory process of biliary origin [69, 70]. It therefore induces inflammatory changes, like oxidative and nitrosative stress [71, 72] and impaired defense against oxidant injury [73], portal tract edema [74] and recruitment of inflammatory cells, particularly neutrophilic infiltration of the liver periductular regions [75]. Hence liver fibrosis is like a wound healing process characterized by the accumulation of extracellular matrix proteins, especially collagen [67, 68, 69, 76]. Although all the hepatic cells may have fibrogenic potential [77, 78], hepatic stellate cells are the main collagen-producing cells in the liver [79, 80]. The profibrogenic liver evolution in long-term (6-9 weeks) extrahepatic cholestasis in rodents makes this experimental model very useful for studying the reversibility of liver fibrosis [81].

In addition, the liver of rats with microsurgical extrahepatic cholestasis shows a significantly higher infiltration by mast cells. In particular, in the liver of these rats, there was an accumulation of mast cells in portal spaces and in the fibrous septa, close to both, fibrosis and bile proliferation [82]. Fibrosis progression is strictly related to the underlying cause of chronic liver disease and four distinct patterns of fibrosis progression have been identified that are related to the "topographic site" of tissue injury, the involvement of different populations of hepatic myofibroblast-like cells and the predominant profibrogenic mechanisms [83-85].These four types of liver fibrosis have been termed: bridging fibrosis, typically found in chronic viral hepatitis; perisinusoidal/pericellular fibrosis, typically found in non-alcoholic steatohepatitis (NASH); centrilobular fibrosis, secondary to venous outflow, as in chronic liver failure; and biliary fibrosis [86].

Biliary fibrosis is a pattern sustained by concomitant proliferation of reactive bile ductules and periductular hepatic myofibroblast-like cells at the interface between portal areas and parenchyma, leading to the characteristic development of portal-portal fibrotic septa [86]. Cholangiopathies in adult and pediatric patients are characterized by cholestasis, necrotic or apoptotic loss of cholangiocytes, cholangiocyte proliferation, that is, ductular reaction, as well as portal/periportal inflammation and fibrosis [87]. In particular, liver fibrosis and cirrhosis are histological characteristics in patients with advanced stage primary biliary cirrhosis, but are rarely reported in murine primary biliary cirrhosis models. Recently published results in human primary biliary cirrhosis showed that Th1 profile is predominant in the liver and NKT and TLR3 (toll like receptor) activation contributes to the liver fibrosis in murine models of primary biliary cirrhosis [88]. On the other hand, Th17 elevation, Treg disminution and NK cell elevation are characteristics essential for pathogenesis in primary biliary cirrhosis, but their significance in liver fibrosis is still unclear [89, 90].

The complexity in the natural history and etiology of liver fibrosis has made it difficult to suggest any standard treatment modalities. To date many anti-fibrotic therapeutic targets have been proposed for, or used in, clinical trials [91], but their effect is limited to control the pathological development and has thus far fallen short of a cure [90].

The current knowledge on the potential efficacy of antifibrotic agents is currently limited to animal models of liver fibrosis, including extrahepatic cholestasis. In the human clinical area it could be detrimental to treat patients with antifibrotic agents without treating the primary cause of damage [92]. Thus in bile duct-ligated rats the reconstruction of bile flow leads to an orchestrated fibrinolytic program that results in near complete reversal of advanced fibrosis. Because of the peak of connective tissue remodeling and the fibrolytic activity associated with massive apoptosis of cholangiocytes and their phagocytic clearance by macrophages, it has been considered that macrophages could upregulate metalloproteinases and become fibrolytic effector cells in experimental biliary fibrosis [93]. Due to the different phenotypes that macrophages can adopt, however, hepatic macrophage migration, mediated by the chemokine receptor CCR8, promotes hepatic inflammation and fibrosis in bile duct- ligated rats [94]. Macrophages and the factors they express, with their potential to act in both a pro- and antifibrotic capacity as well as their ability to regulate the activation of resident and recruited myofibroblasts, is therefore integrated in all stages of the fibrotic process [95].

The Th2 cytokines, IL-4 and IL-13 like TGF-β1, directly stimulate collagen synthesis in mouse and human fibroblasts. Like fibroblast and myofibroblasts, macrophages respond to Th2 cytokines and numerous studies have implicated IL-4/IL-13-stimulated macrophages in the pathogenesis of fibrosis [95-97].Therefore, the partial reversibility of the liver fibrosis in rats with microsurgical extra-hepatic cholestasis after stem mesenchymal cell administration could be attributed to their anti-inflammatory ability [98]. There is increasing evidence that stem cells themselves, specifically mesenchymal stem cells, secrete a variety of pro-inflammatory and anti-inflammatory cytokines and that these cytokines may directly act to limit deleterious, sustained endogenous inflammation [99]. Clearly mesenchymal stem cells seem to possess anti-inflammatory properties, specifically through cytokine expression and infiltration of inflammatory cells, but these effects may not influence all aspects of innate immunity. Specifically, mesenchymal stem cells suppressed T lymphocyte proliferation, altered cytokine secretion and induced a more anti-inflammatory phenotype [100]. Mesenchymal stem cell-mediated immunosuppression is not exclusively the result of a direct inhibitory effect but involves the recruitment of other regulatory networks. Mesenchymal stem cells act in concert with monocytes. By a crosstalk between mesenchymal stem cells and the environment, inflammatory monocytes "license" mesenchymal stem cells to acquire their immunosuppressive properties. Furthermore, mesenchymal stem cells can also activate and expand regulatory T cells (Tregs) [101]. In this way, mesenchymal stem cells could act in the hepatic wound repair secondary to extrahepatic cholestasis in a similar way as in cutaneous wound healing. One should then consider that mesenchymal stem cells can interact with inflammatory cells, including T cells and natural killer cells to promote a more anti-inflammatory and tolerant phenotype [100, 102, 103].

The induction of a tolerogenic microenvironment by mesenchymal stem cells could consequently favor tissue regeneration and, therefore, would reduce fibrosis. In particular, mesenchymal-to-epithelial transition (MET) is a phenomenon by which a cell changes from a mesenchymal phenotype to an epithelial phenotype, an important process during embryonic development, wound healing and tissue regeneration [104]. It has also been suggested that hepatocytes may undergo epithelial-to-mesenchymal transition (EMT) after injury by cholestasis and that the resolution to fibrosis or a healthy outcome depends on the reverse process (MET) [105].

Besides their use to modulate immune responses [106] mesenchymal stem cells have been employed to promote tissue repair [101, 107, 108]. Mesenchymal stem cells may influence positively the recovery from injury *via* paracrine factors that promote tissue repair [109]. Stem cells transplanted into injured tissue express paracrine signaling factors. These include cytokines, chemokines and growth factors that favor angiogenesis, decrease inflammation and activate antiapoptosis signaling systems. These stem cells could differentiate into target areas of injury, alter the extracellular matrix resulting in more favorable tissue remodeling and finally, may activate neighboring resident tissue stem cells [109-112]. Adult stem cell therapy has already been used to treat liver disease [113]. Mesenchymal stem cells have recently been shown to promote liver repair in cases of liver damage. Transplantation of mesenchymal stem cells isolated from human umbilical cords, adipose tissue, bone marrow or rat bone marrow improved the liver function of rodents undergoing acute liver damage by carbon tetrachloride treatment [108]. Infusion of hepatocyte-like cells, which were differentiated *in vitro* from mesenchymal stem cells, also improved liver function following acute injury [114, 115]. Since acute liver failure models were studied, a reduction of serum liver enzymes was shown. On the contrary, in rats with microsurgical extrahepatic cholestasis, improved liver function was shown by monitoring the level of albumin in the serum. This result was quite important for the research on pro-liver effects of mesenchymal stem cell therapy during chronic liver damage, since to date, all other results have been quite discouraging. Furthermore, increasing evidence suggests that mesenchymal stem cells may promote liver fibrosis and cirrhosis. For example, in mouse models of liver cirrhosis, exogenous mouse and human mesenchymal stem cell populations promoted the emergence of myofibroblasts, which are involved in the fibrotic response [116, 117]. Two primary mechanisms have been proposed to explain the therapeutic effects of mesenchymal stem cells or mesenchymal stem cell-derived hepatocytes in liver injury. First, mesenchymal stem cells could generate cells that function as normal hepatocytes. Following engraftment in the liver, transplanted cells express markers of donor hepatocytes. Differentiation towards the hepatocytic lineage, therefore, must occur in the parenchymal microenvironment for mesenchymal stem cell-derived hepatocyte-like cells or mesenchymal stem cells [114, 115, 118].

The second mechanism by which mesenchymal stem cells could promote liver repair is indirect. Soluble factors secreted by mesenchymal stem cells facilitate liver recovery in response to acute damage. Transplantation studies support the cell autonomous role of mesenchymal stem cells in liver repair. Mesenchymal stem cells secrete numerous proteins, but it is unclear which factors facilitate liver recovery [108, 119]. Thus mesenchymal stem cell-mediated liver therapy is a highly promising field with many unanswered questions, for example, which populations are most therapeutic, *i.e.* mesenchymal stem cells, mesenchymal-stem cell-derived hepatocytes, or mesenchymal stem cell-secreted factors, and what types of liver injury are amenable to the above-mentioned therapies [108].

Mesenchymal stem cells represent an alternate cell source to substitute primary hepatocytes in hepatocyte transplantation because of their multiple differentiation potential and nearly unlimited availability. Depending on the underlying liver disease their mode of action is either to replace the diseased liver tissue or to support liver regeneration through their anti-inflammatory, anti-apoptotic and their proliferative action [120]. Cells, isolated either from peritoneal or subcutaneous adipose tissue, expressed mesenchymal stem cell surface markers and featured multiple lineage differentiation. Under conditions favoring hepatocyte differentiation mesenchymal stem cells from human adipose tissue, gained hepatocytic function *in vitro* including urea formation, glycogen synthesis, cytochrome P450 enzyme activity, and expression of hepatocyte-specific transcripts of carbamoyl phosphate synthetase, albumin and cytochrome P450 type 3A4 [121]. Adipose derived mesenchymal stem cells, carrying the similar characteristics to bone marrow mesenchymal stem cells, only much more abundant and easier to obtain, may be a promising treatment for liver fibrosis [122, 123].

Adipose derived mesenchymal stem cells have a therapeutic effect against CCl4-mediated (carbon tetrachloride) liver fibrosis, after intraportal transplantation that could be a better pathway than tail vein transplantation [122].

Adipose-derived stem/stromal cells (ASCs) or adipose mesenchymal stem cells, describe the multipotent, plastic adherent, cell type isolated from adipose tissue [124]. ASCs have a high potential for banking as an alternative or complement to cord blood banking for several of the potential therapeutic applications in which mesenchymal stem cells could be used [125, 126]. Most research and academic work is focused on tissue remodeling and differentiation of ASCs into specialized somatic cell types to replace damaged organs and tissues including the liver [127, 128]. ASCs can be easily isolated from routine liposuction (lipoaspirate) and reconstructive surgery (lipectomy) waste materials [129]. Seo *et al.* demonstrated for the first time that ASCs can differentiate into hepatocyte-like cells by a one-step protocol using hepatocyte growth factor (HGF), oncostatin(OSM) and dimethy sulfoxide (DMSO) [130].

At present, the molecular mechanisms underlying the plasticity of ASCs towards a hepatocyte-like phenotype remain poorly understood. To date, studies on animal models have reported the beneficial effects of ASCs in promoting liver regeneration. In this sense, transplantation of ASCs into extrahepatic cholestatic rats with chronic liver failure revealed that predifferentiated ASCs were able to engraft into the liver and improve its function. ASC transplant in cholestatic rats may allow to recover many biological functions exerted by hepatocytes, including protein metabolism, innate immune response regulation and biodegradation of toxic compounds [131].

Hepatocytes are polarized cells and through the apical surface, secrete bile and detoxification products into bile canaliculi. Moreover, their unique structure, along with the various enzymes expressed, is involved in protein synthesis, transformation of carbohydrates, synthesis of cholesterol, bile salts and phospholipids and detoxification and activation of exogenous substances [124]. Therefore, in the microsurgical extrahepatic cholestatic rats, ASCs reduce the pro-inflammatory response and consequently fibrosis, favor the growth of the hepatocytic population and would promote the function characteristics of this specialized type of epithelial cell *i.e.* the hepatocytes. In summary, the experimental transplant of ASCs in extrahepatic cholestasis would allow the partial recovery of the hepatocytic functions, increasing the animal survival and to achieve extra time to opt for other more aggressive treatments for chronic cholestatic liver disease. Thus ASC transplant may be tried in patients with severe liver insufficiency where surgery is not possible. This therapeutic ability of the mesenchymal stem cells has also been proposed in patients with acute and chronic graft-*vs.*-host disease and other autoimmune disorders, where surgery is also not indicated [132].

Chronic liver disease is a systemic disorder in which multi-organs, such as the kidney and brain, could be involved as a result of the extensive inflammatory response [76]. Additionally, alterations of hematopoietic cells could also be detected. In the later stage of experimental cirrhosis (12 weeks of CCl_4 treatment) a decrease of bone marrow sinusoid and a considerable amount of scattered necrotic cells and apoptosis has been demonstrated. These changes showed that the sinusoidal endothelium lesions of bone marrow and the accompanied changes in hematopoietic cells are intensified with the persistence of liver fibrosis/cirrhosis [133]. Bone marrow-derived cells are known to play important roles in parenchymal regeneration and liver fibrosis. Carbon tetrachloride (or thioacetamide) is reported to stimulate the direct differentiation of bone marrow derived cells to hepatic stellate cells and myofibroblasts and induce liver fibrosis. In bile duct ligation induced liver fibrosis models, collagen-producing fibrocytes were also recruited from the bone marrow. In addition, excess alcohol consumption stimulates both the homing of hepatic stellate cells from the bone marrow and their profibrogenic cytokine production in a mouse model of alcohol-induced fatty liver disease [134].

In order to initiate a bone marrow response, the injured liver must signal to the responding cell types. Stromal-derived factor 1 (SDF-1 or CXC4) has been one of the better characterized stem cell chemoattractants. In the liver, SDF-1 is upregulated in the bile ducts in the liver with injury and plays a role in recruiting extrahepatic stem and progenitors cells to the site of the injury. Furthermore, the receptor to SDF-1, CXCR4, is expressed by a number of different stem cell populations within the bone marrow, including mesenchymal stem cells. The injured liver has also been shown to secrete hepatocyte growth factor (HGF) in order to recruit bone marrow cells. This resulted in an augmented rate of engraftment, potentially caused by an observed increase in SDF-1 expression by biliary epithelial cells which could also be involved in the increased liver density of mast cells found after extrahepatic microsurgical cholestasis [82, 135]. Many of the genes upregulated with injury in the liver after bile duct ligation included cytokines, chemokines and growth factors, including SDF-1 and HGF. Therefore, factors secreted by the cholestatic liver led to the recruitment of bone marrow stem cells [135, 136].

This liver-bone marrow axis that contributes to liver development, liver homeostasis and liver pathology could be based on the liver hematopoietic function from the third week of gestation until shortly after birth [137]. Recapitulation of some of these hematopoietic signals during liver diseases could explain why bone marrow is called upon as a further response to severe liver injury [135, 138].

Several groups have used autologous bone marrow cells as a treatment for cirrhosis. A variety of infusion routes have been used, with some using direct portal vein or hepatic artery infusion and others using peripheral stem cell infusion. However, animal studies have suggested that the route may not be important [138, 139]. Hepatocytes derived from bone marrow cells could be formed by three primary mechanisms. First, bone marrow could theoretically harbor specialized endodermal stem cells that are capable of producing hepatocytes and other epithelial cells. These cells would be analogous to the mesenchymal stem cells. Secondly, a single stem cell population could give rise to the blood and hepatocyte lineages. And thirdly, in contrast with differentiation, bone marrow-derived hepatocytes could be derived by cell fusion [108]. Therefore, in the cases of severe liver insufficiency, the impairment that the bone marrow suffers would prevent its key function of replacing the diseased hepatocyte population [133]. However, mesenchymal stem cell therapy could use the mediators (SDF-1, HGF and others) released by the diseased liver into the peripheral blood and in the Disse space, thus favoring the homing of the grafted cells to the liver [138].

Mesenchymal stem cell transplantation in cholestatic rats not only induces the expansion of the liver hepatocytic subpopulation, but also reduces fibrosis and bile ductular proliferation. This therapeutic effect of the mesenchymal stem cells can be attributed to their ability to decrease the hepatic inflammatory response related to extrahepatic cholestasis, which could involve injured tissue dedifferentiation [140].

The ductular reaction in extrahepatic cholestasis was proposed to correspond to the end stages of cholangiocytic metaplasia or dedifferentiation [141] of hepatocytes, resulting in the activation of existing liver progenitor cells or in *de novo* generation of liver progenitor cells or both [142]. In essence, hepatic ductular reactions occur in "ductal plate" configurations. Ductal plates are primitive forms of intrahepatic bile ducts during embryologic development of the liver corresponding to a double perforated slit-like lumen [141, 143]. Most ductular reactions occur in the form of small or mini-ductal plates, composed of a small central blood vessel, surrounded by a small amount of mesenchyma derived from the original Disse space, and a double layer of biliary type epithelial cells lining a circular, nearly virtual luminal cleft between both layers. Often a tubular dilatation is seen at one or more sites along the luminal perimeter. This configuration corresponds to the double-layered embryonic ductal plates in an early remodeling stage [141]. Indeed, a so-called cholangiocytic metaplasia of hepatocytes could represent a dedifferentiation towards a more primitive cell type [144]. The dedifferentiation concept is supported by several observations in literature. Hepatocyte dedifferentiation is a reversible consequence of a specific signaling network triggered by the extracellular matrix [145].

Ductular reaction type I is predominant in acute complete bile duct obstruction that occurs in microsurgical extrahepatic cholestasis. It results from proliferation of pre-existing cholangiocytes, resulting in elongation, branching and luminal widening of biliary tubes [141]. Elongation, dilation and branching of ducts in bile duct obstruction and inflammation adapt the three-dimensional structure of the tubes to the expansion of the portal mesenchymal caused by edema and inflammation [141]. Ductular reaction 2A has been interpreted as "ductular metaplasia of hepatocytes" and involves a change in secretory polarity. It is typically observed in periportal areas, most characteristically, in chronic cholestatic conditions. The cholestatic hepatocytes activate hepatic stellate cells into a myofibroblastic phenotype responsible for an increased production of the connective tissue matrix. These ductular reaction types 1 and 2A are reversible when the causative trigger is eliminated, excess tubular structures disappear by apoptosis, and the associated fibrosis regresses to considerable extent. Such reversibility illustrates the plasticity of tissues and cells [141]. Ductular reaction type 2A develops in long-term microsurgical extrahepatic cholestatic rats, creating an additional canalicular outlet and a larger cholangiocytic resorbing surface favoring chole-hepatic cycling in chronic cholestasis [82, 141].

The ductular reaction type 2A, as occurs in extrahepatic cholestatic rats, has ductal plate configuration and this structure could be similar to those in the embryonic liver, although in this case it could correspond to the end stages of cholangiocytic dedifferentiation [142]. If so, we can propose treating cholestatic rats with mesenchymal stem cells, since they reduce the ductular reaction, have a pro-differentiation liver effect and therefore favor hepatocytic specialization.

The microsurgical model of extrahepatic cholestasis used in this experimental study could be of interest for studying the pathophysiological mechanisms involved in ductal plate malformations in adults, in particular, congenital hepatic fibrosis [146].

Congenital hepatic fibrosis is a form of ductal plate malformation with characteristic histologic features of aberrant interlobular bile duct proliferation and periductal fibrosis [147]. Portal hypertension is usually the presenting feature of congenital hepatic fibrosis, with varices. Although in most patients the disorder is diagnosed during adolescence or early adulthood, it can also manifest in early childhood or in fifth to sixth decade of life [146, 147].

However, the hypothesized ability of the mesenchymal stem cells for reverting the biliary impairments related to experimental extrahepatic cholestasis and, consequently the associated pathology to ductal plate malformations, allows to consider their transplant as an efficient therapeutical measure for this frequent disease [148, 149].

The mechanisms that can be involved in the dedifferentiation process induced in the cholestatic liver of the rat by the mesenchymal stem cells could also be similar to those described during the early phases of the embryonic development. Hepatocytes and cholangiocytes are derived from common embryonic liver precursor cells, which are referred to as hepatoblast. The liver develops as a tissue bud derived from a diverticulum of the ventral foregut endoderm, which extends into the septum transversum, a structure located between the pericardial and peritoneal cavities [150]. The ventral foregut endoderm develops two protrusions - the cranial part leads to the formation of the intrahepatic bile ducts, while the caudal part generates the extrahepatic biliary tree [151, 152].

During embryonic development, a subset of hepatoblasts aligns itself adjacent to the portal mesenchyma and begins to express several markers of the biliary lineage including SOX9, osteopotin and CK19 [153]. This sheet of cells, known as the "ductal plate" forms primitive ductal structures. This proceeds *via* an intermediate stage in which ductal plate cells adopt a symmetric gene expression pattern. Those adjacent to the portal vein express biliary markers including SOX9, whereas cells adjacent to the parenchyma express the hepatoblast marker HNF4α. Hepatoblasts adjacent to the parenchyma differentiate into the biliary lineage and become histologically indistinguishable from the periportal precursor cells in the nascent ductular structures [154]. Ductal plate cells give rise to periportal hepatocytes and to cholangiocytes lining the interlobular bile ducts, the intralobular ductules and the canals of Hering, but not pericentral hepatocytes [155]. These results provide compelling evidence that both the biliary cells in the canal of Hering and oval cells are derived from the ductal plate [154, 155]. The ductal plate in embryonic liver therefore gives rise to cholangiocytes lining all segments of the intrahepatic bile ducts, as well as to periportal hepatocytes and hepatic progenitor cells [155].

In summary, the results of the current research study allow to suggest that the adipose-derived mesenchymal stem cell transplant in the cholestatic liver of rats could induce a differentiation process similar to that of embryonic development. If so, periportal hepatocytes could be developed at the expense of a ductal plate malformation, *i.e.* ductular reaction post-cholestasis obstruction. Then the function of these new hepatocytes could reduce the impairments related to the cholestatic liver failure. In addition, this mechanism of hepatic regeneration could reduce the intensity of the systemic and splanchnic inflammatory response, which would also reduce the portal hypertension and portosystemic collateral circulation development.

ACKNOWLEDGEMENTS

We would like to thank Maria Elena Vicente for preparing the manuscript, Elizabeth Mascola for translating it into English and librarians of Complutense University Medical School, particularly the Director, Francisco Javier Jorge García-Reyes, and Manuela Crego and María José Valdemoro and B. Braun Surgical S.A. for their technical assistance.

This study was carried out in part with grants from Mutua Madrileña Research Foundation (Ref. nº PA 3077/2008 and AP5966/2009), MICINN PSI2010-19348 and with the special collaboration of the INEUROPA (Instituto de Neurociencias del Principado de Asturias).

CONFLICT OF INTEREST

The author(s) confirm that this chapter content has no conflict of interest.

REFERENCES

[1] Friedenstein AJ, Gorskaja JF, Kulagina NN. Fibroblast precursors in normal and irradiated mouse hematopoietic organs. Exp Hematol 1976; 4: 267-274.

[2] Hoogduljn MJ, Crop MJ, Peeters AM, *et al.* Human heart, spleen and peripheral fat-derived mesenchymal stem cells have immunomodulatory capacities. Stem Cells Dev 2007; 16: 597-604.

[3] Williams JT, Southerland SS, Souza J, Calcutt AF, Cartledge RG. Cells isolated from adult human skeletal muscle capable of differentiating into multiple mesodermal phenotypes. Am Surg 1999; 65: 22-26.

[4] De Bari C, Dell'Accio F, Tylzanowski P, Luyten FP. Multipotent mesenchymal stem cells from adult human synovial membrane. Arthritis Rheum 2001; 44: 1928-1942.

[5] In't Anker PS, Scherjon SA, Kleijburg-van der Keur C, *et al.* Amniotic fluid as a novel source of mesenchymal stem cells for therapeutic transplantation. Blood 2003; 102: 1548-1549.

[6] Gronthos S, Mankani M, Brahim J, Robey PG, Shi S. Postnatal human dental pulp stem cells (DPSCs) *in vitro* and *in vivo*. Proc Natl Acad Sci USA 2000; 97: 13625-12630.

[7] Kadiyala S, Young RG, Thiede MA, Bruder SP. Culture expanded canine mesenchymal stem cells possess osteochondrogenic potential *in vivo* and *in vitro*. Cell Transplant 1997; 6: 125-134.

[8] Erices A, Conget P, Minguell JJ. Mesenchymal progenitor cells in human umbilical cord blood. Br J Haematol 2000; 109: 235-242.

[9] Zuk PA, Zhu M, Ashjian P, *et al.* Human adipose tissue is a source of multipotent stem cells. Mol Biol Cell 2002; 13: 4279-4295.

[10] Pittenger MF, MacKay AM, Beck SC, *et al.* Multilineage potential adult human mesenchymal stem cells. Science 1999; 284: 143-147.

[11] Dominici M, Paolucci P, Conte P, Horwitz EM. Heterogeneity of multipotent mesenchymal stromal cells: from stromal cells to stem cells and viceversa. Transplantation 2009; 87: S36-S42.

[12] Dominici M, Le Blanc K, Mueller I, *et al.* Minimal criteria for defining multipotent mesenchymal stromal cells. The International Society for Cellular Therapy position statement. Cytotherapy 2008; 8: 15-17.

[13] Phinney DG, Prockop DJ. Concise review: mesenchymal stem/multipotent stromal cells: the state of transdifferentiation and modes of tissue repair-current views. Stem Cells 2007; 25: 2896-2902.

[14] Prockop DJ. "Stemness" does not explain the repair of many tissues by mesenchymal stem/multipotent stromal cells (MSCs). Clin Pharmacol Ther 2007; 82: 241-243.

[15] Shyu KG, Wang BW, Hung HF, Chang CC, Shih DT. Mesenchymal stem cells are superior to angiogenic growth factor genes for improving myocardial performance in the mouse model of acute myocardial infarction. J Biomed Sci 2006; 13: 47-58.

[16] Hung SC, Pochampally RR, Chen SC, Hsu SC, Prockop DJ. Angiogenic effects of human multipotent stromal cell conditioned medium activate the PI3K-Akt pathway in hypoxic endothelial cells to inhibit apoptosis, increase survival, and stimulate angiogenesis. Stem Cells 2007; 25: 2363-2370.

[17] Spees JL, Olson SD, Whitney MJ, Prockop DJ. Mitochondrial transfer between cells can rescue aerobic respiration. Proc Natl Acad Sci USA 2006; 103: 1283-1288.

[18] Lyechty KW, Mackenzie TC, Shaaban AF, *et al.* Human mesenchymal stem cells engraft and demonstrate site-specific differentiation after in utero transplantation in sheep. Nat Med 2000; 6: 1282-1286.

[19] Almeida-Porada G, Porada CD, Tran N, Zanjani ED. Cotransplantation of human stromal cell progenitors into preimmune fetal sheep results in early appearance of human donor cells in circulation and boosts cell levels in bone marrow at later time points after transplantation. Blood 2000; 95: 3620-3627.

[20] Bartholomew A, Sturgeon C, Siatskas M, *et al.* Mesenchymal stem cells suppress lymphocyte proliferation *in vitro* and prolong skin graft survival *in vivo*. Exp Haematol 2002; 30: 42-48.

[21] Di Nicola M, Carlo-Stella C, Magni M, *et al.* Human bone marrow stromal cells suppress T-lymphocyte proliferation induced by cellular or non specific mitogenic stimuli. Blood 2002; 99: 3838-3843.

[22] Lee ST, Jang JH, Cheong JW, *et al.* Treatment of high-risk acute myelogenous leukemia by myeloablative chemoradiotherapy followed by co-infusion of T cell-depleted haematopoietic stem cells and culture expanded marrow mesenchymal stem cells from a related donor with one fully mismatched human leukocyte antigen haplotype. Br J Haematol 2002; 118: 1128-1131.

[23] Djouad F, Plence P, Bony C, *et al.* Immunosuppressive effect of mesenchymal stem cells favors tumor growth in allogeneic animals. Blood 2003; 102: 3837-3844.

[24] Devine SM, Cobbs C, Jennings M, Bartholomew A, Hoffman R. Mesenchymal stem cells distribute to a wide range of tissues following systemic infusion into nonhuman primates. Blood 2003; 101: 2999-3001.

[25] Zappia E, Casazza S, Pedemonte E, *et al.* Mesenchymal stem cells ameliorate experimental autoinmune encephalomyelitis inducing T-cell anergy. Blood 2005; 106: 1755-1761.

[26] Ge W, Jiang J, Baroja ML, *et al.* Infusion of mesenchymal stem cells and rapamycin synergize to attenuate alloimmune responses and promote cardiac allograft tolerance. Am J Transplant 2009; 9: 1760-1772.

[27] Yagi H, Soto-Gutierrez A, Parekkadan B, *et al.* Mesenchymal stem cells: Mechanisms of immunomodulation and homing. Cell Transplant 2010; 19: 667-679.

[28] De Miguel MP, Fuentes-Julian S, Blazquez-Martinez A, *et al.* Immunosuppressive properties of mesenchymal stem cells: advances and applications. Curr Mol Med 2012; 12: 574-581.

[29] Bernardo ME, Zaffaroni N, Novara M, *et al.* Human bone marrow-derived mesenchymal stem cells do not undergo transformation after long-term *in vitro* culture and do not exhibit telomere maintenance mechanisms. Cancer Res 2007; 67: 9142-9149.

[30] Miura M, Miura Y, Hesed M, *et al.* Accumulated chromosomal instability in murine bone marrow mesenchymal stem cells leads to malignant transformation. Stem Cells 2006; 24: 1095-1103.

[31] Dwyer RM, Potter-Beirne SM, Harrington KA, *et al.* Monocyte chemotactic protein-1 secreted by primary breast tumors stimulates migration of mesenchymal stem cells. Clin Cancer Res 2007; 13: 5020-5027.

[32] Wang H, Cao F, De A, *et al.* Trafficking mesenchymal stem cell engraftment and differentiation in tumor-bearing mice by bioluminescence imaging. Stem Cells 2009; 27: 1548-1558.

[33] Kid S, Spaeth E, Dembinski JL, *et al.* Direct evidence of mesenchymal stem cell tropism for tumor and wounding microenvironments using *in vivo* bioluminescent imaging. Stem Cells 2009; 27: 2614-2623.

[34] Kucerova L, Matuskova M, Hiubinova K, Altanerova V, Altaner C. Tumor cell behavior modulation by mesenchymal stem cells. Mol Cancer 2010; 9: 129.

[35] Munn HD, Mellor AL. Indoleamine 2, 3-dioxygenase and tumor-induced tolerante. J Clin Invest 2007; 117: 1147-1154.

[36] Razmakhah M, Javeripour M, Erfani N, Habilagahi M, Talei AR, Ghaderi A. Adipose derived stem cells (ASCs) isolated from breast cáncer tissue express IL-4, IL-10 and TGF-β1 and upregulate expression of regulatory molecules on T cells; do they protect breast cancer cells from the immune response? Cell Immunol 2011; 266: 116-122.

[37] Lopez-Iglesias P, Blazquez-Martinez A, Fernández-Delgado J, Regadera J, Nistal M, De Miguel MP. Human adipose-derived stem cells fate after short and long term subcutaneous injection in immunodeficient mice. WJSC 2011; 6: 53-62.

[38] Jung KH, Song SU, Yi T, *et al.* Human bone marrow-derived clonal mesenchymal stem cell inhibit inflammation and reduce acute pancreatitis in rats. Gastroenterology 2011; 140: 998-1008.

[39] Sbano P, Cuccia A, Mazzanti B, *et al.* Use of donor bone marrow mesenchymal stem cells for treatment of skin allograft rejection in a preclinical rat model. Arch Dermatol Res 2008; 300: 115-124.

[40] Han KH, Kang HG, Gil HJ, Lee EM, Ahn C, Yang J. The immunosuppressive effect of embryonic stem cells and mesenchymal stem cells on both primary and secondary alloimmune responses. Transpl Immunol 2010; 23: 141-146.

[41] Ding Y, Xu D, Feng G, Bushell A, Muschel RJ, Wood KJ. Mesenchymal stem cells prevent the rejection of fully allogenic islet grafts by the immunosuppressive activity of matrix metalloproteinase-2 and -9. Diabetes 2009; 58: 1797-1806.

[42] Kim YH, Wee YM, Choi MY, Lim DG, Kim SC, Han DJ. IL-10 induced by CD11b+cells and IL-10 activated regulatory T cells play a role in immune modulation of mesenchymal stem cells in rat islet allograft. Mol Med 2011; 17: 697-708.

[43] Casiraghi F, Azzollini N, Cassis P, *et al.* Pretransplant infusion of mesenchymal stem cells prolongs the survival of a semiallogenic heart transplant through the generation of regulatory T cells. J Immunol 2008; 181: 3933-3946.

[44] Eggenhofer G, Steinmann JF, Renner P, *et al.* Mesenchymal stem cells together with mycophenolate mofetil inhibit antigen presenting cell and T cell infiltration into allogeneic heart grafts. Transpl Immunol 2011; 24: 157-163.

[45] Ge W, Jiang J, Arp J, Liu W, Garcia B, Wang H. Regulatory T-cell generation and kidney allograft tolerante induced by mesenchymal stem cells associated with indoleamine 2, 3-dioxygenase expression. Transplantation 2010; 90: 1312-1320.

[46] Li H, Guo Z, Jiang X, Zhu H, Li X, Mao N. Mesenchymal stem cells alter migratory property of T and dendritic cells to delay the development of murine letal acute graft-*vs.*-host disease. Stem Cells 2008; 26: 2531-2541.

[47] Polchert D, Sobinsky J, Douglas GW, *et al.* IFN-γ activation of mesenchymal stem cells for treatment and prevention of graft *vs.* host disease. Eur J Immunol 2008; 38: 1745-1755.

[48] Ren G, Zhang L, Zhao X, *et al.* Mesenchymal stem cell-mediated immunosuppression occurs *via* concerted action of chemokines and nitric oxide. Cell Stem Cell 2008; 2: 141-150.

[49] Yañez R, Lamana ML, García-Castro J, Colmenero I, Ramírez M, Bueren JA. Adipose tissue-derived mesenchymal stem cells have *in vivo* immunosuppressive properties applicable for the control of the graft-*vs.*-host disease. Stem Cells 2006; 24: 2582-2591.

[50] Yañez R, Oviedo A, Aldea M, Bueren JA, Lamana ML. Prostaglandin E2 plays a key role in the immunosuppressive properties of adipose and bone marrow tissue-derived mesencymal stromal cells. Exp Cell Res 2010; 316: 3109-3123.

[51] Min CK, Kim BG, Park G, Cho B, Oh IH. IL-10-transduced bone marrow mesenchymal stem cells can attenuate the severity of acute graft-*vs.*-host disease after experimental allogeneic stem cell transplantation. Bone Marrow Transplant 2007; 39: 637-645.

[52] Prigozhina TB, Khitrin S, Elkin G, Eizik O, Morecki S, Slavin S. Mesenchymal stromal cells lose their immunosuppressive potential after allotransplantation. Exp Hematol 2008; 36: 1370-1376.

[53] Gerdoni E, Gallo B, Casazza S, *et al.* Mesenchymal stem cells effectively modulate pathogenic immune response in experimental autoimmune encephalomyelitis. Ann Neurol 2007; 61: 219-227.

[54] Urbán VS, Kiss J, Kovács J, *et al.* Mesenchymal stem cells cooperate with bone marrow cells in therapy of diabetes. Stem Cells 2008; 26: 244-253.

[55] Tögel F, Hu Z, Weiss K, Isaac J, Lange C, Westenfelder C. Administered mesenchymal stem cells protect against ischemic acute renal failure through differentiation-independent mechanisms. Am J Physiol Renal Physiol 2005; 269: F31-F42.

[56] González MA, Gonzalez-Rey E, Rico L, Büscher D, Delgado M. Treatment of experimental arthritis by inducing immune tolerance with human adipose-derived mesenchymal stem cells. Arthritis Rheum. 2009; 60: 1006-1019.

[57] Lee RH, Seo MJ, Reger RL, *et al.* Multipotent stromal cells from human marrow home to and promote repair of pancreatic islets and renal glomeruli in diabetic NOD/scid mice. Proc Natl Acad Sci USA 2006;103:17438-17443.

[58] Liu Y, Mu R, Wang S, *et al.* Therapeutic potential of human umbilical cord mesenchymal stem cells in the treatment of rheumatoid arthritis. Arthritis Res Ther 2010;12:R210.

[59] Arnalich-Montiel F, Pastor F, Blázquez-Martínez A, *et al.* Adipose-derived stem cells are a source for cell therapy of the corneal stroma. Stem Cells 2008; 26: 570-579.

[60] English K, French A, Wood KJ. Mesenchymal stromal cells: facilitators of successful transplantation? Cell Stem Cell 2010; 7: 431-442.

[61] Le Blanc K, Rasmusson I, Sundberg B, *et al.* Treatment of severe acute graft-*vs.*-host disease with third party haploidentical mesenchymal stem cells. Lancet 2004; 363: 1439-1441.

[62] Prasad VK, Lucas KG, Kleiner GI, *et al.* Efficacy and safety of *ex vivo* cultured adult human mesenchymal stem cells (prochymal) in pediatric patients with severe refractory

acute graft-*vs.*-host disease in a compassionate use study. Biol Blood Marrow Transplant 2011; 17: 534-541.

[63] Ringden O, Uzunel M, Rasmusson I, *et al.* Mesenchymal stem cells for treatment of therapy-resistant graft-*vs.*-host disease. Transplantation 2006; 81: 1390-1397.

[64] Fang B, Song Y, Liao L, Zhang Y, Zhao RC. Favorable response to human adipose tissue-derived mesenchymal stem cells in steroid-refractory acute graft-*vs.*-host disease. Transplant Proc 2007;39:3358-3362.

[65] Le Blanc K, Frassoni F, Ball L, *et al.* Mesenchymal stem cells for treatment of steroid-resistant, severe, acute graft-*vs.*-host disease: a phase II study. Lancet 2008; 371: 1579-1586.

[66] Lee, S.S, Girod, C, Braillon A, Hadengue A, Lebrec D. Hemodynamic characterization of chronic bile duct-ligated rats: effect of pentobarbital sodium. Am J Physiol 1986; 251: G176-G180.

[67] Sanchez-Patan F, Anchuelo R, Corcuera MT, *et al.* Biliary fibrosis in microsurgical extrahepatic cholestasis in the rat. Microsurgery 2008; 28: 361-366.

[68] Aller MA, Arias JL, García-Domínguez J, Arias JI, Durán M, Arias J. Experimental obstructive cholestasis: the wound-like inflammatory liver response. Fibrogenesis Tissue Repair 2008; 1: 6.

[69] Kershenobich Stalnikowitz D, Weissbrod AB. Liver fibrosis and inflammation. A review. Ann Hepatol. 2003;2:159-163.

[70] Li MK, Crawford JM. The pathology of cholestasis. Semin Liver Dis 2004; 24: 21-41

[71] Britton RS, Bacon BR. Role of free radicals in liver diseases and hepatic fibrosis. Hepato-gastroenterology 1994; 41: 343-348.

[72] Huang YT, Hsu YC, Chen CJ, Liu CT, Wei YH. Oxidative-stress-related changes in the livers of bile-duct-ligated rats. J Biomed Sci 2003; 10: 170-178.

[73] Singh S, Shackleton G, Ah-Sing E, Chakraborty J, Bailey ME. Antioxidant defenses in the bile duct-ligated rat. Gastroenterology 1992;103:1625-1629.

[74] Isayama F, Hines IN, Kremer M, *et al.* LPS signaling enhances hepatic fibrogenesis caused by experimental cholestasis in mice. Am J Physiol Gastrointest Liver Physiol. 2006;290:G1318-328.

[75] Saito JM, Maher JJ. Bile duct ligation in rats induces biliary expression of cytokine-induced neutrophil chemoattractant. Gastroenterology 2000; 118: 1157-1168.

[76] Bataller R, Brenner DA. Liver fibrosis. J Clin Invest 2005; 115: 209-218;

[77] Sedlaczek N, Jia JD, Bauer M, *et al.* Proliferating bile duct epithelial cells are a major source of connective tissue growth factor in rat biliary fibrosis. Am J Pathol 2001; 158: 1239-1244.

[78] Friedman SL, Roll FJ, Boyles J, Bissell DM. Hepatic lipocytes: the principal collagen-producing cells of normal rat liver. Proc Natl Acad Sci USA 1985; 82: 8681-8685.

[79] Canbay A, Higuchi H, Bronk SF, Taniai M, Sebo TJ, Gores GJ. Fas enhances fibrogenesis in the bile duct ligated mouse: a link between apoptosis and fibrosis.Gastroenterology 2002; 123: 1323-1330.

[80] Siller-López F, Sandoval A, Salgado S, *et al.* Treatment with human metalloproteinase-8 gene delivery ameliorates experimental rat liver cirrhosis. Gastroenterology 2004; 126: 1122-1133.

[81] Xia JL, Dai C, Michalopoulos GK, Liu Y. Hepatocyte growth factor attenuates liver fibrosis induced by bile duct ligation. Am J Pathol 2006; 168: 1500-1512.

[82] Aller MA, Ortega L, Sanchez-Patan F, *et al.* Microsurgical extrahepatic cholestasis in the rat: A histopathological liver study. Open Pathology Journal 2008; 2: 71-77.

[83] Pinzani M, Rombouts K. Liver fibrosis: from the bench to clinical targets. Dig Liver Dis 2004; 36: 231-242.

[84] Parola M, Marra F, Pinzani M. Myofibroblast - like cells and liver fibrogenesis: Emerging concepts in a rapidly moving scenario. Mol Aspects Med 2008; 29: 58-66.

[85] Cassiman D, Libbrecht L, Desmet V, Denef C, Roskams T. Hepatic stellate cell/myofibroblast subpopulations in fibrotic human and rat livers. J Hepatol 2002; 36: 200-209.

[86] Parola M, Pinzani M. Hepatic wound repair. Fibrogenesis Tissue Repair 2009; 2: 4.

[87] Friedman SL. Mechanisms of hepatic fibrogenesis. Gastroenterology 2008; 134: 1655-1669.

[88] Wu SJ, Yang YH, Tsuneyama K, *et al.* Innate immunity and primary biliary cirrhosis: activated invariant natural killer T cells exacerbate murine autoimmune cholangitis and fibrosis. Hepatology 2011; 53: 915-925.

[89] Chuang YH, Lian ZX, Tsuneyama K. Increased killing activity and decreased cytokine production in NK cells in patients with primary biliary cirrhosis. J Autoimmun 2006; 26: 232-240.

[90] Ahmad A, Ahmad R Understanding the mechanism of hepatic fibrosis and potential therapeutic approaches.Saudi J Gastroenterol. 2012;18:155-167.

[91] Friedman SL, Rockey DC, Bissell DM. Hepatic fibrosis 2006: report of the Third AASLD Single Topic Conference. Hepatology 2007; 45: 242-249.

[92] Pinzani M, Rosselli M, Zuckerman M. Liver cirrhosis. Best Pract Res Clin Gastroenterol 2011; 25: 281-290.

[93] Popov Y, Sverdlov DY, Bhaskar KR, *et al.* Macrophage-mediated phagocytosis of apoptotic cholangiocytes contributes to reversal of experimental biliary fibrosis. Am J Physiol Gastrointest Liver Physiol 2010; 298: G323-G334.

[94] Heymann F, Hammerich L, Storch D. Hepatic macrophage migration and and differentiation critical for liver fibrosis is mediated by the chemokine receptor C-C motif chemokine receptor 8 in mice. Hepatology 2012; 55: 898-909.

[95] Wynn TA, Barron L. Macrophages: Master regulators of inflammation and fibrosis. Semin Liver Dis 2010; 20: 245-257.

[96] Duffield JS, Forbes SJ, Constandinou CM, *et al.* Selective-depletion of macrophages reveals distinct, opposing roles during liver injury and repair. J Clin Invest 2005; 115: 56-65.

[97] Edwards JP, Zhang X, Frauwirth KA, Mosser DM. Biochemical and functional characterization of three activated macrophage populations. J Leukoc Biol 2006; 80: 1298-1307.

[98] Guo J, Lin GS, Bao CY, Hu ZM, Hu MY. Anti-inflammation role for mesenchymal stem cells transplantation in myocardial infarction. Inflammation 2007; 30: 97-104.

[99] Burchfield JS, Dimmeler S. Role of paracrine factors in stemand progenitor cell mediated cardiac repair and tissue fibrosis. Fibrogenesis Tissue Repair 2008; 1: 4.

[100] Aggarwal S, Pittenger MF. Human mesenchymal stem cells modulate allogenic immune cell responses. Blood 2005; 105: 1815-1822.

[101] Trento C, Dazzi F. Mesenchymal stem cells and innate tolerance: Biology and clinical applications. Swiss Med Wkly 2010; 140: w13121.

[102] Branski LK, Gauglitz GG, Herndon DN, Jeschke MG. A review of gene and stem cell therapy in cutaneous wound healing. Burns 2009; 35: 171-180.

[103] Lau K, Paus R, Tiede S, Day P, Bayat A. Exploring the role of stem cells in cutaneous wound healing. Exp Dermatol 2009; 18: 921-933

[104] Otto WR, Wright NA. Mesenchymal stem cells: from experiment to clinic. Fibrogenesis Tissue Repair 2011; 4: 20.

[105] Bridle KR, Popa C, Morgan M, *et al.* Rapamycin inhibits hepatic fibrosis in rats by attenuating multiple profibrogenic pathways. Liver Transpl 2009; 15: 1315-1324.

[106] Shi Y, Su J, Roberts AI, Shou P, Rabson AB, Ren G. How mesenchymal stem cells interact with tissue immune responses. Trends Immunol 2012; 33:136-143.

[107] Adams B, Xiao QX, Xu Q. Stem cell therapy for vascular diseases. Trends Cardiovasc Med 2007; 17: 246-251.

[108] Duncan AW, Dorrell C, Grompe M. Stem cells and liver regeneration. Gastroenterology 2009; 137: 466-481.

[109] Crisostomo PR, Markel TA, Wang Y, Heldrum DR. Surgically relevant aspects of stem cell paracrine effects. Surgery 2008; 143: 577-581.

[110] Oertel M, Shafritz DA. Stem cell, cell transplantation and liver repopulation. Biochim Biophys Acta 2008; 1782: 61-74.

[111] Kuroda Y, Kitada M, Wakao S, *et al.* Unique multipotent cells in adult human mesenchymal cell populations. Proc Natl Acad Sci U S A 2010; 107:8639-8643.

[112] De Miguel MP, Fuentes-Julian S, Alcaina Y. Pluripotent stem cells: origin, maintenance and induction. Stem Cell Rev 2010; 6: 633-649.

[113] Burra P, Tomat S, Villa E, *et al.* Experimental hepatology applied to stem cells. Dig Liver Dis 2008; 40: 54-61.

[114] Kuo TK, Hung SP, Chuang CH, *et al.* Stem cell therapy for liver disease: parameters governing the success of using bone marrow mesenchymal stem cells. Gastroenterology 2008; 134: 2111-2121.

[115] Banas A, Teratani T, Yamamoto Y, *et al.* Rapid hepatic fate specification of adipose-derived stem cells and their therapeutic potential for liver failure. J Gastroenterol Hepatol 2009; 24: 70-77.

[116] Russo FF, Alison MR, Bigger BW, *et al.* The bone marrow functionally contributes to liver fibrosis. Gastroenterology 2006; 130: 1807-1821.

[117] di Bonzo LV, Ferrero I, Cravanzola C, *et al.* Human mesenchymal stem cells as a two-edged sword in hepatic regenerative medicine: engraftment and hepatocyte differentiation *vs.* profibrogenic potential. Gut 2008; 57: 223-231.

[118] Abdel Aziz MT, Atta HM, Mahfouz S, *et al.* Therapeutic potential of bone marrow-derived mesenchymal stem cells on experimental liver fibrosis. Clin Biochem 2007; 40: 893-899.

[119] Van Poll D, Parekkadau B, Cho CH, *et al.* Mesenchymal stem cell-derived molecules directly modulate hepatocellular death and regeneration *in vitro* and *in vivo*. Hepatology 2008; 47: 1634-1643.

[120] Christ B, Stock P. Mesenchymal stem-cell derived hepatocytes for functional liver replacement. Front Immunol 2012; 3: 168.

[121] Aurich H, Spodda M, Kailtwasser P, *et al.* Hepatocyte differentiation of mesenchymal stem cells from human adipose tissue *in vitro* promotes hepatic integration *in vivo*. Gut 2009; 58: 570-581.

[122] Wang Y, Lian F, Li J, *et al.* Adipose derived mesenchymal stem cells transplantation *via* portal vein improves microcirculation and ameliorates liver fibrosis induced by CCl4 in rats. J Transl Med 2012; 10: 133.
[123] Ouyang J, Shao J, Zou H, Lou Y, Yu Y. Hepatic differentiation of rat mesenchymal stem cells by a small molecule. Chem Med Chem 2012;7:1447-1452.
[124] Al Battah F, De Kock J, Vanhaecke T, Rogiers V. Current status of human adipose-derived stem cells. Scientific World Journal 2011; 11: 1568-1581.
[125] Detante O, Moisan A, Dimastromatteo J, *et al.* Intravenous administration of ^{99m}Tc-HMPAO-labeled human mesenchymal stem cells after stroke: *in vivo* imaging and biodistribution. Cell Transplant 2009; 18: 1369-1379.
[126] Oishi K, Noguchi H, Yukama H, y cols. Differential ability of somatic stem cells. Cell Transplant 2009; 18: 581-589.
[127] Meirelles LD, Nardi NB. Methodology, biology and clinical applications of mesenchymal stem cells. Front Biosci 2009; 14: 4281-4298.
[128] Tremolada C, Palmieri G, Ricordi C. Adipocyte transplantation and stem cells: Plastic surgery meets regenerative medicine. Cell Transpl 2010; 19: 1217-1223.
[129] Zuk PA, Zhu M, Mizuno H, *et al.* Multilineage cells from human adipose tissue: implications for cell-based therapies. Tissue Eng 2001; 7: 211-228.
[130] Seo MJ, Suh SY, Bae YC, Jung JS. Differentiation of human adipose stromal cells into hepatic lineage *in vitro* and *in vivo*. Biochem Biophys Res Commun 2005; 328: 258-264.
[131] Dhawan A, Puppi J, Hughes RD, Mitry RR. Human hepatocyte transplantation: current experience and future challenges. Nat Rev Gastroenterol Hepatol 2010; 7: 288-298.
[132] Ringden O, Le Blanc K. Mesenchymal stem cells for treatment of acute and chronic graft-*vs.*-host disease, tissue toxicity and hemorrhages. Best Pract Res Clin Haematol 2011; 24: 65-72.
[133] Zhao S, Fu Y-M, Li XF, *et al.* Alterations of bone marrow sinusoidal endothelium in rat and patients with cirrhosis. Dig Dis Sci 2010; 55: 654-661.
[134] Fujimiya T, Liu J, Kojima H, Shirafuji S, Kimura H, Fujimiya M. Pathological roles of bone marrow-derived stellate cells in a mouse model of alcohol-induced fatty liver. Am J Physiol Gastrointest Liver Physiol 2009; 297: G451-G460.
[135] Eckersley-Maslin MA, Warner FJ, Grzelak CA, McCaughan GW, Shackel NA. Bone marrow stem cells and the liver: are they relevant? J Gastroenterol Hepatol 2009; 24: 1608-1616.
[136] Kallis K, Alison M, Forbes SJ. Bone marrow stem cells and liver disease. Gut 2007; 56: 716-724.
[137] Collardeau-Frachon S, Scoazec J-Y. Vascular development and differentiation during human liver organogenesis. Anat Record 2008; 291: 614-627.
[138] Gilchrist ES, Plevris JN. Bone marrow-derived stem cells in liver repair: 10 years down the line. Liver Transplant 2010; 16: 118-129.
[139] Lyra AC, Soares MB, da Silva LF *et al.* Infusion of autologous bone marrow mononuclear cells through hepatic artery results in a short-term improvement of liver function in patients with chronic liver disease: a pilot randomized controlled study. Eur J Gastroenterol Hepatol 2010; 22: 33-42.
[140] Aller MA, Blanco-Rivero J, Arias JI, Balfagon G, Arias J. The wound-healing response and upregulated embryonic mechanisms: bothers-in-arms forever. Exp Dermatol 2012; 21: 497-503.

[141] Desmet VJ. Ductal plates in hepatic ductular reactions. Hypothesis and implications. I. Types of ductular reaction reconsidered. Virchows Arch 2011; 458: 251-259.
[142] Desmet VJ. Ductal plates in hepatic ductular reactions. Hypothesis and implications. II Ontogenic liver growth in childhood. Virchows Arch 2011; 458: 261-270.
[143] Van Eyken P, Sciot R, Callea F, Van der Steen K, Moerman P, Desmet VJ. The development of intrahepatic bile ductus in man: a keratin-immunohistochemical study. Hepatology 1988; 8: 1586-1595.
[144] Desmet VJ, Roskams T, Van Eyken P. Ductular reactions in the liver. Pathol Res Pract 1995; 191: 513-524.
[145] Godoy P, Hengstler JG, Ilkavets I, *et al.* Extracellular matrix modulates sensitivity of hepatocytes to fibroblastoid dedifferentiation and transforming growth factor beta-induced apoptosis. Hepatology 2009; 49: 2031-2043.
[146] Ma C, Brunt EM. Histopathologic evaluation of liver biopsy for cirrhosis. Adv Anat Pathol 2012; 19: 220-230.
[147] Venkatanarasimha N, Thomas R, Armstrong EM, Shirley JF, Fox BM, Jackson SA. Imaging features of ductal plate malformations in adults. Clin Radiol 2011; 66: 1086-1093.
[148] Erlinger S. Ductal plate malformations: a morphogenetic classification based on genetic defects. Clin Res Hepatol Gastroenterol 2011; 35:604-606.
[149] Raynaud P, Tate J, Callens C, *et al.* A classification of ductal plate malformations based on distinct pathogenic mechanisms of biliary dysmorphogenesis. Hepatology 2011; 53: 1959-1966.
[150] Lemaigre FP. Mechanisms of liver development: concepts for understanding liver disorders and design of novel therapies. Gastroenterology 2009; 137: 62-79.
[151] Raynaud P, Carpentier R, Antoniou A, Lemaigre FP. Biliary differentiation and bile duct morphogenesis in development and disease. Int J Biochem Cell Biol 2011; 43: 245-256.
[152] Strazzabosco M, Fabris L. Development of the bile ducts: Essentials for the clinical hepatologist. J Hepatol 2012; 56: 1159-1170.
[153] Lemaigre FP. Molecular mechanisms of biliary development. Prog Mol Biol Transl Sci 2010; 97: 103-126.
[154] Greenbaum LE. The ductal plate: a source of progenitors and hepatocytes in the adult. Gastroenterology 2011; 141: 1152-1155.
[155] Carpentier R, Suñer ER, Van Hul N, *et al.* Embryonic ductal plate cells give rise to cholangiocytes, periportal hepatocytes, and adult liver progenitor cells. Gastroenterology 2011; 141: 1432-1438

Send Orders for Reprints to reprints@benthamscience.net
Surgical Inflammation, 2013, 277-308

CHAPTER 10

Inflammation Meets Evo-Devo

María-Angeles Aller[1], Natalia Arias[2], Sherezade Fuentes-Julian[3], Alejandro Blazquez-Martinez[3], Salvador Argudo[4], Maria-Paz de Miguel [3], Jorge-Luis Arias[2] and Jaime Arias[1,*]

[1]Surgery Department, School of Medicine, Complutense University of Madrid, Madrid, Spain; [2]Neurosciences Laboratory, Psychobiology Department, School of Psychology, University of Oviedo, Asturias, Spain; [3]Cell Engineering Laboratory, La Paz Hospital, Autonoma University of Madrid Madrid, Spain and [4]General Surgery Unit, Sudeste Hospital, Arganda del Rey, Madrid, Spain

Abstract: Inflammation integrates diverse mechanisms that are associated not only with pathological conditions, such as cardiovascular diseases, type 2 diabetes, obesity, neurodegenerative diseases and cancer, but also with physiological processes like reproduction *i.e.*, oogenesis and embryogenesis as well as aging. In the current review, we propose that the inflammatory response could also recapitulate the phylogenia and the ontogenia. Highly conserved inflammatory mechanisms that play a main role in the evolutive development of different animal species, both invertebrates as well as vertebrates are identified. In this way, inflammation could represent a key tool used by nature to modulate organisms according to the environmental conditions in which these develop. Thus inflammation could be the pathway by which the environmental conditions could be related to the evolutionary development. The hypothetical consideration of inflammation as recapitulation of phylogenia and ontogenia could make it possible to integrate the pathophysiological mechanisms of these diverse chronic pathological conditions.

Keywords: Surgical inflammation, evo-devo, phylogenia, ontogenia, acute phase response, ischemia, hydration, catabolism, lipoprotein-related metabolism, vitellogenesis, metaflammation.

INTRODUCTING THE INFLAMMATION

Nowadays, inflammation is considered a highly beneficial and adaptive response that is triggered by noxious stimuli and conditions, such as infection and tissue

***Address correspondence to Jaime Arias:** Cátedra de Cirugía, Facultad de Medicina, Universidad Complutense, Pza. de Ramón y Cajal s.n., 28040 MADRID, Spain; Tel: +34 91 394 1389; Fax: +34 91 3947115; E-mail: jariasp@med.ucm.es

Jaime Arias, Maria-Angeles Aller and Jose-Ignacio Arias (Eds)

injury [1, 2]. However, this standard view of inflammation as a reaction to injury or infection might need to be expanded to account for the inflammatory processes induced by other types of adverse conditions [1]. The human diseases that are associated with these conditions, including atherosclerosis, asthma, type 2 diabetes and neurodegenerative diseases are all characterized by chronic low-grade inflammation and this adaptive response, since being intermediate between basal and inflammatory states, has been termed para-inflammation [1].

Furthermore, human aging can be explained by the emerging concept of para-inflammation-driven inflammaging, *i.e.*, a combination of inflammation and aging [3-5]. Inflammaging seems to favor the onset of typical age-related diseases like atherosclerosis, dementia, osteoporosis and cancer [6, 7] (Fig. **1**).

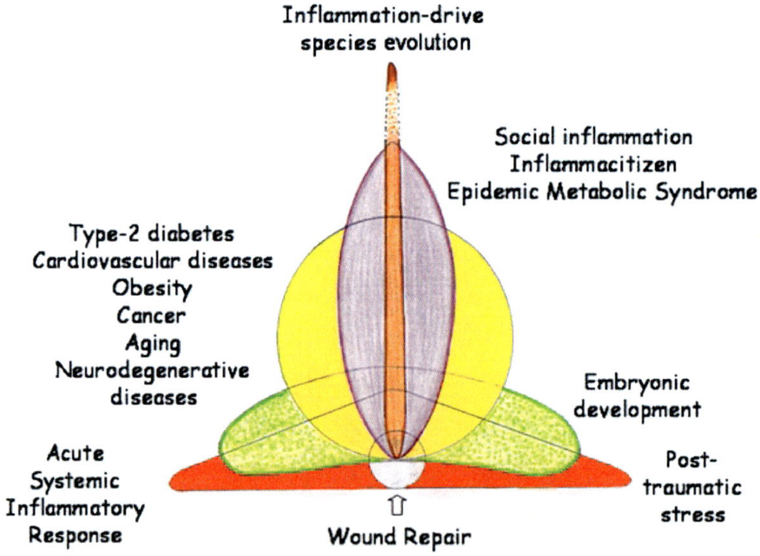

Figure 1: Schematic representation of inflammation like a process underlying numerous physiological as well as pathological phenomena.

However, a key adaptive characteristic of inflammation, whether acute, chronic or acute-on-chronic, is that it produces tissue, organ or even organism remodeling [8, 9]. In this way, it has been proposed that the inflammatory response has features in common with tissue development, which requires involution of pre-existing tissue elements [8-10]. The ability of the tissues to involute or dedifferentiate could represent a return to early stages of development [11]. Therefore, it could form an effective defense mechanism to escape death after injury since it could make retracing a well-known route possible, *i.e.* the initial phases of the embryonic development during the evolution of the inflammatory response [8, 10, 11]. The correlation that can be established between the embryonic and the inflammatory events suggests that the results obtained from the research regarding both great fields of knowledge must be interchangeable to obtain the maximum advantage [11].

In the adult body, many pathways that play an essential role during embryological development are inactivated later in life, although some of them may be transiently expressed during adult repair processes [11, 12]. This ability of the tissues to involute or dedifferentiate could constitute an effective solution against any type of injury, since it allows to cells, tissues, organs and organisms to remodel according to the new environmental situations that are imposed upon them.

Nonetheless, the inflammatory response also seems to compile mechanisms that have a great value from a phylogenetic point of view. It would be explained how similarly mechanisms are shared in essence by the diverse types of the inflammatory response, from acute high-grade to chronic low-grade inflammation.

PHYLOGENETICS AND ONTOGENIC MECHANISMS IN INFLAMMATION

Some of the fundamental mechanisms of the systemic inflammatory response to the injury are similar to those mechanisms that are expressed by the different animal species during their development. This is the reason why we have proposed the hypothesis that the inflammatory response could recapitulate phylogeny and ontogeny through the successive expression of pathophysiological mechanisms of increasing complexity that have a trophic meaning to the injured body [13].

The systemic inflammatory response that is induced in the injured organism could be described as a succession of three overlapped phases, during which the phenotypes of metabolic progressive complexity related to the use of oxygen are expressed.

In the first phase of the inflammatory response, hydroelectrolytic alterations stand out, with edema secondary to the ischemia-reperfusion phenomenon and nutrition by diffusion, which predominates. In the following phase, the metabolic response is characterized by hypermetabolism and enzymatic stress associated with immunological and endocrinologic responses [14]. The incorrect use of oxygen persists in this phase and the systemic alterations produced are referred collectively as the acute phase response (APR) [15]. Enzymatic stress favors extracellular (fermentation) and intracellular (phagocytosis) digestion [8].

The last phase of the inflammatory response is characterized by the capacity to use the oxygen in oxidative metabolism, *i.e.* oxidative phosphorylation. In this phase, patients recover their capillary function, and therefore, nutrition is mediated by them. This type of metabolism is characterized by a large production of ATP, which is used to drive specialized multiple cellular processes, and would determine the onset of the healing [8, 14].

Since these trophic mechanisms are of increasing complexity, progressing from anoxia to total specialization in the use of oxygen to obtain usable energy, it could be speculated that they represent the successive reappearance of the stages that took place during the evolution of life without oxygen on Earth from ancient times. In this sense, the inflammatory response not only could recapitulate ontogeny [11], but also phylogeny, through the successive expression of phenotypes that have a trophic meaning.

The great ubiquity of the basic mechanisms that manage the inflammatory response suggests that they are inseparably ligated to life evolution and, therefore, would be integral part of it. In this way, said mechanisms possibly bury their roots into the origin of eukaryotic life.

Some of the fundamental mechanisms of inflammation, both acute and chronic, can be recognized in the origin and evolutive development of different animal species and, for this reason, in the current article we are aiming at establishing a corresponding relation between both of them. Thus the functions that characterize each phase of the inflammatory response of the body to the injury or to stress could represent regression to remote stages of the species evolution.

Ischemia and Hydration: The Beginning

The inflammatory response irrespective of the specific cause, *i.e.* allergic, infections, ischemia, toxins or stress, could have basic mechanisms shared by all of these types of diseases. We have previously proposed that whatever the cause of the inflammatory response is, its principal objective could be to provide nutrition to the injured tissues [8, 16]. Particularly, the inflammatory response related to surgery and trauma, also named surgical inflammation, seems to recapitulate diverse trophic mechanisms related to developmental processes [11].

The interstitial space always seems to be the battle field for inflammation, whether it is due to trauma [8, 10], infection [17] or tumors [18, 19]. The successive pathophysiological mechanisms that develop in the interstitial space of tissues when they undergo surgical inflammation are considered increasingly complex trophic functional systems for using oxygen because they go from ischemia to the development of an oxidative mechanism [16]. Therefore, a correlation between the increased organism complexity and the development of the use of the atmospheric oxygen could be established [20, 21]. This correlation seems to exist in the evolutive phases of the surgical inflammatory response since progressive cellular and tissue complexity occurs parallel to a gradual oxygenation process from ischemia after severe traumatic injury, to progressive reoxygenation until the correct revascularization by capillarogenesis occurs in the injured organism [14].

A successive molecular and cellular infiltration of the interstitial space is produced during the evolution of the surgical inflammatory response [10, 14]. This space is occupied by the extracellular matrix that is not an inert substance [22]; rather it plays a significant role in different physiological processes and disease conditions [22-24]. Phylogenetic data obtained from recently completed genome sequencing projects have shown that the molecules of the extracellular matrix, especially those related to cell-matrix adhesion are "ancient and exquisitely conserved in multicellular animals" [23, 25]. Perhaps this is the reason why the extracellular matrix performs a key role in both the evolution of surgical inflammation and the early stages of animal development.

The inflammatory mechanisms that drive the successive molecular and cellular infiltration of the interstitial space recall some of the fundamental mechanisms of the distinct steps of the early stages of invertebrate and vertebrate development. Perhaps, first we should highlight hydration because it is a prime and initial step of inflammation [14], and development as well [26- 29] (Fig. **2**).

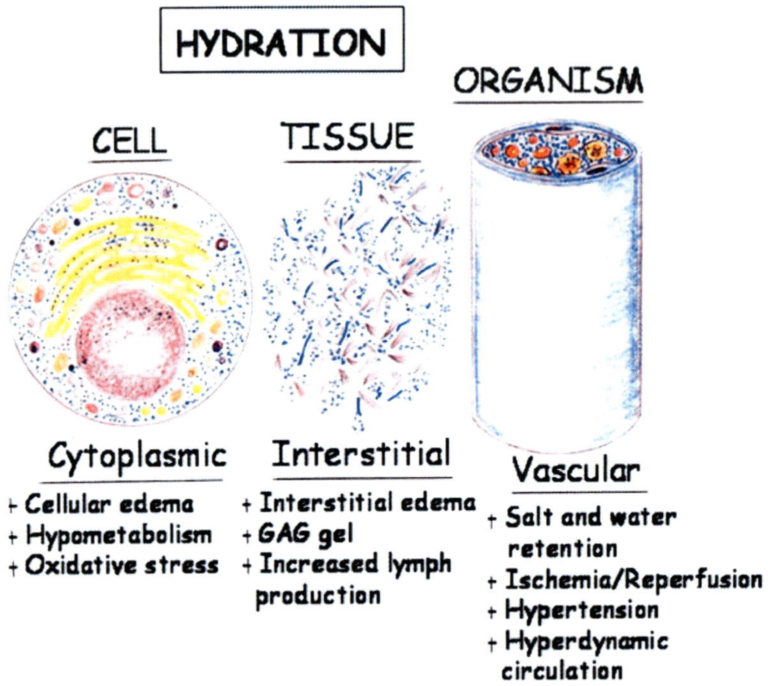

Figure 2: Local, regional and systemic hydroelectrolytic changes associated to the early phase of the inflammatory response. The hydroelectrolytic alterations would induce diverse pathological mechanisms depending on the site in which they are expressed. GAG: glycosaminoglycans.

Hydration is a fundamental step of inflammation and development, probably because it favors nutrition by diffusion in both cases. In injured tissue hydration, *i.e.* cellular and interstitial edema, is secondary to ischemia-revascularization phenomenon with oxidative and nitrosative stress [14]. Increased degradation of the extracellular matrix with accumulation of fragments of glycosaminoglycans has been proposed as an important mechanism for edema formation because of the hydrophilic properties of glycosaminoglycans and particularly of hyaluronan [30]. Glycosaminoglycans attract and entrap water and ions, thereby forming hydrated gels, while permitting the flow of cellular nutrients and favoring edematous infiltration of the tissue as well as the interstitial fluid flow and the tissue lymph pressure gradient [31].

In several animal species hydration is one of the initial events in development. Thus in lepidoptera dormant follicles, which include a single oocyte and seven nurse cells encased in an epithelium of follicle cells, they become active when they suffer an increase in turgor pressure and are visibly swollen [26]. The follicle cells, as an epithelium, have a system of intercellular channels containing a matrix of sulfated glycosaminoglycans that enable hemolymph to reach the oocyte [26]. In fish, fertilized eggs are activated by exposure to fresh water. After activation, the zona radiata or acellular eggshell, takes up water, gains resistance to breakage and can support up to 100 times more weight than oviductal eggs [32]. In marine fish, the final volume of the egg is acquired during oocyte maturation due to water uptake. During oocyte hydration and maturation, amino acids derived from yolk protein hydrolysis are osmotic effectors but hydration of oocyte also depends on the accumulation of ions like K^+, Mg^{2+}, Ca^{2+}, Cl^- and ammonium (NH_4^+) [28]. Early preimplantation mouse embryos also require intracellular accumulation of glycine to provide osmotic support and thus control cell volume [27] (Table **1**).

Table 1: Related factors involved in the inflammatory response and in development.

Inflammatory Response	**Development**
- Innate immune response	* ***Oviparous animals:***
- Acute phase response	-Vertebrate and Invertebrate-vitellogenin genes
. Pentraxins	- Pentraxins
. C-reactive protein-bind to LDL	
. Fibrinogen	- Vitellogenesis
. Serum amyloid A increases the ability of	- Fat body
HDL to accept cholesterol	
- Hydrolysis of adipose tissue	
- Increased lymph production	- Hemolymph lipids from the fat body
- Coagulation	- Melanin
- Factor XIIIa	- Transglutaminase
- IL-6-induced changes in the lipoprotein	- Vitellin (glycolipoprotein)
Profile	
- Mast cell activation	- Granulocyte/Hemocyte activation

Table 1: continued

- Apolipoprotein-B-containing particles	- Apolipoprotein B
. LDL	
. VLDL	
- Corticoids-Aldosterone: oxidative stress- fibrogen	- Steroid producing follicle cells
	- Oenocyte accumulation of lipid droplets
* ***Mammalian embryos:***	
- Atherogenic dyslipidemia	- Accumulation of cholesterol
- Hepatic steatosis	- Accumulation of lipids into the yolk sac
- Insulin resistance - Embryo environment rich in g glucose:	
. Lipid synthesis	
. Cell growth and division	
- Obesity	
- Metabolic Syndrome	

IL: Interleukin; LDL: Low density lipoprotein; HDL: High density lipoprotein; VLDL: Very low density lipoprotein.

The liquid that is accumulated in the interstitial space of the inflamed tissues or organs, and which infiltrates the extracellular matrix, progressively adopts some of the properties that have been described in the hemolymph [33, 34]. The circulatory system depending on whether blood and interstitial fluid mix can be divided into two major groups: the open circulatory system and the closed circulatory system. In this last system, the blood circulates only within the internal lumen of the blood vessels and does not mix with interstitial fluid. On the contrary, in the phyla with the open circulatory system such as *Arthropoda*, the blood can freely blend into the interstitial fluid to generate hemolymph [35]. The internal organs in these animals are submerged within an internal cavity called the hemocoel and directly receive oxygen and nutrients, and deposit metabolic wastes [35, 36]. Therefore, it could be considered that in the inflamed tissue the closed circulatory system suffers a switch to acquire some of the characteristics of the open circulatory system and perhaps of the hemolymph. In this way, the inflammatory exudate bathes the cells of the injured tissues and organs, due to the quick infiltration of the extracellular matrix [14].

The open circulatory system in the inflamed tissue, like in insects, permits coagulation to be more exuberant to quickly seal wounds, limit fluid loss, entrap microbes at wound sites and restore the tissue [34]. The great increase of the endothelial permeability in the inflamed organs also allows selective diffusion through the interstitial space of circulating substances in the blood that have been released as a neuroendocrine system response to stress *i.e.* the hypothalamic-pituitary-adrenal and sympathetic-adrenal medullary or sympathetic nervous system [14]. This selectivity in the localization of the inflammatory response that induces interstitial edema could also favor the interstitial accumulation of substances derived from the acute phase response (APR) [37].

However in this initial phase of the systemic inflammatory response in mammals, it could be considered that hypometabolism, anaerobic glycolysis, low temperature and a decrease in energy expenditure [14] reduce the expression of specialized functions with a high energetic expense for the traumatized organism, drive the catabolism and therefore, favor its deconstruction (Fig. **3**).

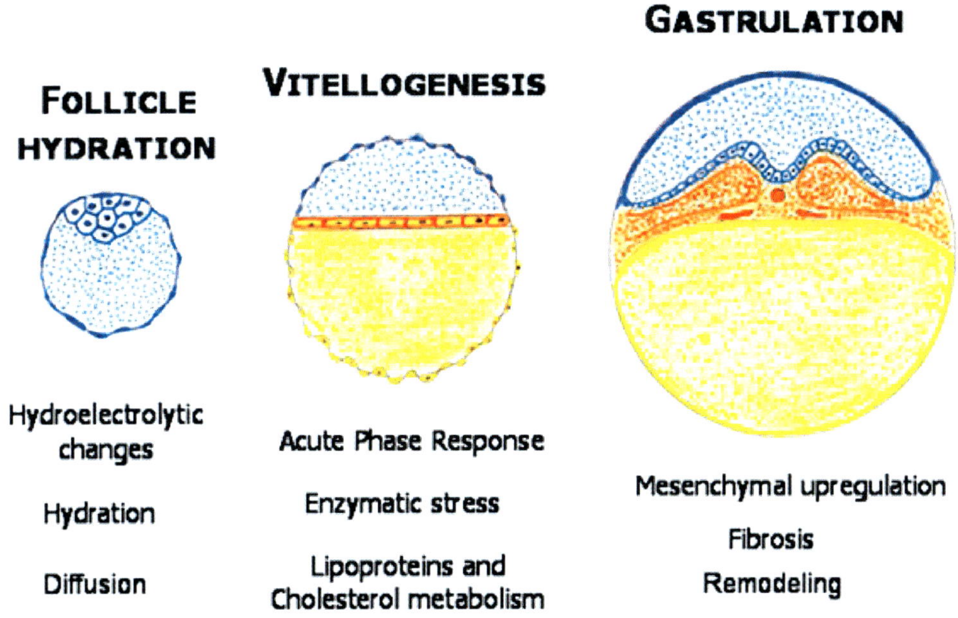

Figure 3: Schematic representation of the mechanisms characteristic of the different phases of the inflammatory response that also participate in diverse steps of the evolutive development of animal species, both invertebrates and vertebrates, *i.e.* follicle hydration, vitellogenesis and gastrulation. In essence, the basic mechanisms involved in follicle hydration, vitellogenesis and gastrulation, could be identified through the acute or chronic evolution of inflammation.

Vitellogenesis and Acute-Phase Response: The Lipoprotein-Related Metabolism

In oviparous animals, accumulation of yolk materials into oocytes during oogenesis and their mobilization during embryogenesis are key processes for successful reproduction [26, 28, 32]. All oviparous species, including insects, provide their eggs with vitellin as a major yolk storage glycolipoprotein [38]. The precursor vitellogenin is synthesized by the fat body, the main organ of the intermediate metabolism of insects [38]. Moreover, the majority of proteins of the hemolymph are synthesized in the fat body. In this organ vitellogenin is modified to facilitate the transport of carbohydrates, lipids and other nutrients into oocyte during vitellogenesis. In fact, it has been suggested that the lipid would be used as an energy source for oogenesis, in addition to being incorporated with the oocytes in the vitellogenesis process [38] (Fig. **2**).

Vitellogenins are stored in oocytes as vitellin, a reserve food-source for the future embryo [38]. In the insects, vitellogenins are involved in the regulation of hormonal dynamics, antioxidant activity, immune defense, longevity and social behavior [38, 39]. Furthermore, it has been postulated, based on phylogenetic studies, that the entire vitellogenin sequence should be used when searching for phylogenetic inferences [38]. Vitellogenins are part of a multi-gene family that includes insect apolipophorins and human apolipoprotein B [38] (Table **1**).

Vitellogenesis in fish also describes the incorporation of vitellogenin protein carbohydrates and lipids by the oocyte. The lipids accumulating within the oocyte originate from plasma - very low density lipoproteins (VLDL) and from vitellogenins [28]. Lipids could be sequestered from the plasma VLDL by the binding to apolipoprotein B [28, 32]. The ability to transport fat, in the form of lipoprotein, through the circulatory system by eukaryotes is one of their most significant functions right from the beginning of existence [32].

The reason and functional basis for the vitellogenin transport system initially evolved provide information about how energy in the form of fat can be distributed. Thus the evolutionary advancement of storing energy in the form of fat has provided organisms with an enormous advantage in adapting to environmental and developmental changes [32]. Comparative studies based on amino acid sequences and gene organization support the hypothesis of a common evolutionary origin of the vertebrate and invertebrate vitellogenin genes [32, 40].

An isoform of apolipoprotein B, and apopB_{48} particles, are chylomicrons, which transport dietary cholesterol and triglycerides from the intestine to sites of storage and utilization within the body, such as the adipose tissue, skeletal and cardiac muscle and the liver [41]. However, during cardiovascular inflammation, cholesterol esters may be transferred from high density lipoprotein (HDL) to apolipoprotein B-containing particles, such as low-density lipoprotein (LDL cholesterol) or VLDL [42]. Trapping of apolipoprotein B containing particles within the arterial wall is unquestionably the essential initiating event for the development of complex atherosclerotic lesions [41]. Hepatic steatosis results from increased hepatic uptake of free fatty acids derived mainly from the hydrolysis of adipose-tissue triglycerides, increased because of insulin resistance, but also from dietary chylomicrons and hepatic biogenesis [43]. Hepatic steatosis in turn might play a key role in the pathogenesis of cardiovascular disease through the systemic release of several inflammatory mediators and/or through the production of insulin resistance and atherogenic dyslipidemia [43, 44].

The acute phase response is a core part of the innate immune response and produces changes in more than 200 proteins grouped as either positive or negative acute phase proteins [37, 45]. Positive acute phase proteins include C-reactive protein, fibrinogen, haptoglobin, α_2-macroglobulin, α_1-acid glycoprotein, transferrin, ceruloplasmin and serum amyloid A [45]. IL-6, produced in response to tissue damage and infection, is a central mediator of the immune system inducing the liver acute-phase response [46].

Inflammation and the concomitant acute phase response induce significant changes in the lipoprotein profile [47]. Likewise, IL-6 and acute phase proteins, particularly C-reactive protein, have been correlated to disease severity and outcome in most of the chronic low-grade inflammatory conditions like cardiovascular diseases, obesity, metabolic syndrome, type-2 diabetes, and non-alcoholic fatty liver disease (NAFLD), which includes a large spectrum that ranges from fatty liver, non-alcoholic steatohepatitis and cryptogenetic cirrhosis and depression [43, 44, 48-51].

There are conflicting results as to whether IL-6 is a beneficial or harmful cytokine [52]. There is, however, increasing evidence to show that IL-6 has a protective role during neural and liver injury [46]. In this context, it has been suggested that IL-6 favors hepatic secretion of VLDL triglyceride by increasing the availability of apoB and thereby, reducing hepatic lipid content by increased triglyceride export [52]. In addition, acute phase proteins, particularly the lipoprotein serum amyloid A, increase the ability of acute phase HDL to serve as an acceptor for cellular cholesterol efflux promoting the removal of excess cholesterol from macrophages as well as increasing the availability of cellular free cholesterol [47, 53].

The predominance of the lipid metabolism with accumulation of cholesterol within embryos [26, 32] as well as in the chronic inflamed tissue [43, 44], could also be attributed to it being a precursor molecule of many hormones, like aldosterone, corticoids, progesterone, androgens and estrogen [28]. Particularly, endogenous sex steroids have been implicated in the pathology of, and protection against, a limited number of inflammatory disorders. Indeed estrogens limit while androgens could increase wound inflammation [54]. Also mineralocorticoids, *i.e.* aldosterone and glucocorticoids, are involved in the pathophysiology of inflammation because they produce oxidative stress, insulin resistance and fibrogenesis, as well as the promotion of adipogenesis [55]. Maybe due to the imperious need of this hormone potential, the developing oocyte is located in the centre of the follicle and is surrounded by steroid producing follicle cells [32]. It has also been considered that endogenous lipid stores in fish oocytes and early embryos could be used as an energy substrate [56].

Mammalian embryos, however, have a changing pattern of energy metabolism, *i.e.* ATP generation, during early development. The most abundant energetic substrates in the embryo environment are glucose, pyruvate, lactate and glutamine [57]. For most mammalian proliferative cells the fundamental molecules catabolized are glucose and glutamine. This means that glucose and glutamine supply most of the carbon, nitrogen and free energy and reduce equivalents necessary to support cell growth and division [58]. Particularly interesting is the fact that some glucose is diverted to macromolecular precursor such as acetyl-CoA for fatty acids. Glutamine uptake also appears to be critical for lipid synthesis in that it supplies carbon in the form of mitochondrial oxaloacetate to maintain citrate production in the first step of tricarboxylic acid [58].

The close relationship between lipid metabolism and inflammation has been emphasized in obesity. Thus, it has been suggested that current life style trends in modern society, characterized by excess of nutrients, reduced physical activity and increased lifespan could alter immune signaling and produce a chronic low-grade inflammatory state [59]. Because obesity-associated inflammation is considered a novel form of inflammation triggered by metabolic cues, the term of *"metaflammation"* has been proposed for it [59, 60].

The acute phase response is a pervasive physiological response of the body to injury [61]. Acute-phase changes may be divided into changes in the concentrations of many plasma proteins, known as the acute phase proteins and a large number of behavioral, physiologic, biochemical, and nutritional changes [37]. In nearly all animal species, albumin represents the major negative acute-phase protein which, during the acute phase response, decreases in blood concentration and increases in the inflammatory interstitial space [45]. Proteolysis during the acute phase response favors a protein-switch, because the resulting increase of amino acids is used for the synthesis of positive acute phase proteins, between which pentraxins *i.e.* serum amyloid P and C-reactive protein, stand out [61, 62].

Pentraxins are a super-family of multifunctional conserved proteins, some of which are components of the humoral arm of innate immunity and behave as functional ancestors of antibodies [62, 63]. Pentraxins are ancient proteins with high phylogenetic conservation. They are considered highly conserved acute phase innate immune proteins [61-64]. The classic short pentraxins, C-reactive protein and serum amyloid P component, are produced in the liver in response to inflammatory signals, most prominently IL-6 [62].

C-reactive protein circulates as a disc shaped pentamer and is dissociated by exposure of bioactive lipids on activated cell membrane and exhibits anti-inflammatory properties [63]. After dissociation, monomeric C-reactive protein could deposit in the inflamed tissue and represents an *"activation signal"* for inflammatory cells [63], but may also be able to minimize inflammation while enhancing apoptotic cell clearance [64]. Serum amyloid-P is closely related to C-reactive protein [64] and could promote anti-inflammatory responses [65].

C-reactive protein and serum amyloid-P are considered the main acute-phase reactants in humans, but also in arthropods different forms of C-reactive protein and serum amyloid-P are abundant constituents of the hemolymph [62]. In addition, it is noteworthy that C-reactive protein can bind to LDL and co-localize with LDL in human atherosclerotic lesions [62].

The long pentraxin PTX3 may play a regulatory role in inflammation but is also required for cumulus matrix organization [66]. Cumulus cells are closely connected to the oocyte during follicular development and ovulation, forming a reciprocal functional interconnection [67, 68]. Therefore, PTX3 that allows the formation of a highly organized hyaluronan-rich cumulus matrix favors ovulation and subsequent fertilization [62, 66, 68, 69]. It has been proposed that PTX3 could have a similar function in hyaluronic acid-enriched inflammatory tissues [62, 69].

PTX3 also plays an important role in humoral innate immunity and inflammation [70]. Levels of circulating PTX3 increase in humans during systemic inflammatory response syndrome, myocardial infarction or septic shock [71]. In this inflammatory context, the high levels of PTX3 found associated with macrophages and endothelial cells in atherosclerotic plaques acting as a natural angiogenic inhibitor stand out [71, 72].

Because both invertebrates and vertebrates detect and respond to microbial antigens, it is likely that a system recognizing these epitopes emerged at a very early stage in the evolution of animal species. In invertebrates, hemolymph coagulation and melanin formation are prominent as such responses [33]. Transglutaminase appears to be a common coagulation factor because it is involved in coagulation in arthropods and also acts as vertebrate clotting factor XIIIa [34]. The clots of large insects first form as a soft, initial, *"primary"* clot that is subsequently melanized [34]. Coagulation in insects contributes to wound healing and both processes depend on hemocytes, also called granulocytes [33,

34]. In humans, activation of factor XIII is involved in atherogenesis and polymorphisms are related to the risk of coronary artery disease, atherothrombotic ischemic stroke and peripheral artery disease [73]. Procoagulant factors, *i.e.* plasminogen activator inhibitor I (PAI-1), fibrinogen and factor VII are also highest in patients with NAFLD, which explains the risk of the incidence of cardiovascular events among these patients [43].

Granulocytes may be close to the most ancient precursor of mast cells in invertebrates. In ascidians, the basophil/mast cells like granular hemocytes have been considered a potential mast cell progenitor and some granular hemocytes in *arthropoda* also closely approximate the ultra-structure of modern mast cells [74]. During evolution mast cells might have lost their potential to circulate in the blood once differentiated into sessile, tissue-homing cells [74].

Mast cells, strategically located in the interstitial space, could be among the first responders to orchestrate mechanical and biochemical stimuli that initiate inflammation [75]. Mast cells have the ability to produce vasoactive amines, enzymes *i.e.* proteases, cytokines, chemokines and growth factors through degranulation. This plasticity of the mast cells, which is the base for the known *"mast cell heterogeneity"* [75] suggests that mast cells can also show diverse responsiveness during the successive phases of the inflammatory response [11]. Mast cells stimulated through Toll-like receptors (TLRs) express "surgical" cytokine responses consisting mainly of IL-4, IL-8, tumor necrosis factor (TNF)-α and IL-6 [74, 76]. In turn, IL-6, not only is the major mediator for the hepatocyte secretion of most of the acute phase proteins, but actually is also considered the major cytokine produced by activated mast cells, as well as a key factor that can trigger mast cell differentiation [77]. The acute phase response in the intestine resembles that seen in the liver. Indeed IL-6 mRNA is increased in the intestine during inflammation [78-80]. Among the cytokines produced during inflammation in the gut-liver axis, IL-6 is particularly important because of its multiple biological effects both in the liver, intestine and other organs and tissues, including thermogenesis, stimulation of the hypothalamic-pituitary-adrenal axis and stimulation of growth hormone secretion [80]. Moreover, the pro-inflammatory cytokine IL-6 is critically involved in the pathophysiology of various aspects of NAFLD. Particularly, serum levels of this cytokine correlate remarkably well with the presence of insulin resistance and IL-6 has been shown to regulate hepatic insulin resistance [81].

Mast cells have well established roles as mediators of allergic, fibrotic and angiogenic diseases [14] and increasing evidence has implicated these cells in atherosclerotic plaque development [82, 83]. Mast cells also produce serine proteases that could activate metalloproteinase leading to extracellular matrix remodeling [74, 82]. The tissue distribution of mast cells containing serine proteases varies across animal species and the large number of functions described to these enzymes clearly indicates their importance in mast cell biology [74]. In this way, serine proteases appear to be a major link between innate immunity and tissue remodeling [74]. This is one of the reasons why it has been proposed that the mast cell phylogenetic progenitor is evolved from a primitive local innate immunity cell into a tissue regulatory and remodeling cell [74].

White adipose tissue may represent an important source of mast cells in physiological and pathological situations [84]. Moreover, homeostasis of lipid metabolism is essential for mast cell survival and dysregulation of lipid metabolism, with oxysterols accumulation, the derivates of cholesterol, which may induce mast cell apoptosis [85].

Oenocytes, kind of specialized hepatocyte-like cells [86], are found in a wide range of insects [87]. The presence of densely packed smooth and rough endoplasmic reticulum, together with other morphological features characteristic of mammalian steroidogenic cells and hepatocytes, indicates that oenocytes are cells with specialized secretory functions [87]. Oenocytes accumulate large numbers of lipid droplets specifically during fasting. As this is a hallmark of hepatocytes, the possibility is raised that insect oenocytes might process lipids in a similar way to the mammalian liver [86]. Analogous to the mammalian adipose-liver axis, lipid mobilization from the fat body, the main organ of the intermediate metabolism of insects [39] during starvation produces lipid droplet accumulation in *Drosophila* oenocytes, a metabolic change resembling hepatic steatosis [86, 88] (Table **1**).

Increasingly sophisticated approaches are required to understand the critical roles of energy homeostasis. Several disorders have comparable syndromes in lower metazoans, like worms, flies and zebrafish [88]. Unbiased methods have been used to identify more genes where mutation in lower metazoans leads to phenotypes that are comparable to human syndromes of altered energy homeostasis like NAFLD, diabetes mellitus and obesity [88]. In this context, it has been speculated that *Drosophila* may prove useful, not only for modeling hepatic steatosis, but also for the regulation of body fat content [89]. Indeed multiple genes have been identified that either positively or negatively regulate whole fly triglyceride levels when targeted specifically in neurons, the fly liver *i.e.* oenocytes, the fat body or muscle cells. Since more than 60% of the candidate genes with strong lipid storage regulatory potential linked with regulation of adiposity are conserved across animal phyla to humans, screening genes is considered a unique starting point to the elucidation of novel regulatory modalities in mammals [89].

Metamorphosis and Remodeling: Gastrulation Dictates Their Rules

When talking about metamorphosis the caterpillar-to-butterfly and tadpole-to-frog transition immediately come to mind. However, most metazoan phyla metamorphose: for example, in cnidarians, flat worms or mollusks [90]. It has also been considered that all chordates have a homologous metamorphosis stage during their post-embryonic development. Vertebrate metamorphosis has been molecularly well characterized only in anurans, which could be probably for historical, anthropocentric, epistemological as well as technical reasons [90].

We have hypothesized that the phylogenetic evolution of our body is written in the successive phases which make up the acute inflammatory response. Therefore, it could be considered that when evolution of a serious traumatized patient is favorable, he could first undergo a dedifferentiation followed by a process of differentiation or specialization which would represent a complete metamorphosis program, which occurs with lepidoptera [91]. This specialization would require the return of the prominence of oxidative metabolism and angiogenesis in the affected tissues and epithelial organs to create the capillary bed that would make the repair possible [8].

Nutrition mediated by blood capillaries is established because of angiogenesis. The new functional properties of microcirculation include the exchange of oxygen, nutrients and waste products. This oxygen support induces oxidative metabolism, an efficient method for extracting energy from blood molecules, which begins with the Krebs cycle and ends with oxidative phosphorylation [8]. Oxygen and oxidative metabolism is an excellent combination through which cells can obtain an abundant energy supply for tissue repair by specialized cells, but this combination has the inconvenience that it produces energetic stress [14] (Fig. **3**).

Nonetheless little is known about the capacity of eukaryotic cells to monitor the redox state for supporting specialized functions [92]. Although NF-κB acts mainly as an initiator of inflammation, recent studies suggest that it also functions in the equally complex process of resolution of inflammation [93]. Obviously, the mechanisms that promote tissue structure and restoring of functions also include the mechanisms involved in the resolution of inflammation [94]. In particular, endogenous pro-resolving lipid mediators, *i.e.* lipoxins, resolvins and protectins, have been the most studied. In essence, pro-resolution factors revert back the pro-inflammatory phenotype to its prior physiological state and therefore the microcirculatory functions of tissues and organs return to homeostasis [95].

A common complication of the post-natal inflammatory response in mammals is fibrosis. Scar formation and fibrosis are processes incompatible with tissue regeneration [96]. It has been suggested that molecular and cellular mechanisms are involved in gastrulation during embryo development return when the activation of a fibrotic process occurs, whether by local remodeling *i.e.* wound repair, or systemic remodeling *i.e.* aging [11].

Gastrulation is a developmental phase that delineates the three embryogenic germ layers: ectoderm, endoderm and mesoderm [97]. Although the details of gastrulation differ among different species, the cellular mechanisms involved in gastrulation are common to all animals ([97]. The molecular and cellular contribution to gastrulation may be made by the two halves of the egg and early embryo structures: The amnion or *"animal"* side, thus named because it suggests movement and activity, which has the egg nucleus and the central nervous system form from *"animal"* cells; and the yolk sac or *"vegetal"*, because it suggests sluggishness, which is filled with yolk material (*vitellum)* for nutrition [98].

Moreover, the amnion could be considered as an embryonic functional axis with the ability to manage the embryo interstitial fluid, as well as with a strong neurogenic phenotype [99, 100]. In regards to the yolk sac, it could be considered, not only a yolk deposit for nutrition but also a hematopoietic-angiogenic axis with a strong immune-endocrine potential phenotype [11, 101].

In essence, during gastrulation it could be considered that the extraembryonic mesoderm with its amniotic and yolk-sac-derived functions internalizes to form the primary mesenchyma [11]. Afterwards this is followed by mesenchymal-epithelial transition to create secondary epithelium [102]. The vast arrangement of the mesenchyma around and between the developing amniotic and yolk sac cavities suggests an important role of the mesenchyma in orchestrating embryo development. Mesenchymal stem cells are a versatile group of cells derived from mesodermal progenitors and can be found in several fetal and adult tissues [103]. The concept that fibroblasts are simple residual embryonic mesenchymal cells explains the incorrect and often interchangeable substitution of the term *"fibroblast"* for *"mesenchymal"* [104]. However, this hypothetical internalization process of the plurifunctional extraembryonic mesoderm to form the mesenchyma could explain the amazing quick capacity of the fibroblast not only to transform in epithelial cells but also to create a heterogeneous population capable to express neuro (contractile cells *i.e.* smooth muscle cells and pericytes), immune (myofibroblasts), endocrine (adipocytes) as well as remodeling (profibrogenic cells) phenotypes [11].

This amazing property of the mesenchymal or stromal cells to conserve a memory of its early embryonic origin undergoing reprogramming events could allow them post-injury to re-enter the embryonic programs of tissue formation and obtain regeneration [105]. Generally, while the monopotent and tissue-committed stem cells were described in the adult tissue, stem cells with a pluripotent/multipotent capacity were thought to be restricted to the early embryonic stages. However, recent evidence challenged this idea by confirming the presence of pluripotent/multipotent stem cells in adult tissues and organs [106]. Particularly, adult human mesenchymal cell populations contain distinctly multipotent stem cells. These stem cells have the ability to generate the multiple cell types of the three germ layers, like ectodermal, endodermal and mesodermal lineage cells [107].

During vertebrate gastrulation, the cell behavior is strictly coordinated in time and space by various signaling pathways. In vertebrates, the non-canonical Wnt/planar cell polarity (Wnt/PCP) pathway is a key regulator of convergence and extension movements also involved in the internalization of mesodermal cells and their migration [108]. Wnt represents a large morphogenic family of secreted lipid-modified glycoproteins that during embryogenesis controls multiple developmental processes [108, 109] and during adult life regulates tissue maintenance and remodeling [109, 110]. At the cellular level, Wnt signals coordinate changes in cellular metabolism favoring either a “quiescent metabolism” or a “proliferating metabolism” [109, 110]. This is why it is tempting to speculate that common alterations in metabolic programming may accompany embryonic and/or stem cell differentiation and these may also be involved in adult tissue development and/or remodeling [109].

Moreover, synthesis and deposition of extracellular matrix are key features of fibroblasts [111]. Components of the extracellular matrix, including fibronectin, laminin and collagen are essential regulators of cell migration, adhesion and polarity during both normal vertebrate development [112] and the progression of diseases, such as age-related diseases [113]. It has been suggested that the extracellular matrix network should be present during zebrafish gastrulation and that this network should be positioned to affect, at a minimum, the polarized behavior of mesodermal cells [112]. Furthermore, age-related changes in cell behavior and morphology of fibroblasts appear to be linked to alterations [113]. In chronically inflamed tissues there is increasing evidence to suggest that aberrant expression of extracellular matrix molecules and fragments of the extracellular matrix that are derived from tissue-remodeling processes can influence immune cell activation, differentiation and survival [22].

CHRONIC LOW-GRADE METABOLIC INFLAMMATION-RELATED EVO-DEVO: THE ATTEMPT TO INTEGRATE THE AMNION-VITELLOGENIC-GASTRULATION PHENOTYPES

Today, evo-devo research is characterized by a dialectical approach that, on the one hand, looks at how developmental systems have evolved and, on the other hand, probes the consequences of these historically established systems for organism evolution [114]. A further question is how evolutionary developmental interactions relate to environmental conditions [114]. In this context, it could be hypothesized that, since inflammation is a hypothetical re-capitulator response of the fundamental mechanisms that govern the phylogeny and the ontogeny, it would constitute a useful tool of nature to integrate both processes (Fig. **4**).

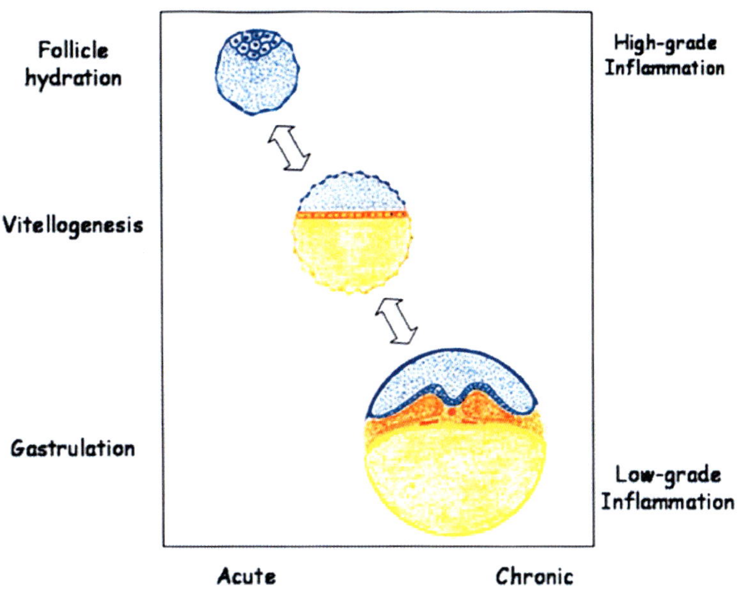

Figure 4: Diagram showing the hypothetical correlation between follicle hydration, vitellogenesis and gastrulation and the different types of the inflammatory response, depending of time (acute or chronic) and degree (high- or low-grade).

The inflammatory response, because of its supposed ability to recreate primitive or ancestral evolutive states of animal life, could also exploit the possibility to induce genetic and epigenetic regulations to create a new developmental context in accordance with today's environmental factors. In this way, under the inflammatory influence, chromatin can not only undergo changes in its conformation in response to various cellular metabolic demands [115], but can also undergo epigenetic regulation, in which case, the same genotype can produce different phenotypes in response to the actually external conditions [114, 115].

In addition, through the recovery of ancient evolutive phenotypes during the inflammatory response, the body could have the chance of choosing the most appropriate phenotype to survive according to the harmful circumstances that fall upon it. The equivalent pathological response of a population could be explained by this mechanism when similar harmful factors fall upon it, such as chronic psychosocial stress, sedentary style of life, a westernized diet, alcohol intake or smoking. In this way, it could be considered that the metabolic syndrome, which due to nuclear underlying pathophysiological processes leading to its development, and the confusion between the conceptual definitions, continues to be a source of medical controversy [116].

The metabolic syndrome refers to the clustering of cardiovascular risk factors that include dyslipidemia, obesity, diabetes and hypertension [116, 117]. However, youths that are overweight and obesity in youth is also a worldwide public health problem. Overweight and obesity in childhood and adolescents affects many systems, resulting in clinical conditions such as metabolic syndrome, early atherosclerosis, dyslipidemia, type-2 diabetes and hypertension [118, 119]. Due to the high incidence of this complex syndrome, both among children and adolescents as well as in aging people, it has been proposed that this disease spreads like an epidemic and, therefore it indeed must be scrutinized for an infectious cause [120] (Fig. **5**).

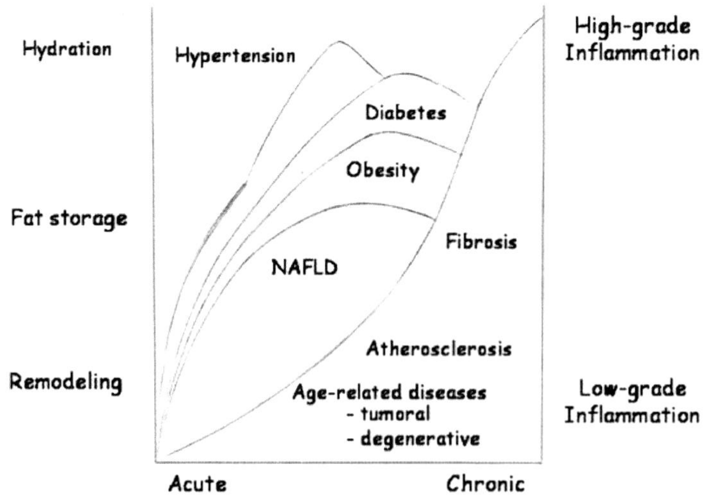

Figure 5: Hypothetical distribution of the diverse conditions integrated in the metabolic syndrome in the westernized populations

Furthermore obesity may exaggerate the inflammatory response to stressors [121] and there is also a robust association between metabolic syndrome, obesity, NAFLD and encephalopathy-associated depression [13, 121]. The inflammatory mediators have the capacity to induce depression, sleep and appetite disturbances and fatigue, which characterize depression, and they are part of a cytokine-triggered syndrome termed "sickness behavior", that also occurs when an organism has a wound or an infection [51, 121].

In turn, this vicious cycle, that seems to be generated around inflammation, seems to close when it is assumed that the psychophysiological stress- originating from the masterfully created human mind with biological, social, behavioral, psychological, transcendental and religious components- is a risk factor for cardiovascular and metabolic diseases [122]. In this way, it has been suggested that inflammation could be a psychophysiological biomarker in chronic psychosocial stress, generated by example by low socioeconomic status, job stress/burnout, childhood adversity and life event stress, caregiver stress and loneliness [123]. In this way, the individual with an inflammatory pathology secondary to the conditions of life imposed upon him by the Western society could be considered an "*inflammacitizen*". If so, it is possible that the Society, composed of these people sensitized by inflammation, cannot avoid their modulator influence. Particularly, obesity is considered from a global population perspective as an epidemic condition [124].

Chronic low-grade inflammation, also named metabolic inflammation or "metaflammation" [60] is believed to be a key pathogenic mechanism of several metabolic disorders including metabolic syndrome and their related diseases mentioned above [50, 59]. The metabolic inflammation hypothesis has gained popularity with the demonstration of the central involvement of the stress-activated protein kinases JNK1 and IKKβ in their pathogenesis [48, 50]. These enzymatic complexes in turn are situated at the focal points of different signaling pathways involved in innate immunity, inflammation and stress [50].

Nonetheless, the association of diseases shared by the same key pathogenic mechanism, *i.e.* inflammation, in the metabolic syndrome, could be also the result of the tissue, organic and systemic recapitulation of ancestral phylogenic ontogenic mechanisms. Through the expression of old mechanisms regulating: 1. the interstitial hydroelectrolytic distribution with cell hydration; 2. vitellogenesis related to the acute-phase-response and 3. gastrulation with mesenchymal remodeling, the basic physiopathological mechanisms leading to the development of different conditions would be established in the animal body (Fig. **4**). In addition, the expression of these three pathological phenotypes could be distributed between all the individuals that constitute the westernized society depending on their genetic polymorphism. If so, these three basic mechanisms could be related with the development of the different conditions associated with the metabolic syndrome, such as hypertension, type 2 diabetes, dyslipidemia, NAFLD, sickness behavior, depression, atherosclerosis, and aging-related diseases, *i.e.* profibrotic degenerative and tumoral diseases (Fig. **5**).

In this context, the use of inflammation by the body could represent the camouflaged expression of efficient mechanisms of evolution and development that would allow survival although the drastic environmental conditions are imposed upon it. Maybe this is the reason that the body attempts to inhibit certain types of the inflammatory response, particularly when chronic, are very difficult or unsuccessful, since their mechanisms would take root in their own mechanisms of adaptive survival.

If the different types of inflammatory response, both acute and chronic, marking the life of human beings, integrate evolutive ancestral mechanisms, it could also be considered that through research we could "trace" the biochemical origins of our life, as if we were carrying out an archaeological dig. On the contrary, we could ask ourselves with respect to the role that inflammation could play in our future evolution. Since the final objective of this amazing response always seems to be a remodeling of the organism in harmony with the correlative environmental conditions, which are partially modulated by the human being, we are indeed sculpting the future of our species.

It is most likely that this set of diseases suffered by our Western society represents the distribution of the abovementioned phenotypes among those individuals who form part of this society. In this case, it should be considered that this set of diseases would represent a true "Social Inflammatory Syndrome". This hypothetical social approach of the inflammatory response would imply the existence of individual groups who suffer a similar pathology, and at the same time, this common pathological characteristic would define them as true pathological bodies of the society they belong to. Therefore, the set of pathologies considered, if grouped based on the different and hypothetical phylogenic or ontogenic phenotype expressed (*i.e.* hypertensive, arterial, pulmonary or portal pathology with sodium and water retention, oxidative stress, increased hydrostatic pressure and hemodynamic alterations; lipoprotein related pathology with hyperinsulinemia, due to resistance to insulin, dyslipidemia, enzymatic stress, obesity, NAFLD and early atherosclerosis; and age-related pathology with profibrotic alterations, degenerative stress and tumoral pathology) would represent three pathological phenotypes that integrate, in turn, a social body with a great transforming capacity potential of the society they make up.

Overall, these supposed social groups, through the expression of different inflammatory phenotypes, would integrate a megaorganism that would possess a great biotransforming capacity. At the same time, the distribution of different inflammatory phenotypes among individuals that make up a natural grouping could be a good system for their social integration. Therefore, this hypothesis could possibly facilitate a future demonstration of the real role that the individuals, differentiated due to their *"modus vivendi",* have in social organisms. This social pro-inflammatory behavior would therefore imply the activation of stressful and archaic activity directed at the excessive and competitive obtaining of specific trophic supports that favor a lipid metabolism and megaorganism proliferation. In essence, the behavior of this occidental megaorganism would be similar to that of a tumor that uses the inflammatory response in order to survive, which is its priority [18, 19]. This egoistic behavior of Western societies would be similar to malignant tumors since they impoverish and induce cachexia in the environment in which they live, they distance themselves from their potential competitors and, like tumoral metastasis they invade new territories.

Lastly, if the different types of the inflammatory response, both acute and chronic, that mark the life of the human beings, integrate ancestral evolutive mechanisms, it is possible that through careful and intentional research, we could trace the biochemical origins of life. In this sense, perhaps inflammation represents an archaeological tool of unsuspected usefulness. On the contrary, we could also ask ourselves in terms of the role that inflammation could be playing regarding our future evolution as an animal species. Since the final objective of this amazing response seems to be to make the organism survive, whether individual or socially, in harmony with the correlative environmental conditions, perhaps we could try to foresee our immediate future if we were able to discover the laws that govern the predominating expression of the different phenotypes composing the inflammatory response.

ACKNOWLEDGEMENTS

We would like to thank Maria Elena Vicente for preparing the manuscript, Elizabeth Mascola for translating it into English and librarians of Complutense University Medical School, particularly the Director, Francisco Javier Jorge García-Reyes, and Manuela Crego and María José Valdemoro and B. Braun Surgical S.A. for their technical assistance.

This study was carried out in part with grants from Mutua Madrileña Research Foundation (Ref. nº PA 3077/2008 and AP5966/2009), MICINN PSI2010-19348 and with the special collaboration of the INEUROPA (Instituto de Neurociencias del Principado de Asturias).

CONFLICT OF INTEREST

The author(s) confirm that this chapter content has no conflict of interest.

REFERENCES

[1] Medzhitov R. Origin and physiological roles of inflammation. Nature 2008; 454: 428-35.
[2] Smale ST. Selective transcription in response to an inflammatory stimulus. Cell 2010; 140: 833-44.
[3] Franceschi, C., Bonafe, M., Valensin, S., *et al.* Inflamm-aging. An evolutionary perspective on immunosenescence. Ann N Y Acad Sci 2000; 908: 244-254.
[4] Franceschi, C., Capri, M., Monti, D., *et al.* Inflammaging and anti-inflamming: A systemic perspective on aging and longevity emerged from studies in humans. Mech Ageing Dev 2007; 128: 92-105.
[5] Goto, M. Inflammaging (inflammation + aging): A driving force for human aging based on an evolutionarily antagonistic pleiotropy theory? Biosci Trends 2008; 2: 218-230.

[6] Caruso, C., Lio, D., Cavallone, L., Franceschi, C. Aging, longevity, inflammation and cancer. Ann N Y Acad Sci 2004; 1028: 1-13.
[7] Bürkle, A., Caselli, G., Franceschi, C., *et al.* Pathophysiology of ageing, longevity and age related diseases. Immun Aging 2007; 4: 4.
[8] Aller, M.A., Arias, J.L., Nava, M.P., Arias, J. Post-traumatic inflammation is a complex response based on the pathological expression of the nervous, immune, and endocrine functional systems. Exp Biol Med (Maywood) 2004a; 229: 170-181.
[9] Nathan, C., Ding, A. Non resolving inflammation. Cell 2010; 140: 871-882.
[10] Aller, M.A., Arias, J.L., Sanchez-Patan, F., Arias, J. The inflammatory response: An efficient way of life. Med Sci Monit 2006; 12: RA225-234.
[11] Aller, M.A., Arias, J.I., Arias, J. Pathological axes of wound repair: Gastrulation revisited. Theor Biol Med Model 2010; 7: 37.
[12] Selman, M., Pardo, A., Kaminski, N. Idiopathic pulmonary fibrosis: Aberrant recapitulation of developmental programs? Plos Medicine 2008; 5: e62.
[13] Aller, M.A., Arias, J.L., Arias, J.I., Sanchez-Patan, F., Arias, J. The inflammatory response recapitulates phylogeny through trophic mechanisms to the injured tissue. Med Hypotheses 2007; 68: 202-209.
[14] Aller, M.A., Arias, J.I., Alonso-Poza, A., Arias, J. A review of metabolic staging in severely injured patients. Scand J Trauma Resusc Emerg Med 2010; 17: 18-27.
[15] Cone, J.B. Inflammation. Am J Surg 2001; 182: 558-562.
[16] Aller, M.A., Arias, J.L., Arias, J. Post-traumatic inflammatory response: perhaps a sucesión of phases with a nutricional purpose. Med Hypotheses 2004b; 63: 42-46.
[17] Arias, J.I., Aller, M.A., Arias, J. Surgical inflammation: a pathophysiological rainbow. J Transl Med 2009; 7: 19.
[18] Arias, J.I., Aller, M.A., Arias, J. The use of inflammation by tumor cells. Cancer 2005; 104: 223-228.
[19] Arias, J.I., Aller, M.A., Arias, J. Cancer cell: using inflammation to invade the host. Mol Cancer 2007; 6: 29.
[20] Raymond, J., Segre, D. The effect of oxygen on biochemical networks and the evolution of complex life. Science 2006; 311: 1764-1767.
[21] Acquisti, C., Klefe, J., Collins, S. Oxygen content of transmembrane proteins over macroevolutionary time scales. Nature 2007; 445: 47-52.
[22] Sorokin, L. The impact of the extracellular matrix on inflammation. Nature Rev Immunol 2010; 10: 712-723.
[23] Rhodes, J.M., Simons, M. The extracellular matrix and blood vessels formation: not just a scaffold. J Cell Mol Med 2007; 11: 176-205.
[24] Dhar, A., Ray, A. The CCN family proteins in carcinogenesis. Exp Oncol 2010; 32: 2-9.
[25] Hynes, R.O., Zhao, Q. The evolution of cell adhesion. J Cell Biol 2000; 150: F89-F96.
[26] Telfer, W.H. Egg formation in Lepidoptera. J Insect Sci 2009; 9: 1-21.
[27] Baltz, J.M., Tartia, A.P. Cell volume regulation in oocytes and early embryos: connecting physiology to successful culture media. Hum Reprod Update 2010; 16: 166-176.
[28] Lubzens, E., Young, G., Bobe, J., Cerda, J. Oogenesis in teleosts: How fish eggs are formed. Gen Comp Endrocrinol 2010; 165: 367-389.
[29] Skoblina, M.N. Hydration of oocytes in bony-fishes. Ontogene 2010; 41: 5-18.
[30] Jiang, D., Liang, J., Noble, P.W. Hyaluronan in tissue injury and repair. Ann Rev Cell Dev Biol 2007; 23: 435-461.

[31] Chen, B., Fu, B. A model for charged molecule transport in the interstitial space. Conf Proc IEEE Eng Med Biol Sci 2005; 1: 55-58.

[32] Arukwe, A., Goksϕyr, A. Eggshell and egg yolk proteins in fish: hepatic proteins for the next generation: oogenetic, population, and evolutionary implications of endocrine disruption. Comp Hepatol 2003; 2: 4.

[33] Muta, T., Iwanaga, S. The role of hemolymph coagulation in innate immunity. Curr Opin Immunol 1996; 8: 41-47.

[34] Dushay, M.S. Insect hemolymph clotting. Cell Mol Life Sci 2009; 66: 2643-2650.

[35] Jin, S-W., Patterson, C. The opening act. Vasculogenesis and the origins of circulation. Arterioscler. Tromb Vasc Biol 2009; 29: 623-629.

[36] Wasserthal, L.T. *Drosophila* flies combine periodic heartbeat reversal with circulation in the anterior body mediated by a newly discovered anterior pair of ostial valves and "venous" channels. J Exp Biol 2007; 210: 3707-3719.

[37] Gabay, C., Kushner, I. Acute-phase proteins and other systemic responses to inflammation. N Engl J Med 1999; 340: 448-454.

[38] Tufail, M., Takeda, M. Molecular characteristics of insect vitellogenins. J Insect Physiol 2008; 54: 1447-1458.

[39] Münch, D., Amdam, G.V. The curious case of aging plasticity in honey bees. FEBS Lett 2010; 584: 2496-503

[40] Davis, R.A. Evolution of processes and regulators of lipoprotein synthesis: from birds to mammals. J Nutr 1997; 127: 7955-8005.

[41] Sniderman, A., Couture, P., De Graaf, J. Diagnosis and treatment of apolipoprotein B dyslipoproteinemias. Nat Rev Endocrinol. 2010; 6: 335-46.

[42] Natarajan, P., Ray, K.K., Cannon, C.P. High-density lipoprotein and coronary heart disease. J Am Coll Cardiol 2010; 55: 1283-1289.

[43] Targher, G., Day, C.P., Bonora, E. Risk of cardiovascular disease in patients with nonalcoholic fatty liver disease. N Engl J Med 2010; 363: 1341-1350.

[44] Tarantino, G., Savastano, S., Colao, A. Hepatic steatosis, low-grade chronic inflammation and hormone/growth factor/adipokine imbalance. World J Gastroenterol 2010; 16: 4773-4783.

[45] Cray, C., Zaias, J., Altman, N.H. Acute phase response in animals: A review. Comp Med 2009; 59: 517-526.

[46] Kopf, M., Bachmann, M.F., Marsland, B.J. Averting inflammation by targeting the cytokine environment. Nature Rev Drug Discov 2010; 9: 703-718.

[47] Jahangiri, A. High-density lipoprotein and the acute phase response. Curr Opin Endrocrinol Diabetes Obes 2010; 17: 156-160.

[48] Czaja, M.J. JNK regulation of hepatic manifestation of the metabolic syndrome. Trends Endocrinol Metab 2010; 21:707-13.

[49] Marsland, A.L., McCaffery, J.M., Muldoon, M.F., Manuck, S.B. Systemic inflammation and the metabolic syndrome among middle-aged community volunteers. Metabolism. 2010; 59:1801-8.

[50] Solinas, G., Karin, M. JNK1 and IKKβ: molecular links between obesity and metabolic dysfunction. FASEB J 2010; 24: 2596-2609.`

[51] Wager-Smith, K., Markou, A. Depression: A repair response to stress-induced neuronal microdamage that can grade into a chronic neuroinflammatory condition? Neurosci Biobehav Rev 2010; 35:742-64.

[52] Sparks, J.D., Cianci, J., Jokinen, J., Chen, L.S., Sparks, C.E. Interleukin-6 mediates hepatic hypersecretion of apolipodrotein B. Am J Physiol Gastrointest Liver Physiol 2010; 299: G980-G989.

[53] Van der Westhuyzen, D.R., De Beer, F.C., Webb, N.R. HDL cholesterol transport during inflammation. Curr Opin Lipidol 2007; 18: 147-151.

[54] Gilliver, S.C. Sex steroids as inflammatory regulators. J Steroid Biochem Mol Biol 2010; 120: 105-115.

[55] Whaley-Connell, A., Johnson, M.S., Sowers, J.R. Aldosterone: Role in the cardiometabolic syndrome and resistant hypertension. Prog Cardiovasc Dis 2010; 52: 401-409.

[56] Sturmey, R.G., Reis, A., Leese, H.J., McEvory, T.G. Role of fatty acids in energy provision during oocyte maturation and early embryo development. Reprod Domest Anim 2009; 44: 50-58.

[57] Dumollard, R., Carroll, J., Duchen, M.R., Campbell, K., Swann, K. Mitochondrial function and redox state in mammalian embryos. Semin Cell Dev Biol 2009; 20: 346-353.

[58] Vander Heiden, M.G., Cantley, L.C., Thompsson, C.B. Understanding the Warburg effect: The metabolic requirements of cell proliferation. Science 2009; 324: 1029-1033.

[59] Hummasti, S., Hotamisli̇gil, G.S. Endoplasmic reticulum stress and inflammation in obesity and diabetes. Circ Res 2010; 107: 579-591.

[60] Hotamisligil, G.S. Inflammation and metabolic disorders. Nature 2006; 444: 860-867.

[61] Bayne, C.J., Gerwick, L. The acute phase response and innate immunity of fish. Dev Comp Immunol 2001; 25: 725-743.

[62] Bottazzi, B., Garlanda, C., Salvatori, G., Jeannin, P., Manfredi, A., Mantovani, A. Pentraxins as a key component of innate immunity. Curr Opin Immunol 2010; 18: 10-15.

[63] Martinez de la Torre, Y., Fabbri, M., Jaillon, S., *et al.* Evolution of the pentraxin family: the new entry PTX4. J Immunol 2010; 184: 5055-5064.

[64] Litvack, M.L., Palaniyar, N. Soluble innate immune pattern-recognition proteins for clearing dying cells and cellular components: implications on exacerbating or resolving inflammation. Innate Immun 2010; 16: 191-200.

[65] Castaño, A.P., Lin, S-L., Surowy, T., *et al.* Serum amyloid P inhibits fibrosis through FcγR-dependent monocyte-macrophage regulation *in vivo*. Sci Transl Med 2009; 1: 1-11.

[66] Inforzato, A., Rivieccio, V., Morreale, A.P., *et al.* Structural characterization of PTX3 disulfide bond network and its multimeric status in cumulus matrix organization. J Biol Chem 2008; 283: 10147-10161.

[67] Cillo, F., Brevini, T.A.L., Antonini, S., Paffoni, A., Ragni, G., Gandolfi, F. Association between human oocyte developmental competente and expression levels of some cumulus genes. Reproduction 2007; 134: 645-650.

[68] Pisani, L.F., Antonini, S., Pocar, P., *et al.* Effects of pre-mating nutrition on mRNA levels of developmentally relevant genes in sheep/oocytes and granulosa cells. Reproduction 2008; 136: 303-312.

[69] Scarchilli, L., Camaioni, A., Bottazzi, B., *et al.* PTX3 interacts with Inter-α-trypsin inhibitor. Implications for hyaluronan organization and cumulus oophorous expansion. J Biol Chem 2007; 282: 30161-30170.

[70] Deban, L., Jaillon, S., Garlanda, C., Bottazzi, B., Mantovani, A. Pentraxis in innate immunity: lessons from PTX3. Cell Tissue Res. 2010; 343: 237-49.

[71] Rusnati, M., Camozzi, M., Moroni, E., *et al.* Selective recognition of fibroblast growth factor-2 by the long pentraxin PTX3 inhibits angiogenesis. Blood 2004; 104: 92-99.

[72] Leali, D., Alessi, P., Coltrini, D., Rusnati, M., Zetta, L., Presta, M. Fibroblast growth factor-2 antagonist and antiangiogenic activity of long-pentraxin 3-derived synthetic peptides. Curr Pharm Des 2009; 15: 3577-3589.

[73] Muszbek, L., Bereczky, Z., Bagoly, Z., Shemirani, A.H., Katona, E. Factor XIII and atherothrombotic diseases. Semin Thromb Hemost 2010; 36: 18-33.

[74] Crivellato, E., Ribatti, D. The mast cell: an evolutionary perspective. Biol Rev 2010; 85: 347-360.

[75] Galli, S.J., Kalesnikoff, J., Grimbaldeston, M.A., Piliponsky, A.M., Williams, C.M.M., Tsai, M. Mast cells as "tunable" effector and immunoregulatory cells: Recent advances Ann Rev Immunol 2005; 23: 749-786.

[76] Bachelet, I., Levi-Schaffer, F. Mast cells as effector cells, a costimulating question. Trends Immunol 2007; 28: 360-365.

[77] Hu, Z-Q., Zhao, W-H., Shimamura, T. Regulation of mast cell development by inflammatory factors. Curr Top Med Chem 2007; 14: 3044-3050.

[78] Molmenti, E.P., Ziambaras, T., Perlmutter, D.H. Evidence for an acute phase response in human intestinal epithelial cells. J Biol Chem 1993; 288: 14116-14124.

[79] Wang, Q., Wang, J.J., Boyce, S., Fischer, J., Hasseigren, P.O. Edotoxemia and IL-1β stimulate mucosal IL-6 production in different parts of the gastrointestinal tract. J Surg Res 1998; 76: 27-31.

[80] Pritts, T., Hungness, E., Wang, Q., Robb, B., Hershko, D., Hasselgren, P-O. Mucosal and enterocyte IL-6 production during sepsis and endotoxemia-role of transcription factors and regulation by the stress response. Am J Surg 2002; 183: 372-383.

[81] Tilg, H. The role of cytokines in non-alcoholic fatty liver disease. Dig Dis 2010; 28: 179-185.

[82] Bui, Q.T., Prempeh, M., Wilensk, R.L. Atherosclerotic plaque development. Int J Biochem Cel Biol 2009; 41: 2109-2113.

[83] Yeong, P., Ning, Y., Xu, Y., Li, X., Yin, L. Tryptase promotes human monocyte-derived macrophage from cell formation by suppressing LXRα activation. Biochem Biophys Acta 2010; 1801: 567-576.

[84] Poglio, S., De Toni-Costes, F., Arnaud, E., Laharrague P, Espinosa E, Casteilla L, Cousin B. Adipose tissue as a dedicated reservoir of functional mast cell progenitors. Stem Cell Stem Cells. 2010; 28: 2065-72.

[85] Fukunaga, M., Nunomura, S., Nishida, S., *et al.* Mast cell death induced by 24(S), 25-epoxycholesterol. Exp Cell Res 2010; 316: 3272-3281.

[86] Gutierrez E, Wiggins D, Fielding B, Gould AP. Specialized hepatocyte-like cells regulate Drosophila lipid metabolism. Nature 2007; 445:275-80.

[87] Gould, A.P., Elstob, P.R., Brodu, V. Insect oenocytes: a model system for studying cell-fate specification by Hox genes. J Anat 2001; 199: 25-33.

[88] Schlegel, A., Stainier, D.Y.R. Lessons from "lower" organisms: What worms, flies and zebrafish can teach us about human energy metabolism. Plos Genet 2007; 3: e199.

[89] Pospisilik, J.A., Schramek, D., Schnidar, H., *et al. Drosophila* genome-wide obesity screen reveals hedgehog as a determinant of brown *versus* white adipose cell fate. Cell 2010; 140: 148-160.

[90] Paris, M., Laudet, V. The history of a developmental stage: Metamorphosis in chordates. Genesis 2008; 46: 657-672.

[91] Aller, M.A., Arias, J.L., Nava, M.P., Arias, J. Evolutive trophic phases of the systemic acute inflammatory response, oxygen use mechanisms and metamorphosis. Psicothema 2004c; 16: 369-372.

[92] Agarwal, A.K., Auchus, R.J. Minireview: Cellular redox state regulates hydroxysteroid dehydrogenase activity and intracellular hormone potency. Endocrinology 2005; 146: 2531-2538.

[93] Ghosh, S., Hayden, M.S. New regulators of NF-κB in inflammation. Nature Rev 2008; 8: 837-849

[94] Serhan, C.N., Brain, S.D., Buckley, C.D., *et al.* Resolution of inflammation: state of the art, definitions and terms. FASEB J 2007; 21: 325-332.

[95] Lawrence, T., Gilroy, D.W. Chronic inflammation: a failure of resolution? Int J Exp Path 2007; 88: 85-94.

[96] Buchanan, E.P., Longaker, M.T., Lorenz, H.P. Fetal skin wound healing. Adv Clin Chem 2009; 48: 137-161.

[97] Mikawa, T., Poh, A.M., Kelly, K.A., Ishii, Y., Reese, D.E. Induction and patterning of the primitive streak, and organizing center of gastrulation in the amniote. Develop Dynamics 2004; 229: 422-432.

[98] Elinson, R.P., Beckham, Y. Development in frogs with large eggs and the origin of amniotes. Zoology 2002; 105: 105-117.

[99] Bellini, C., Boccardo, F., Bonioli, E., Campisi, C. Lymphodynamics in the fetos and newborn. Lymphology 2006; 39: 110-117.

[100] Chang, Y.J., Hwang, S.M., Tseng, C.P., *et al.* Isolation of mesenchymal stem cells with neurogenic potentials from the mesoderm of the amniotic membrane. Cells Tissues Organs 2010; 192: 93-105.

[101] De Miguel, M.P., Arnalich-Montiel, F., Lopez-Iglesias, P., Blázquez-Martinez, A., Nistal, M. Epiblast-derived stem cells in embryonic and adult tissue. Int J Dev Biol 2009; 53: 1529-1540.

[102] Acloque, H., Adams, M.S., Fishwick, K., Bronner-Fraser, M., Nieto, M.A. Epithelial-mesenchymal transitions: the importance of changing cell state in development and disease. J Clin Invest 2009; 119: 1438-1449.

[103] Feng, B., Chen, L. Review of mesenchymal stem cells and tumors: Executioner or conspirator? Cancer Biother Radiopharm 2009; 24: 717-721.

[104] Kalluri, R., Neilson, *E.G.* Epithelial-mesenchymal transition and its implications for fibrosis. J Clin Invest 2003; 112: 1776-1782.

[105] Kragl, M., Knapp, D., Nacu, E., *et al.* Cells keep a memory of their tissue origin during axo to limb regeneration. Nature 2009; 460: 60-65.

[106] Zuba-Surma, E.K., Kucia, M., Ratajczak, J., Ratajczak, M.Z. "Small stem cells" in adult tissues: very small embryonic-like stem cells (VSELs) stand up. Cytometry 2010; 75: 4-13.

[107] Kuroda, Y., Kitada, M., Wakao, S., *et al.* Unique multipotent cells in adult human mesenchymal cell populations. PNAS 2010; 107: 8639-8643.

[108] Roszko, I., Sawada, A., Solnica-Krezel, L. Regulation of convergent and extension movements during vertebrate gastrulation by the Wnt/PCP pathway. Semin Cell Develop 2009; 20: 986-997.

[109] Sethi, J.K., Vidal-Puig, A. Wnt signalling and the control of cellular metabolism. Biochem J 2010; 427: 1-17.

[110] Li, L., Clevers, H. Coexistance of quiescent and active adult stem cells in mammals. Science 2010; 327: 542-545.

[111] Krenning, G., Zeisberg, E.M., Kalluri, R. The origin of fibroblasts and mechanism of cardiac fibrosis. J Cell Physiol 2010; 225: 631-637.

[112] Latimer, A., Jessen, J.R. Extracellular matrix assembly and organization during zebrafish gastrulation. Matrix Biol 2010; 29: 89-96.

[113] Wolfson, M., Budovsky, A., Tacutu, R., Fraifeld, V. The signaling hubs at the cross road of longevity and age-related disease networks. Int J Biochem Cell Biol 2009; 41: 516-520.

[114] Muller, G.B. Evo-devo: extending the evolutionary synthesis. Nature Rev Genet 2007; 8: 943-949.

[115] Choudhuri, S., Cui, Y., Klaassen, C.D. Molecular targets of epigenetic regulation and effectors of environmental influences. Toxicol Appl Pharmacol 2010; 245: 378-393.

[116] Duvnjak, L., Duvnjak, M. The metabolic syndrome-An ongoing story. J Physiol Pharmacol 2009; 60: 19-24.

[117] Grundy SM, Adams-Huet B, Vega GL.Variable contributions of fat content and distribution to metabolic syndrome risk factors. Metab Syndr Relat Disord 2008; 6:281-8.

[118] Halpern, A., Mancini, M.C., Magalhães, M.E., *et al.* Metabolic syndrome, dyslipidemia, hypertension and type 2 diabetes in youth: from diagnosis to treatment. Diabetol Metab Syndr. 2010; 2: 55.

[119] Blüher, M. Fat tissue and long life. Obesity Facts 2008; 1: 176-182.

[120] Nathan, C. Epidemic inflammation: Pondering obesity. Mol Med 2008; 14: 485-492.

[121] Kiecolt-Glaser, J.K., Gouin, J.P., Hantsoo, L. Close relationships, inflammation and death. Neurosci Biobehav Rev 2010; 35: 33-38.

[122] Hamer, M., Malan, L. Psychophysiological risk markers of cardiovascular disease. Neurosci Biobehav Rev 2010; 35: 76-83.

[123] Hänsel, A., Hong, S., Camara, R.J.A., Von Kämel, R. Inflammation as a psychophysiological biomarker in chronic psychosocial stress. Neurosci Biobehav Rev 2010; 35: 115-121.

[124] Hansen CH, Gilman AP, Odland JO. Is thermogenesis a significant causal factor in preventing the "globesity" epidemic? Med Hypotheses 2010;75: 250-6.

Send Orders for Reprints to reprints@benthamscience.net
Surgical Inflammation, 2013, 309-343

CHAPTER 11

Experimental Models of Surgical Inflammation

Maria-Angeles Aller[1], Natalia de las Heras[2], Natalia Arias[3], Isabel Prieto[4], Laureano Lorente[1], Maria-Paz Nava[5], Luis Santamaria[6], Jorge-Luis Arias[2], Vicente Lahera[2] and Jaime Arias[1,*]

[1]Department of Surgery, School of Medicine, Complutense University of Madrid, Madrid, Spain; [2]Physiology Department, School of Medicine, Complutense University of Madrid, Madrid, Spain; [3]Neurosciences Laboratory, Department of Psychobiology, School of Psychology, University of Oviedo, Oviedo, Asturias, Spain; [4]Department of Surgery, La Paz Hospital, Autonoma University of Madrid, Madrid, Spain; [5]Physiology Department (Animal Physiology II), Biology School, Complutense University of Madrid, Spain and [6]Cellular Biology and Morphological Sciences Department, School of Medicine, Autonoma University of Madrid, Madrid, Spain

Abstract: Prehepatic portal hypertension induces a splanchnic low-grade inflammatory response that could switch to high-grade inflammation with the development of severe and life-threatening complications when associated with chronic liver disease. The extraembryonic origin of the portal system may determine the regression to an extraembryonic phenotype *i.e.*, vitellogenic and amniotic, during the evolution of both types of portal hypertension. Thus prehepatic portal hypertension, or compensated hypertension by portal vein ligation in the rat, is associated with molecular mechanisms related to vitellogenesis, where hepatic steatosis and splanchnic angiogenesis stand out. In turn, extrahepatic cholestasis in the rat induces intrahepatic portal hypertension, or decompensated hypertension, with ascites and hepatorenal syndrome. The splanchnic interstitium, the mesenteric lymphatic system, and the peritoneal mesothelium seem to create an inflammatory pathway that could have a key pathophysiological relevance in the production of ascites. The hypothetical comparison between the ascitic and the amniotic fluid also allows for translational investigation. The induced regression of the splanchnic system to extraembryonic functions by portal hypertension highlights the great relevance of the extraembryonic structures even during post-natal life.

Keywords: Portal hypertension, microsurgery, extrahepatic cholestasis, ascites, mini-brain, high grade inflammation, fetal development, amniotic fluid, lymph flow, hepatic steatosis, mast cell, splanchnic system.

***Address correspondence to Jaime Arias:** Department of Surgery, School of Medicine, Complutense University, Ramón y Cajal Square, 28040 MADRID, Spain; Tel: +34 91 394 1389; Fax: +34 913947115; E-mail: jariasp@med.ucm.es

INTRODUCTION

Portal hypertension is defined as a pathological increase in portal vein pressure and it is diagnosed when the hepatic venous pressure gradient is above the normal range [1]. It has been proposed that low-grade inflammation related to portal hypertension switches to high-grade inflammation with the development of severe and life-threatening complications when associated with chronic liver disease [2].

It could be considered that the underlying central theme in low-grade portal hypertensive inflammation is the disturbance in splanchnic and systemic hemodynamics [1, 2]. This splanchnic and systemic hemodynamic response would be aggravated during the progression of the chronic liver disease [2, 3]. Thus a critical state is produced in which the appearance of noxious factors during the progressive evolution of chronic liver disease would favor the development of a high-grade splanchnic and systemic inflammatory response [2, 4,5].

The portal system includes all veins which carry blood from the abdominal part of the alimentary tract, the spleen, pancreas and gallbladder [6]. This venous system transports the splanchnic venous flow through the portal vein to the liver [1, 6]. The afferent venous circulation of the liver as well as its efferent venous system, *i.e.*, the hepatic veins, derives from an extraembryonic venous system, the vitelline venous system, which transports blood from the yolk sac to the heart at the end of the 3rd week of gestation [7]. This extraembryonic origin of the portal system perhaps determines some of the pathological evolutive characteristics when it suffers hyper-pressure.

Hence it is important to keep in mind that a common characteristic of mammals is the development of extraembryonic supporting tissues and organs that are required for embryonic implantation, survival and development "in utero" [8]. Particularly, in the earliest stage of the embryonic development, the vitelline system as well as that of the amnion, stand out [7, 8] (Fig. **1**).

The portal system, derived from the extraembryonic vitelline venous system continues to perform a vital trophic role for post-natal organism survival and development, although based on its new metabolic needs [2, 7]. However, when the portal system suffers an aggression, *i.e.*, portal hypertension, perhaps a regression to the underlying or original embryonic functions could be induced by inflammatory mechanisms [9].

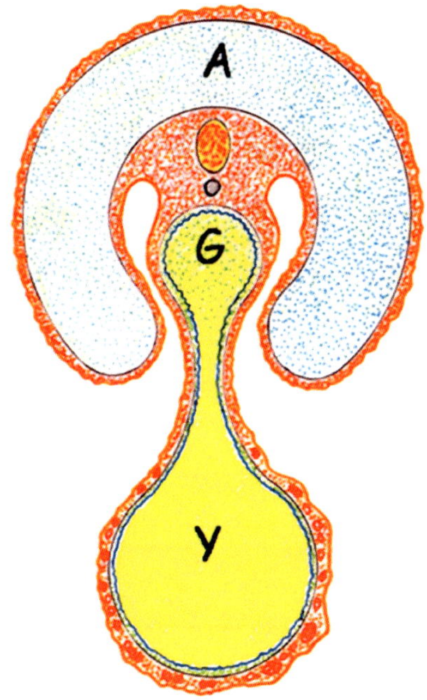

Figure 1: Schematic transverse representation of mammal embryo. The amniotic cavity surrounds the embryo and the amniotic fluid flows through the gut. The yolk sac is connected to the mid-gut by a narrow vitelline duct. Amniotic cavity; Y: yolk sac; G: gut.

LOW-GRADE INFLAMMATORY PORTAL HYPERTENSION: THE VITELLINE CONNECTION

Prehepatic portal hypertension by partial portal vein ligation in the rat induces a splanchnic and systemic chronic low-degree inflammatory response that could be developed through the expression of three successive and overlapping phenotypes: ischemia-reperfusion phenotype, immune phenotype and angiogenic phenotype [2, 3]. Thus, it has been already proposed that these phenotypes could represent the expression of trophic functional systems with increasing metabolic complexity [2, 10]. Therefore, in the portal hypertensive rat it could be considered that the body adapts the support, *i.e.*, the trophic system, to the metabolic needs characteristic of each inflammatory phenotype. In turn, the metabolic activity of each inflammatory phenotype would be determined by the mechanisms used for cellular energy production [9] (Table **1**).

The ischemia-reperfusion phenotype secondary to the hyperdynamic syndrome could represent oxidative and nitrosative stress with edema, which favors diffusion through the inflamed tissues and organs [2, 10]. Hyperdynamic circulation stands out among the splanchnic and systemic alterations related to portal hypertension [1, 11-15]. It has been suggested that the splanchnic and systemic vasodilation is the initial step leading to the hyperdynamic syndrome or progressive vasodilatory syndrome [12, 16]. Multiple organ failure in portal hypertensive chronic liver disease is in large part attributable to this syndrome [14, 16]. Furthermore, hyperdynamic circulation could favor the initiation and maintenance of an inflammatory response. First, the pathological increase of the portal pressure that occurs in the hyperdynamic splanchnic circulation could favor a disturbed splanchnic venous flow with shear stress mediated by non-laminar flow [12]. The disturbed or non-laminar flow with associated reciprocating low shear stress has profound effects on the biology of the vascular wall, particularly the vascular endothelium, and could stimulate inflammation [17, 18]. Second, both the increase in blood flow speed and the opening of arteriovenous shunts that induces the splanchnic hyperdynamic circulation would reduce oxygen tissue availability. This fact would produce tissue hypoxia and therefore chronicity of the inflammatory response [19].

It is widely understood that the gastrointestinal tract functions in a state of low-grade inflammation because of the constant exposure to potentially inflammatory stimuli [19]. Therefore, in portal hypertension hypoxia-related with disturbed intestinal blood flow could aggravate this low-grade inflammatory state, favoring the hyperactivation of hypoxia-inducible factor (HIF) and the IκB/nuclear factor (NF)-κB system, both endogenous alarm signals for the presence of mucosal gastrointestinal inflammatory disease [19]. In this way, the gastrointestinal tract often represents the source for the development of systemic inflammation with multiple organ dysfunctions [20, 21]. The association of mucosal hypoxia, splanchnic hyperemia and development of portal-systemic collaterals bypassing the liver in portal hypertension also suggests that the gastrointestinal tract could play a key role in the induction and maintenance of a low-grade inflammatory response [2, 3].

During the expression of the ischemia-reperfusion phenotype through the progression of the interstitial edema, the lymphatic circulation could be simultaneously activated. This circulatory switch increases mesenteric lymph flow and favors gut-derived factors that could reach the systemic circulation avoiding the liver filter [22, 23].

Since the evolutionary symbiosis between gut, *i.e.*, enteric nervous system considered as a "mini-brain" [24], and the Central Nervous System, it is possible to hypothesize the contributory role of altered bidirectional gut-brain neural, noradrenergic, cholinergic and nitrergic communications resulting from damaged intestinal mucosal integrity to the development of a systemic inflammatory response [25]. More recently, multiple studies have shown a potentially important neural pathogenic role in the portal hypertension-induced hyperdynamic circulation [1]. Vagal afferent nerves may be the signaling pathway from the hypertensive gastrointestinal tract to the central nervous system [26]. Also, although in portal hypertension there is a global overactivity of the adrenergic system, a splanchnic sympathetic nerve regression, which may contribute to aggravating splanchnic vasodilation, is produced [1].

It has been considered that homeostatic mechanisms attempt to correct the progressive hyperdynamic circulatory state of portal hypertension, including activation of the sympathetic nervous system and the renin-angiotensin-aldosterone system with renal sodium retention [27]. These homeostatic mechanisms seem to be complementary since increased sodium intake or retention can directly affect the excitability or responsiveness of the rostral ventrolateral medulla neurons to enhance sympathetic reflexes [28].

Hydration by sodium retention is a fundamental step of inflammation [29]. The increase of endothelial permeability in the tissues and organs that suffer inflammation causes interstitial edema [18]. This also allows the selective diffusion into the interstitial space of other circulating substances into the blood. Among those released as a response to the neuro-endocrine system to induced stress, in this case, by portal hypertension, the hypothalamic-pituitary-adrenal axis, the sympathetic-adrenal medullary or sympathetic nervous system and the renin-angiotensin-aldosterone system stand out [27]. This selectivity in the localization of the early inflammatory response that induces interstitial edema could also favor the posterior interstitial storage of substances derived from the acute phase response. In this way, the interstitial space is shaped from the start of the portal hypertensive pathology as the main field where the battle of inflammation takes place.

The expression of the immune phenotype by the splanchnic system which has suffered ischemia and/or reperfusion is coupled with interstitial infiltration by inflammatory cells and by bacteria [30-32]. It has been hypothesized that the symbiosis of inflammatory cells and bacteria for extracellular (fermentation) and intracellular (phagocytosis) could favor tissue trophism [2, 10]. Improper use of oxygen persists in this immune phase and it is associated with enzymatic stress. Compensation of the acute phase response includes the production of positive acute phase proteins that bind proteolytic enzymes and inhibitors of leukocyte and liposomal proteolytic enzymes [33, 34]. Likewise, the natural inhibitors of matrix metalloproteinases (TIMPs) could promote anti-enzymatic stress [3].

Portal hypertension is one factor determining bacterial intestinal translocation to mesenteric lymph nodes [30, 32]. In addition, the increased presence of mast cells in the hypertrophied mesenteric lymph nodes of prehepatic portal hypertensive rats [35, 36] would not only collaborate in the production of mesenteric adenitis, but also it would constitute a source of inflammatory mediators located between the intestine and systemic blood circulation [37, 38]. The mesenteric lymph nodes are key structures involved in the gut-associated lymphoid tissue (GALT) [39]. GALT constitutes the largest lymphatic organ in the body and has an important function in the maintenance of the intestinal mucosal integrity, as well as in the control of mucosal inflammation [40]. GALT activation in portal hypertensive enteropathy would produce the release of inflammatory mediators. Then these mediators would be transported by the intestinal lymph vessels to the systemic circulation aggravating the inflammatory response [9]. In different conditions related to intestinal ischemia, such as hemorrhagic shock or severe burns, mesenteric lymph node circulation has the priority over portal circulation for transporting inflammatory mediators released in the intestinal wall [41, 42]. This fact suggests that in other conditions that also produce intestinal hypoxia, like portal hypertension, the mesenteric lymph is a regional pro-inflammatory mediator vehicle, that is, a splanchnic one, but with a systemic effect [9, 10].

Prehepatic portal hypertension in the rat, both in the short-(1 month) and in the long-term (1 year) could produce hepatic accumulation of triglycerides and cholesterol [43-46]. The mechanisms by which portal hypertension could induce liver steatosis are not fully understood. Hepatic steatosis, as well as visceral adipose tissue, are metabolic risk factors in mesentery and omentum or visceral fat because their anatomical position drains the venous blood directly to the liver through the portal vein [47]. We speculate that these pathological strategies of the body inducing intra-abdominal fat deposits around the portal venous system could represent ontogenic reminiscences associated with the yolk sac development, or phylogenetical, related to vitellogenesis. In the first case, the liver and particularly the omentum can be thought of as the substitutes of the yolk sac, in which the animal carries out a pathological deposit of lipids. In this hypothetical situation through the expression of inflammatory mediators, *i.e.*, tumor necrosis factor (TNF)-α, IL-6, C-reactive protein and leptin [47] the liver and the omentum would be able to regress to evolutive phases in which the metabolic characteristics were suitable [2]. In the second way, and from an ancestral perspective, the body would adopt the molecular mechanisms related to the vitellogenesis. This is a process by which all oviparous species provision their eggs with vitelline, as a major yolk storage glycolipoprotein, that in turn constitutes a reserve food-source for the future embryo [48] (Fig. **1**).

The ability to transport fat in the form of lipoprotein through the circulatory system by eukaryotes is one of their more significant functions right from the beginning of existence [49]. Thus the evolutionary advancement of storing energy in the form of fat has provided organisms with an enormous advantage in adapting to environmental and developmental changes [49]. An isoform of apolipoprotein B, and apo B_{48} particles, are chylomicrons, which transport dietary cholesterol and triglycerides from the intestine to sites of storage and utilization within the body, such as the adipose tissue, skeletal and cardiac muscle and the liver [50].

Hepatic steatosis results from increased uptake of free fatty acids derived mainly from the hydrolysis of adipose-tissue triglycerides, increased because of insulin resistance, but also from dietary chylomicrons and hepatic biogenesis [51]. Inflammation and the concomitant acute phase response induce marked changes in the lipoprotein profile [52]. Thus in portal hypertensive-rat, hepatic steatosis is associated with the plasmatic increase of low density lipoprotein (LDL) and lipopolysaccharide binding protein (LBP) as well as reduction of high-density lipoproteins (HDL) [43, 45]. In turn, hepatic steatosis might play a key role in the pathogenesis of cardiovascular disease through the systemic release of several inflammatory mediators and/or through the production of insulin resistance and atherogenic dyslipidemia [51, 53].

The acute-phase-response is a core part of the innate immune response and produces changes in more than 200 proteins grouped as either positive or negative acute phase proteins [54, 44]. Positive acute phase protein biomarkers which increase in concentration during the inflammatory response include the classic short pentraxins, *i.e.*, C-reactive protein, serum amyloid P component and serum amyloide A [54, 55]. IL-6 produced in response to tissue damage and infection is a central mediator of the immune system inducing the liver acute-phase-response [56]. IL-6 and positive acute phase proteins, particularly C-reactive protein, have been correlated to disease severity and outcome in most of the chronic low-grade inflammatory conditions like cardiovascular diseases, obesity, metabolic syndrome, type-2 diabetes and non-alcoholic fatty liver disease (NAFLD), which includes a large spectrum that ranges from fatty liver, non-alcoholic steatohepatitis and cryptogenetic cirrhosis [51, 53, 57-59].

However, conflicting results exist as to whether IL-6 is a beneficial or harmful cytokine [60]. There is increasing evidence to show that IL-6 has a protective role during liver injury [56]. Hence, it has been suggested that IL-6 favors hepatic secretion of very low density lipoprotein (VLDL) triglyceride by increasing the availability of apo B and thereby reducing hepatic lipid content by increased triglyceride export [60]. It is also accepted that acute phase proteins, particularly serum amyloid A, inhibits the ability of acute phase HDL to serve as an acceptor for cellular cholesterol efflux. This promotes the removal of excess cholesterol from macrophages, as well as increases the availability of cellular free cholesterol and thereby, increases the development of atherosclerotic lesions [52, 61].

On the contrary, during cardiovascular inflammation cholesterol esters may be transferred from HDL to apolipoprotein B-containing particles, such as LDL or VLDL [62]. Trapping of apolipoprotein B containing particles within the arterial wall is unquestionably the essential initiating event for the development of complex atherosclerotic lesions [50]. Recent evidences support a strong association between NAFLD and cardiovascular diseases. Particularly, NAFLD is considered a risk factor for atherosclerosis [51] and ample evidence indicates that inflammation could be the pathophysiological mechanism linking NAFLD and cardiovascular diseases [51, 63]. In this context, we have found in the long-term (22 months) prehepatic portal hypertensive-rats that liver steatosis is related to an inflammatory aortic response. Particularly, the increased expression of NF-κB, TNF-α, IL-1β and IL-6 in the rat's aortic wall suggests the existence of a chronic inflammatory state [64].

The remodeling by angiogenesis could characterize the third inflammatory phenotype of the portal hypertensive response. Angiogenesis is defined as the growth of new vessels from pre-existing ones [65]. Although the final objective of endothelial growth is to form new vessels for oxygen, substrates and blood cells, other functions, like antioxidative as well as antienzymatic stress properties, could be carried out before the new vessels, *i.e.*, mature capillaries, are formed [2, 9]. During the evolution of chronic liver diseases the establishment of an abnormal splanchnic and systemic angio-architecture, including portosystemic collaterals, stands out [2, 66, 67].

Since in portal hypertension the basic structural alteration found in the gastrointestinal tract is vascular and consists in the increased size and the number of vessels, the very appropriate name of "hypertensive portal intestinal vasculopathy" has been proposed [68]. However, in addition to vascular alterations, histological evidence of non-specific inflammation has been described in the gastroenteropathy associated with portal hypertension [68]. Therefore, angiogenesis plays a key role in development of portal hypertension and represents a potential therapeutic target [69].

Chronic inflammatory infiltration found in the small bowel predominantly consists of mononuclear cells, and it is accompanied by atrophy, a decreased villous/crypt ratio, edema of the lamina propia, fibromuscular proliferation, and thickened *muscularis* mucosa [70, 71]. Since most of the aforementioned characteristics can be explained on the basis of increased levels of mast cell mediators [72], these cells could be involved in the pathogenesis of portal hypertensive chronic enteropathy [35, 36]. Furthermore, in experimental portal hypertensive enteropathy, the increased degree of mast cell infiltration coexists with a higher vessel number in these intestinal layers. Indeed, the number of mast cells shows a positive and statistically significant correlation with the vascular diameter and total microvascular surface [73]. Splanchnic hyperemia, increased splanchnic vascularization, and the development of portal-systemic collateral circulation in experimental portal hypertension are all angiogenic processes that are partly vascular endothelial growth factor (VEGF) dependent [74, 75]. Given that mast cells release many angiogenic factors, including VEGF [72], they possibly are involved in the promotion of the hypertensive portal vasculopathy, as well as of the portal-systemic collateral circulation.

One characteristic of mast cells is their phenotypic heterogeneity. Mast cell heterogeneity is presumably the result of microenvironmental conditions that dictate gene expression and phenotype development [76]. Given the evolutive nature of portal hypertension, the splanchnic mast cell response could be influenced by the predominant phenotype in each evolutive phase.

The splanchnic dependent angiogenic process in portal hypertension could also represent a reminiscence of the extraembryonic vitelline functions. The yolk sac is an extraembryonic vitelline structure not only related with lipid storage, metabolism and transport [48, 49], but also with angiogenesis and hematopoiesis [7, 77]. Endothelial cells and hematopoietic stem cells simultaneously differentiate within the blood islands in the yolk sac [77]. Indeed because hematopoietic stem cells always emerge in close physical association with endothelial cells, a common origin for the two cell types has been proposed [78]. It is generally accepted that hematopoietic stem cells generated in yolk sac blood islands sequentially colonize the embryonic liver, then the aorta-gonads-mesonephros and finally the bone marrow [7]. If so, the excessive splanchnic angiogenic response induced by portal hypertension could be related to the embrionary colonization process by cells bearing a dual hemato-endothelial phenotype. In addition, there is evidence of the association between liver cirrhosis and bone marrow alterations in both rats and patients [79]. Inflammatory mediators may be responsible for increased expression of adhesion molecules in the bone marrow sinusoidal endothelium. However, more investigation is needed to clarify the precise mechanism of how sinusoidal endothelium changes affect the hematopoietic cells [79]. Greater understanding is required pertaining to the relationship of portal hypertension with both processes, *i.e.*, angiogenic and hematopoietic. Thus the mast cell, a plurifunctional bone-marrow-derived cell, could emulate a rudimentary hematopoietic response in the gastrointestinal tract.

HIGH-GRADE INFLAMMATORY PORTAL HYPERTENSION: THE AMNIOTIC CONNECTION

Liver disease could be the most frequent factor for worsening portal hypertensive syndrome. Particularly, chronic liver disease and cirrhosis aggravate this syndrome exceedingly [80]. Hepatic dysfunction related to fibrosis or cirrhosis would aggravate the grade of systemic inflammation characteristic of the chronic portal hypertensive syndrome. Consequently, the vascular dysfunction with both blood and lymphatic hyperdynamic circulation would be favored [9].

Ascites: The Portal Hypertensive Peritoneum

Increased lymph flow is known to occur in diffuse abnormalities of liver architecture such as fibrosis and cirrhosis [81, 82]. The size and number of lymphatics are increased due to the increased hepatic lymph production which is caused by disturbance of the microcirculation typical of portal hypertension [82]. Expansion of lymphatics is also a prominent feature of gastrointestinal inflammation. The dysregulation of lymphatics exacerbates, in turn, gastrointestinal disease [83]. During cirrhotic portal hypertension dilation of esophageal and gastric lymph vessels may be related to the absorption of excess interstitial fluid [84]. However, the main features of liver decompensation in cirrhosis are ascites [85], hepatorenal syndrome [80, 86] and hepatic encephalopathy [80].

Ascites and hepatorenal syndrome are the major challenging complications of cirrhosis and portal hypertension that significantly affect the course of the disease [87]. Hepatorenal syndrome is a serious complication of end-stage disease occurring mainly in patients with advanced cirrhosis and ascites, who have marked circulatory dysfunction [86]. Although ascites can be observed in multiple diseases [88], it is most frequent due to cirrhosis with portal hypertension.

The three major factors involved in the pathogenesis of ascites are portal hypertension, arterial vasodilation and neurohormonal activation, all of them leading to sodium and water retention [87]. Arteriolar vasodilation causes underfilling of systemic arterial vascular space with a decrease in the effective arterial blood volume. Consequently, baroreceptor-mediated activation of renin-angiotensin-aldosterone system, sympathetic and parasympathetic nervous systems and non-osmotic release of antidiuretic hormone occur to restore normal blood homeostasis [87, 89-91]. On the other hand, splanchnic vasodilation increases splanchnic lymph production exceeding the lymph transportation system capacity and leads to lymph leakage into the peritoneal cavity [92]. Persistent renal sodium and water retention, alongside increased splanchnic vascular permeability in addition to lymph leakage into peritoneal cavity play the major role in a sustained ascites formation [90, 92]. Over time the stasis of lymph flow in lymphatic channels of the intestine could lead to lymphangiectasia with an accompanying loss of proteins and lymphocytes [93].

In the past, it was considered that ascites treatment depends on a reduction of lymph formation by indirect *i.e.* dietary restriction of salt and water, and diuretic drugs, or direct *i.e.* portosystemic shunt, portal decompression or, alternatively, and acceleration of an already rapid lymph return (peritoneovenous shunt) to match the high rate of lymph production. Conversely, factors that favor lymph formation *i.e.* mineralocorticoids, exogenous salt, or inhibit lymph return *i.e.* impaired lymphatic contractility or central venous hypertension, intensify lymph imbalance and worsen ascites [92, 94].

Other mechanisms proposed to be involved in ascites formation are based on hepatorenal reflex, secondary to a rapid increase in sinusoidal hepatic pressure [92, 95] and the splenorenal reflex-mediated reduction in renal vascular conductance, which exacerbates sodium and water retention in the kidneys and may eventually contribute to renal dysfunction and, consequently, ascites formation [96].

The development of ascites is a major complication of cirrhosis that induces an impaired quality of life and decreases survival. The most difficult patients to treat are those with refractory ascites, which are characterized by a lack of response to diuretic treatment [97]. Spontaneous bacterial peritonitis is a frequent and severe complication of decompensated cirrhosis [98]. Bacterial translocation is the key mechanism in its pathogenesis and the common causative microorganisms are gram-negative bacteria such as *Escherichia coli* and *Klebsiella pneumoniae* [99]. The clinical manifestations of spontaneous bacterial peritonitis are subtle and require a high index of suspicion and almost always occur in a large volume of ascites in patients with liver cirrhosis. Abdominal pain can be continuous and is different from tense ascites. Ascitic polymorphonuclear leukocyte cell count is essential for diagnosis and management [98, 99]. However, by means of a polymerase chain reaction (PCR)-based method and automated nucleotide sequencing it is possible to detect and identify the presence of fragments of bacterial DNA in patients with culture-negative, non-neutrocytic ascites, indicating the existence of bacterial DNA translocation [100]. Paralytic *ileus*, hypotension and hypothermia are seen in advanced illness, where prognosis may be death and one third of patients will develop renal failure [90, 99].

Secondary bacterial peritonitis is an infrequent complication in cirrhotic patients and presents a significant more severe local inflammatory response than in patients with spontaneous bacterial peritonitis [100, 101]. On the contrary, *"bacteriascites"* is the term used to describe the colonization of ascitic fluid by bacteria in the absence of a local inflammatory reaction, which suggests the concurrent failure of defensive mechanisms [99].

Splanchnic Interstitium, Mesenteric Lymphatics and Peritoneal Mesothelium: A Hypothetically Inflammatory Continuum in the Portal Hypertensive Syndrome

The standard view of inflammation as a reaction to injury or infection might need to be expanded to account for the inflammatory processes induced by other types of adverse conditions [102]. Therefore, the splanchnic and systemic impairments that are produced during the evolution of the syndrome associated with portal hypertension could be considered of an inflammatory nature. If so, and similar to other type of inflammatory response, it would begin in the interstitial space [2, 3, 29] (Table **2**).

The early inflammatory response in portal hypertension could be associated with abnormal ion transport. There is increasing evidence that the conditions characterized by an inflammatory response have alterations in cellular membrane potential with depolarization and abnormal ion transport [103]. In addition, disturbances of ion transport are produced in intra- and extracellular edema. It has been stated that small fluctuations in cell hydration or cell volume act as a potent signal for cellular metabolism and gene expression [104]. Oxidative and nitrosative stress increases degradation of extracellular matrix and causes edema [105]. The accumulation of glycosaminoglycans fragments has been proposed as an important mechanism for edema formation due to its hydrophilic properties [106]. Likewise, while the progression of interstitial edema reduces the blood capillary function, it simultaneously enhances lymphatic circulation, thus producing a circulatory switch in the inflamed tissues and organs.

Furthermore, splanchnic interstitial flow could be relevant for lymphangiogenesis [107]. The interstitial fluid flow associated with edema, even though it can be extremely slow, can have important effects on tissue morphogenesis and function, cell migration and differentiation and matrix remodeling, among other processes [108]. Abnormally increased interstitial flow rates can occur during low-grade inflammation and can also trigger fibroblasts to differentiate or remodel the extracellular matrix, contributing thus to the development of tissue fibrosis [107, 109-112]. Interstitial flow may significantly alter the distribution of metalloproteinases and lymphatic growth factors, inducing lymphatic endothelial cell migration and capillary morphogenesis [107, 110]. Mast cells and lymphatics could be important players in the development of the splanchnic inflammatory process [9]. Thus it has been shown that *in vitro* mast cell degranulation impairs lymphatic contractile activity, probably through activation of H_1 receptors by histamine. It has been suggested that this action could interfere with the expected ability of lymphatic vessels to reduce edema during inflammation [113].

Two of the principal functions of intestinal lymphatics are to assist in the maintenance of interstitial volume within relatively normal limits during alterations in capillary filtration, *i.e.* acute portal hypertension, and the removal of absorbed water and chylomicrons [114]. Unidirectional fluid transport into the initial lymphatics from the splanchnic interstitial space could be facilitated by the primary and secondary valve systems and then by contractile lymphatics [115, 116]. During inflammation the elevation of lymphatic endothelial permeability in an outward direction has two major effects. First, fluid is cleared from the tissue less efficiently. With the increased permeability of the blood vessels already producing more fluid in the tissue than normal, the decreased transport by the lymphatics causes this edema to increase even more [116, 117]. Second, the leaking lymphatics allow inflammatory mediators to remain in the tissue longer increasing thus the inflammatory intestinal response [116] (Fig. **2**)

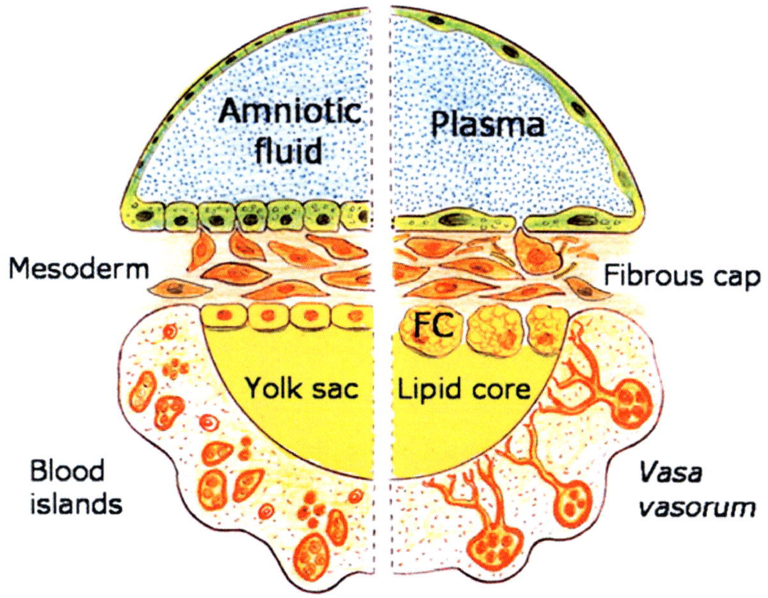

Figure 2: Schematic representation in which a comparison between the embrionary development (gastrulation phase)(left) and the atherosclerotic plaque in the artery wall (right) is made. FC: foam cell.

Mesenteric lymph transports cells (lymphocytes), lipids (chylomicrons), proteins (plasma proteins, immunoglobulins), enzymes (alkaline phosphatase, amylase), hormones (insulin, incretins) and electrolytes (chloride and bicarbonate) to the systemic circulation [115, 118]. The biological role of the mesenteric lymph in the pathogenesis of splanchnic and systemic inflammation is not fully clarified up to date. However, there is now evidence to show that mesenteric lymph plays a key role in the pathogenesis of multiple organ dysfunction in trauma/hemorrhagic shock, burns, reperfusion injury and surgical stress [41, 42, 115, 119-121].

The hemodynamic alterations that portal hypertension imposes on the splanchnic circulation [16, 80] allow considering that changes in the mesenteric lymph flow and composition are also produced [9]. Therefore, the mesenteric lymph could play an etiopathogenic role in the multiple organ dysfunction developed in the portal hypertensive syndrome [16]. Particularly, bacteria and toxins, like bacterial lipopolysaccharide (LPS), and inflammatory mediators with high affinity for chylomicrons, that are lipids, could use the mesenteric lymph vessels to bypass the liver and induce a systemic response [122].

Lymphangiogenesis, the formation of new lymphatic vessels, occurs in several pathological conditions associated with chronic inflammation [123, 124], including portal hypertensive enteropathy [84] and liver cirrhosis [81, 82]. Inflammatory cells, through the secretion of stimulatory factor such as VEGF-C and TNF-α, can stimulate lymphatic endothelial cells [125-127] and consequently regulate gut lymphatic remodeling in portal hypertensive enteropathy. Lymphangiogenesis generally accompanies angiogenesis [128], the basic structural alteration of the hypertensive portal gastroenteropathy [68]. However, pathological lymphangiogenesis may occur in absence of blood vessels [127, 129].

The biological role of lymphangiogenesis in the pathogenesis of gastrointestinal chronic inflammation needs further clarification. Inflammation triggers gut lymphangiogenesis [130-133], and this may be beneficial for the resolution of chronic inflammation since lymphatic vessels remove inflammatory cells and mediators from the inflammation sites, favoring resolution [133-135]. Lymphovenous communications located both in lymphatic vessels and mesenteric lymph nodes [115] could also have a pathophysiological significance in the setting of chronic intestinal inflammation that need to be explored. Furthermore, one highly specialized form of tissue remodeling in chronic inflammation is lymphoid neogenesis, that is, the development of new lymphoid tissue in inflammatory sites [134, 136]. It has been proposed that during chronic inflammation lymphangiogenesis and lymphoid neogenesis would be synergistic processes that mutually amplify each other [136].

Severe hepatic dysfunction related to fibrosis or cirrhosis would aggravate the grade of splanchnic inflammation in portal hypertension, and as a result would increase the incidence of complications. Consequently, the vascular splanchnic dysfunction, with increased blood flow and portal pressure, would get worse and the interstitial hepato-intestinal-lymph flow would be favored. Splanchnic ischemia-reperfusion injury secondary to the acute-on-chronic vascular dysfunction could result in higher renin-angiotensin-aldosterone system activity and excessive interstitial edema and lymph flow [137, 138]. The liver has been assumed to be the likely source of ascites in patients with liver disease [81]. Nevertheless, the cirrhotic liver is not the sole or even the major source of ascites in most patients [89, 94]. Weeping of fluid in great excess from the peritoneal lining and serosal surfaces of the bowel is often striking in portal hypertension as are dilated lymphatics on the surface of the small intestine, in the mesentery and within the retroperitoneal space [94]. Therefore, it is accepted that when lymphatic drainage mechanisms are overwhelmed, excess lymph collects in the peritoneal cavity, thus causing ascites [90, 139, 140] (Fig. **2**).

Nevertheless, peritoneal mesothelial cells would not be considered as a passive barrier for the lymph leakage of splanchnic origin in ascites formation. In the normal peritoneal cavity mesothelial cells play an important role as a source of intraperitoneal phospholipid lubricant [141]. Surfactant proteins have been found to be associated with the phospholipid-containing surfactant-like material that line mesothelial cells and exert anti-inflammatory and immunomodulatory functions [142]. In addition, the overlapped peritoneal mesothelial cells have a surface covered with great number of microvilli and a cytoplasm filled with a greater number of ribosomes, mitochondria, rough endoplasmic reticulum and Golgi apparatus [143]. Particularly, the numerous pinocytic vesicles in the membrane and the cytoplasm indicate active end- and exo- transcytosis in the process of secretion and reabsorption of peritoneal fluid [143]. Peritoneal mesothelial cells by secreting chemokines, cytokines and growth factors such as VEGF [144] could have an active participation in the inflammatory response as a developer in the intestinal wall in portal hypertensive syndrome and, therefore, in ascites formation.

Obstructive Cholestasis in the Rat: A Model of Decompensated Portal Hypertensive Syndrome

Obstructive cholestasis is characterized by jaundice, discolored urine, pale stools and pruritus [145]. The serious repercussions of cholestasis on the liver and on the systemic level have led to the creation of many experimental models so as to better understand its pathogenesis, prophylaxis and treatment [146, 147].

Obstructive cholestasis causes cirrhotic chronic hepatic insufficiency and portal hypertension. Several surgical techniques for developing obstructive cholestasis have been described, especially in the rat. These techniques could be divided into two groups, macrosurgical and microsurgical. Macrosurgical techniques are based on the section of the common bile duct between ligatures. These macrosurgical techniques of obstructive extrahepatic cholestasis are called "bile duct ligation" (BDL) and cause the development of infected biliary pseudocysts by dilation of the bile duct proximal end. As a result an important number of the animals die during the first two weeks of the postoperative period because of sepsis [147, 148]. To avoid these infectious complications we have proposed performing a microsurgical technique which consists in the resection of the extrahepatic biliary tract [146, 147, 149]. The use of broad-spectrum antibiotic and vitamin K allows the long-term evolution of the obstructive cholestatic-rats [146, 147].

In the long-term evolution, between 8 to 10 weeks, microsurgical extrahepatic cholestatic-rats develop hepatomegaly with a marked ductular proliferation and fibrosis [150]. It has been suggested that liver fibrogenesis resembles a wound-healing process leading to scar formation [151-153]. In relation to extrahepatic alterations, jaundice, choluria, portal hypertension with an enlarged spleen and collateral portosystemic circulation, hepatic encephalopathy and ascites stand out [147, 154, 155]. Therefore, experimental extrahepatic cholestasis is not only a good model for studying chronic hepatic disease related to biliary obstruction, but also for studying extrahepatic complications, particularly ascites.

In the rat, chronic liver disease due to obstructive cholestasis produces progressive hemodynamic dysfunction with ascites and hepatorenal syndrome. BDL rats after four weeks of biliary obstruction present an initial disturbance in renal function associated with ascites. Two weeks later, rats with obstructive cholestasis clearly developed hepatorenal syndrome with ascites [156]. In these chronic phases of macrosurgical obstructive cholestasis, high rates of bacterial translocation, with endotoxemia and consecutive systemic inflammatory response, also exist [157, 158].

In rats with obstructive cholestasis, the portal hypertensive syndrome with low-degree splanchnic and systemic inflammation can progress to severe systemic inflammatory response syndrome leading to multiple organ failure. After extrahepatic cholestasis, the rat can suffer the effects of generalized ischemia/reperfusion injury and exacerbation of oxidative and nitrosative stress. It is accepted that there is a strong correlation between experimental obstructive jaundice and oxidative stress [159]. BDL mainly impairs the liver rat ability of antioxidant regeneration especially at the mitochondria level [160]. Thus it has been demonstrated that treatment with antioxidants improves the hepatic cellular redox status [161, 162].

Long-term (6 weeks) microsurgical cholestatic rats show a splanchnic redistribution of cytokines, with an increase of Th_1 (TNFα and IL-1β) and Th2 (IL-4 and IL-10) production in the small bowel and in the mesenteric lymph nodes [163]. It has been proposed that this splanchnic inflammatory response associated with ascites could be mediated, among others factors, by mast cells. Degranulation of splanchnic mast cells, including the mast cells present in the peritoneum, could result in the release of mediators with a potent vasodilator and exudative actions such as histamine, proteases and other enzymes, arachidonic acid metabolites and reactive oxygen and nitrogen species [76] which could cause intense exudation related to an endothelial permeability increase, which could be in turn the cause of swelling, increased splanchnic lymphatic flow and production of peritoneal exudate [9].

The suggested pathophysiological mediator role of the mesenteric lymph in worsening the splanchnic portal hypertensive inflammatory response induced by obstructive cholestasis can be studied by the cannulation of the rat mesenteric lymph duct [164-166]. The mesenteric lymph duct in the rat is observed as a white dyed duct, approximately 10mm above the origin of the left adrenal vein, and is accompanied by the mesenteric artery. Using an operating microscope, the connective tissue surrounding the duct could be carefully cleared. In brief, the cannulation technique is made using a heparinized polyethylene catheter with an outer diameter of 1mm. Then, a ligature is placed around the duct and the catheter. Lastly a small drop of cyanoacrylate glue or tissue adhesive is applied to the duct at the point of entry of the catheter to prevent lymph leakage [164, 166].

The relative distribution profiles of protein functional classes in normal rodent mesenteric lymph differ significantly from that reported for the plasma. The most abundant protein classes in mesenteric lymph are protease inhibitors, immune-related proteins, particularly those implicated in innate immunity, and carrier proteins [167]. Therefore, mesenteric lymph has a unique profile compared with plasma and thus represents more than a simple filtrate [167]. Recent proteomic analyses of post-hemorrhagic shock mesenteric lymph have documented the increase of proteins functionally involved in tissue inflammation [168]. These results provide a starting point for the in-depth investigation of the pathophysiology role of mesenteric lymph in other conditions in which it is considered that the gastrointestinal tract is the driving force behind multiple organ dysfunctions, like the portal hypertensive syndrome. In rats with long-term surgical cholestasis we have shown using the transcription factor LYVE-1, as a marker of lymphangiogenesis [169], the existence of intestinal lymphatic hyperplasia (Fig. **3**). In this experimental model subperitoneal lymphangiogenesis associated with ascites is also developed.

Lastly, ascites produces intra-abdominal hypertension. Elevated intra-abdominal pressure could compresses thin walled mesenteric veins promoting venous hypertension, intestinal interstitial edema, bacterial translocation, sepsis and multiple organ failure [170-172].

Portal Hypertensive Ascites and the Amniotic Way of Life

Ascites is a common manifestation of liver failure, being one of the cardinal signs of portal hypertension [173]. Ascitic fluid formation is not well known pathogenic mechanism. However, ascitic fluid is a bioactive medium containing electrolytes, with high levels of sodium, proteins including albumin and enzymes, as well as cells, including leukocytes [174]. Some of these characteristics make it similar to another bioactive medium, the amniotic fluid [175-177]. Amniotic fluid, the protecting liquid contained in the amnion cavity, is an essential extraembryonic component for fetal development and maturation during pregnancy [176, 178].

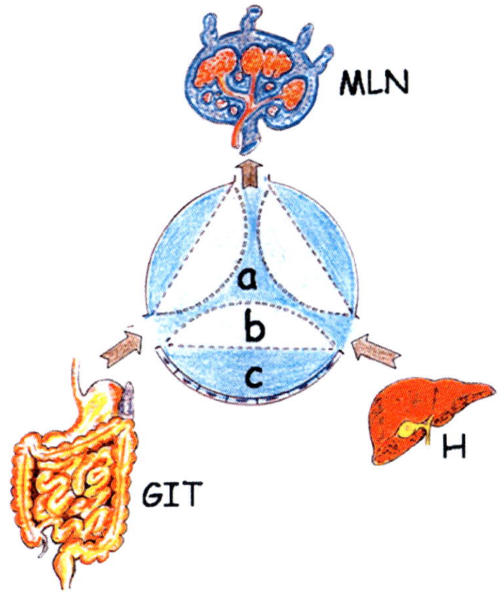

Figure 3: Schematic view of the evolutive phases in the formation of the interstitial-lymphatic-peritoneal mesothelium inflammatory axis in portal hypertensive ascites: a. Splanchnic lymphatic flow resulting from the gastrointestinal tract (GIT) and the hepatic (H) interstitium drained through the mesenteric lymph node (MLN) in physiological situations. b. Chronic-low-grade inflammation in the compensated portal hypertensive syndrome increases mesenteric lymphatic flow. c. Acute-on-chronic splanchnic inflammation in the decompensated portal hypertensive syndrome increases the ascitic fluid.

Body fluid is distributed among three major fluid spaces: intracellular fluid, interstitial fluid and plasma. Nevertheless, the distribution of fluid in each of these compartments is dramatically different in the fetus compared with the adult [179]. Particularly, the amniotic fluid that surrounds the fetus may be considered an extension of the extracellular space of the fetus [178, 179]. Thus, the lymphatic system plays an essential role in the regulation of fluid distribution between the plasma and the interstitial fluid and probably with the amniotic fluid [179]. In patients with portal hypertension and ascites, it could also be hypothesized that the lymphatic splanchnic system plays a key role in the fluid distribution between the plasma and the ascitic fluid. If so, a pathological pathway of increasingly complex structures with a similar function to the management of the extracellular fluid would be formed [9] (Fig. **4**)

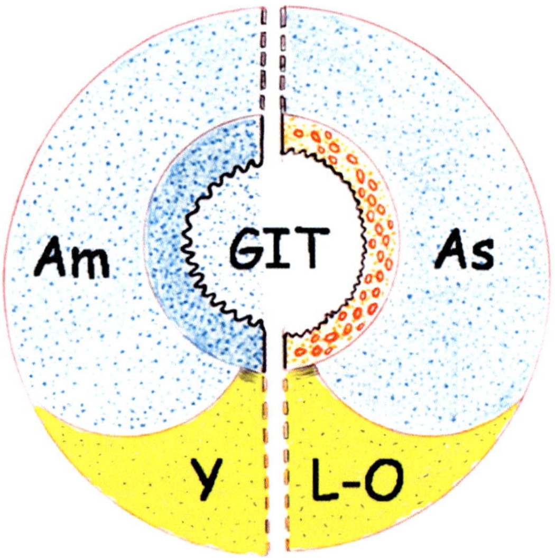

Figure 4: Comparative and schematic representation of the fetal (left) and portal hypertensive (right) gastrointestinal tract. Amniotic fluid through gastrointestinal tract of the embryo favors trophism and maturation. On the contrary, the proposed equivalent fluid, *i.e.* ascitic fluid, in the adult organism is confined within the peritoneal mesothelial cavity. Am: amniotic fluid; As: ascitic fluid; Y: yolk sac; L-O: liver and great omentum; GIT: gastrointestinal tract.

In the early stages of pregnancy, amniotic fluid consists of a filtrate of maternal blood [177, 180]. That is why in this period drugs taken by the mother can enter amniotic fluid by diffusion across the placenta [177, 181]. However, its composition is known to change as pregnancy proceeds [175]. At these stages amniotic fluid is a bioactive medium actively secreted by the cells lining the amniotic cavity and as gestation progresses it includes significant volume of fetal urine [182].

The hypothetical comparison of the characteristics of amniotic and ascitic fluids would oblige raising again the role of peritoneal mesothelial cells in the etiopathogeny of ascites that occurs in the decompensated portal hypertensive syndrome.

The first fluid to enter the gastrointestinal system is amniotic fluid and contributes to fetal nutritional requirements and plays a significant role in gut development and maturation [182]. Thus growth-promoting effects of amniotic fluid are equivalent to human milk [182]. The trophic effect of orally consumed amniotic fluid is attributed in part to its content in growth factors, including epidermal growth factor (EGF), hepatocyte growth factor (HGF), transforming growth factor-alpha (TGF-α), fibroblast growth factor (FGF), insulin-like growth factor (IGF-s) and VEGF [182, 183].

The functional comparison of amniotic and ascitic fluids would imply that in the decompensated portal hypertensive syndrome the abdominal mesothelium acquires properties of the amniotic membrane or amnion. In essence, the body acquires the ability to express functions that correspond to a structure of extra-embrionary origin, the amnion. This hypothesis would imply several suppositions or suggestions. For example, the intestine in the case of portal hypertensive ascites could not benefit from the supposed trophic properties of the ascitic fluid given that the peritoneal cavity-gastrointestinal pathway does not exist in post-natal life. Likewise, the prenatal interruption of the amniotic fluid transit in cases of prenatal intestinal obstruction prevents the fetus from benefiting from its trophic properties and it has been suggested that it contributes to fetal undergrowth [184].

The amniotic membrane is a tissue of particular interest because it possesses cells having characteristic of stem cells with multipotent differentiation ability [185, 186]. Therefore, to explore the possibilities that the "ascitic peritoneum" could be a source of stem cells and growth factors could open new paths of knowledge for the study of its pathogeny. Moreover, the ascitic fluid could be a source of powerful therapies for using its supposedly beneficial properties. The embryonic regression of the peritoneum that induces the inflammatory response induced by portal hypertension also could favor the presence of active antimicrobial components as those described in the amniotic fluid [187]. Thus the resistance to infection of the ascites would be explained, with usual subtle clinical manifestations in cases of secondary bacterial peritonitis [97, 100, 101].

The hypothetical existence of a regression to the prenatal functional mechanisms of the abdominal interstitium-lymphatic-mesothelium axis could serve to integrate the existing knowledge of the decompensated portal hypertensive syndrome. In this hypothesis it is considered that the main objective of this de-repression of "dormant" biochemical functions is the recuperation of the amnion. The major phylogenetic importance that this structure has perhaps lies in that during development it protectively surrounds the embryo and creates a full-filled cavity in which the embryo develops [178]. Its acquisition, that is, the "amniotic egg" was one of the main causes that enabled amniotes to escape the bonds that confined their ancestors to aquatic environments [178, 188]. If so, it could be proposed that there is no better method to escape the sea than taking the sea with us, as an amniotic-mesothelial structure full of saline trophic fluid [188, 189]. Since this ability would be associated in the post-natal life with mesothelial cells, its major spread through the body is not surprising, coating cavities, *i.e.* aracnoides, sinovial, pleura, testicular and vaginal, to create virtual spaces that facing traumatic, infectious or tumoral injury, quickly carry out an exudative response that is simultaneously protecting and trophic. Therefore, although the mesothelial exudative inflammatory response is considered pathological, its proven evolutive and beneficial characteristics should not be forgotten both from the ontogenic and phylogenetic points of view [9].

In summary, the extraembryonic origin of the portal system seems to determine some of its evolutive pathological properties when it suffers hypertension, both compensated, *i.e.* prehepatic, and decompensated, *i.e.* intrahepatic. The partial portal vein ligation, or compensated, and the extrahepatic cholestasis or decompensated, are the experimental models most frequently used to study both types of portal hypertension. Prehepatic portal hypertension by partial portal vein ligation in the rat induces the expression of three overlapping phenotypes, whose pathophysiological mechanisms recall those that are associated with the yolk sac development or vitellogenics. In turn, in obstructive cholestatic-rats the decompensation induced by the severe liver disease would produce ascites. The functional comparison between the ascitic and amniotic fluids would imply that in the decompensated portal hypertensive syndrome the abdominal mesothelium acquires properties of the amnion [190].

The expression of these extraembryonic functions during the evolution of these two types of experimental portal hypertension can be subject to diverse interpretations. Regardless of its meaning, it is important that the re-expression of these extraembryonic functions induced by portal hypertension might be considered today in inflammation. This consideration suggests that the hypothetical comparison between the inflammatory portal hypertensive evolutive types and the evolutive development of extraembryonic systems, *i.e.* vitelline and amniotic, could allow for translational research.

ACKNOWLEDGEMENTS

We would like to thank Maria Elena Vicente for preparing the manuscript, Elizabeth Mascola for translating it into English and librarians of Complutense University Medical School, particularly the Director, Francisco Javier Jorge García-Reyes, and Manuela Crego and María José Valdemoro and B. Braun Surgical S.A. for their technical assistance.

This study was carried out in part with grants from Mutua Madrileña Research Foundation (Ref. nº PA 3077/2008 and AP5966/2009), MICINN PSI2010-19348 and with the special collaboration of the INEUROPA (Instituto de Neurociencias del Principado de Asturias).

CONFLICT OF INTEREST

The author(s) confirm that this chapter content has no conflict of interest.

REFERENCES

[1] Martell M, Coll M, Ezkurda N, Raurell I, Genesca J. Physiopathology of splanchnic vasodilation in portal hypertension. World J Hepatol 2010; 2:208-220.

[2] Aller MA, Arias JL, Cruz A, Arias J. Inflammation: a way to understanding the evolution of portal hypertension. Theor Biol Med Model 2007; 4:44.

[3] Aller MA, Arias JL, Arias J. The mast cell integrates the splanchnic and systemic inflammatory response in portal hypertension. J Transl Med 2007; 5:44.

[4] Cazzaniga M, Dionigi E, Gobbo G, Fioretti A, Monti V, Salerno F. The systemic inflammatory response syndrome in cirrhotic patients: Relationship with their in-hospital outcome. J Hepatol 2009; 51:475-482.

[5] Malik R, Mookerjee RP, Jalan R. Infection and inflammation in liver failure: Two sides of the same coin. J Hepatol 2009; 51:426-429.

[6] Sherlock S. The portal venous system and portal hypertension. In: *Diseases of the Liver and Biliary System.* Edited by Sherlock S. London: Ed. Blackwell Scientific Publications; 1989; 151-207.

[7] Collardeu-Frachon S, Scoazec JY. Vascular development and differentiation during human liver organogenesis. Anat Rec 2008; 291:614-621.
[8] Dobreva MP, Pereira PNG, Deprest J, Zwijsen A. On the origin of amniotic stem cells: of mice and men. Int J Dev Biol 2010; 54:761-777.
[9] Aller MA, Prieto I, Argudo S, De Vicente F, Santamaria L, De Miguel MP, *et al.* The interstitial lymphatic peritoneal mesothelium axis in portal hypertensive ascites: when in danger, go back to the sea. Int J Inflam 2010; 2010:148689.
[10] Aller MA, Nava MP, Duran M, Alvarez E, Arias JL, Sanchez-Patan F, *et al.* Evolutive phases of the experimental prehepatic portal hypertension. J Gastroenterol Hepatol 2007; 22:1127-1133.
[11] Goszmann RJ. Hyperdinamic circulation of liver disease forty years later: pathophysiology and clinical consequence. Hepatology 1994; 20:1359-1363.
[12] Iwakiri Y, Groszmann RJ. The hyperdynamic circulation of chronic liver diseases: from the patient to the molecule. Hepatology 2006; 43:S121-S131.
[13] Moreau R, Lebrec D. Molecular and structural basis of portal hypertension. Clin Liver Dis 2006; 10:445-457.
[14] Rodriguez-Vilarrupla A, Fernandez M, Bosch J, Garcia-Pagan JC. Current concepts on the pathophysiology of portal hypertension. Ann Hepatol 2007; 6:28-36.
[15] La Villa G, Gentilini P. Hemodynamic alterations in liver cirrhosis. Mol Aspects Med 2008; 29:112-118.
[16] Iwakiri Y, Groszmann RJ. Vascular endothelial dysfunction in cirrhosis. J Hepatol 2007; 46:927-934.
[17] Harrison DG, Widder J, Grumbach I, Chen W, Weber M, Searles C. Endothelial mechanotransduction, nitric oxide and vascular inflammation. J Inter Med 2006; 259:351-363.
[18] Chiu J-J, Chien S. Effects of disturbed flow on vascular endothelium: Pathophysiological basis and clinical perspectives. Physiol Rev 2011; 91:327-387.
[19] Colgan SP, Taylor CT. Hypoxia: an alarm signal during intestinal inflammation. Nature Rev Gastroenterol Hepatol 2010; 7:281-287.
[20] Carrico CJ, Meakins JL, Marshall JC, Fry D, Maier RV. Multiple-organ-failure-syndrome: the gastrointestinal tract. The "motor" of MOF. Arch Surg 1986; 121:196-208.
[21] Suliburk J, Helmer K, Moore F, Mercer D. The gut in systemic inflammatory response syndrome and sepsis. Eur Surg Res 2008; 40:184-189.
[22] Deitch EA. Bacterial translocation or lymphatic drainage of toxic products from the gut: What is important in human beings? Surgery 2002; 131:241-244.
[23] Alexander JS, Ganta VC, Jordan PA, Witte MH. Gastrointestinal lymphatics in health and disease. Pathophysiology 2010; 17:315-335.
[24] Gershon MD. Developmental determinants of the independence and complexity of the enteric nervous system. Trends Neurosci 2010; 33:446-454.
[25] Lyte M. Reciprocal gut-brain evolutionary symbiosis provokes and amplifies the postinjury systemic inflammatory response syndrome. Surgery 2009; 146: 950-954.
[26] Liu H, Schuelert N, McDougall JJ, Lee SS. Central neural activation of hyperdynamic circulation in portal hypertensive rats depends on vagal afferent nerves. Gut 2008; 57:966-973.
[27] Schrier RW, Arroyo V, Bernardi M, Epstein M, Henriksen JH, Rodes J. Peripheral arterial vasodilatation hypothesis: a proposal for the initiation of renal sodium and water retention in cirrhosis. Hepatology 1988; 8:1151-1157.

[28] Stocker SD, Madden CJ, Sved AF. Excess dietary salt intake alters the excitabiligy of central sympathetic networks. Physiol Behav 2010; 100:519-524.

[29] Aller MA, Arias JL, Nava MP, Arias J. Post-traumatic inflammation is a complex response based on the pathological expression of the nervous, immune and endocrine functional systems. Exp Biol Med (Maywood) 2004; 229:170-181.

[30] Garcia-Tsao G, Albillos A, Barden GE, West AB. Bacterial translocation in acute and chronic portal hypertension. Hepatology 1993; 17:1081-1085.

[31] Garcia-Tsao G, Wiest R. Gut microflora in the pathogenesis of the complications of cirrhosis. Best Pract Res Clin Gastroenterol 2004; 18:353-372.

[32] Llamas MA, Aller MA, Marquina D, Nava MP, Arias J. Bacterial translocation to mesenteric lymph nodes increases in chronic portal hypertensive rats. Dig Dis Sci 2010; 55:224-254.

[33] Gabay C, Kushner I. Acute-phase proteins and other systemic responses to inflammation. N Engl J Med 1999; 340:448-454.

[34] Cray C, Zaias J, Altman NH. Acute phase response in animals: A review. Comp Med 2009; 59:517-526.

[35] Prieto I, Aller MA, Santamaria L, Nava MP, Madero R, Perez-Robledo JP, *et al*. Prehepatic portal hypertension produces increased mast cell density in the small bowel and in mesenteric lymph nodes in the rat. J Gastroenterol Hepatol 2005; 20:1025-1031.

[36] Moquillaza LM, Aller MA, Nava MP, Santamaria L, Vergara P, Arias J. Partial hepatectomy, partial portal vein stenosis and mesenteric lymphadenectomy increase splanchnic mast cell infiltration in the rat. Acta Histochem 2010; 112:372-82.

[37] McLachlan JB, Hart JP, Pizzo SV, Shelburne CP, Staats HF, Gunn MD, *et al*. Mast cell-derived tumor necrosis factor induces hypertrophy of draining lymph nodes during infection. Nature Immunol 2003; 4:1199-1205.

[38] Bischoff SC. Physiological and pathophysiological functions of intestinal mast cells. Semin Immunopathol 2009; 31:185-205.

[39] Cäruntu FA, Benea L. Spontaneous, bacterial peritonitis: pathogenesis, diagnosis, treatment. J Gastrointest Liver Dis 2006; 15:51-56.

[40] Jung C, Hugot J-P, Barreau F. Peyer's patches: The immune sensors of the intestine. Int J Inflam 2010; 2010:823710.

[41] Magnotti LJ, Deitch EA. Burns, bacterial translocation, gut barrier function, and failure.J Burn Care Rehabil 2005; 26:383-391.

[42] Damie SS, Moore EE, Nydam TL, Banerjee M, Gamboni-Robertson F, Su X, *et al*. Post-shock mesenteric lymph induces endothelial NF-κB activation. J Surg Res 2007; 143:136-140.

[43] Aller MA, Vara E, Garcia C, Nava MP, Angulo A, Sanchez-Patan F, *et al*. Hepatic lipid metabolism changes in short- and long-term prehepatic portal hypertensive rats. World J Gastroenterol 2006; 12:6828-6834.

[44] Alonso MJ, Aller MA, Corcuera MT, Nava MP, Gomez F, Angulo A, *et al*. Progressive hepatocytic fatty infiltration in rats with prehepatic portal hypertension. Hepato-Gastroenterol 2005; 52:541-546.

[45] Sanchez-Patan F, Anchuelo R, Aller MA, Vara E, Garcia C, Nava MP, *et al*. Chronic prehepatic portal hypertension in the rat: is it a type of metabolic inflammatory síndrome? Lipids Health Dis 2008; 7:4.

[46] Kim LJ, Nalls MA, Eiriksdottir G, Sigurdsson S, Launer LJ, Koster A, Chaves PH, Jonsdottir B, Garcia M, Gudnason V, Harris TB; AGES-Reykjavik Study Investigators. Association of visceral and liver fat with the metabolic syndrome across the spectrum of obesity: The AGES-Reykjavik study. Obesity (Silver Spring) 2011; 19: 1265-71

[47] Ibrahim MM. Subcutaneous and visceral adipose tissue: structural and functional differences. Obes Rev 2010; 11:11-18.

[48] Tofail M, Takeda M. Molecular characteristics of insect vitellogenins. J Insect Physiol 2008; 54:1447-1458.

[49] Arukwe A, Goksφyr A. Eggshell and egg yolk proteins in fish; hepatic proteins for the next generation: oogenetic, population, and evolutionary implications of endocrine disruption. Comp Hepatol 2003; 2:4.

[50] Sniderman A, Couture P, De Graaf J. Diagnosis and treatment of apolipoprotein B dyslipoproteinemias. Nat Rev Endocrinol 2010; 6:335-346

[51] Targher G, Day CP, Bonora E. Risk of cardiovascular disease in patients with nonalcoholic fatty liver disease. N Engl J Med 2010; 363:1341-1350.

[52] Jahangiri A. High-density lipoprotein and the acute phase response. Curr Opin Endocrinol Diabetes Obes 2010; 17:156-260.

[53] Tarantino G, Savastano S, Colao A. hepatic steatosis, low-grade chronic inflammation and hormona/growth factor/adipkine imbalance. World J Gastroenterol 2010; 16: 4773-4783.

[54] Eckersall PD,Bell R.Acute phase proteins:Biomarkers of infection and inflammation in veterinary Vet J 2010; 185:23-27

[55] Schreiber G,Tsykin A,Aldred AR, Thomas T, Fung WP,Dickson PW *et al.*The acute phase response in the rodent. Ann N Y Acad Sci 1989; 557:61-85.

[56] Kopf M, Bachmann MF, Marsland BJ. Averting inflammation by targeting the cytokine environment. Nature Rev Drug Discov 2010; 9:703-718.

[57] Tordjman J, Poitou C, Hugol D, Bouillot J-L, Basdevant A, Bedossa P, *et al.* Association between adipose tissue macrophages and liver histopathology in morbid obesity: Influence of glycemic status. J Hepatol 2009; 51:354-362.

[58] Marsland AL, McCaffery JM, Muldoon MF, Manuck SB. Systemic inflammation and the metabolic syndrome among middle-aged community volunteers. Metabolism 2010; 59:1801-1808.

[59] Solinas G, Karin M. JNK1 and IKKβ: molecular links between obesity and metabolic dysfunction. FASEB J 2010; 24:2596-2609.

[60] Sparks JD, Cianci J, Jokinen J, Chen LS, Sparks CE. Interleukin-6 mediates hepatic hypersecretion of apolipodrotein B. Am J Physiol Gastrointest Liver Physiol 2010; 299:G980-G989.

[61] Van der Westhuyzen DR, De Beer FC, Webb NR. HDL cholesterol transport during inflammation. Curr Opin Lipidol 2007; 18:147-151.

[62] Natarajan P, Ray KK, Cannon CP. High-density lipoprotein and coronary heart disease. J Am Coll Cardiol 2010; 55:1283-1289.

[63] Loria P, Lonardo A, Targher G. Is liver fat detrimental to vessels?: intersections in the pathogenesis of NAFLD and atherosclerosis. Clin Sci 2008; 115:1-12.

[64] Cruz A, Heras N, Aller MA, Losada M, Nava MP, Paz A, *et al.* Low-grade aortic inflammation in long-term prehepatic portal hypertensive rats. Br J Surg 2009; 96(Suppl5):5.

[65] Puxeddu I, Ribatti D, Crivallato E, Levi-Schaffer F. Mast cells and eosinophils: A novel link between inflammation and angiogenesis in allergic diseases. J Allergy Clin Immunol 2005; 116:531-536.

[66] Coulon S, Heindryckx F, Geerts A, Van Steenkiste C, Colle I, Van Vlierberghe H. Angiogenesis in chronic liver disease and its complications. Liver Int 2011; 31:146-162.

[67] Thabut D, Shah V. Intrahepatic angiogenesis and sinusoidal remodeling in chronic liver disease: New targets for the treatment of portal hypertension? J Hepatol 2010; 53:976-980.

[68] Viggiano TR, Gostout CJ. Portal hypertensive intestinal vasculopathy: A review of the clinical endoscopic and histopathological features. Am J Gastroenterol 1992; 87:944-954.

[69] Rondonotti E, Villa F, Signorelli C, De Francis R. Portal hypertensive enteropathy. Gastrointest Endosc Clin N Am 2006; 16:277-286.

[70] Nagral AS, Joshi AS, Bhatia SJ, Abraham FP, Vora IM. Congestive jejunopathy in portal hypertension. Gut 1993; 34:694-697.

[71] Misra V, Misra SP, Dwivedi M, Gupta SC. Histomorphometric study of portal hypertensive enteropathy. Am J Clin Pathol 1997; 108:625-657.

[72] Galli SJ, Kalesnikoff J, Grimbaldeston MA, Piliponsky AM, Williams CM, Tsai M. Mast cells as "tunable" effector and immunoregulatory cells: recent advances. Ann Rev Immunol 2005; 23:749-786.

[73] Diez-Arias JA, Aller MA, Palma MD, Arias JL, Muñiz E, Sanchez M, *et al.* Increased duodenal mucosa infiltration by mast cells in rats with portal hypertension. Dig Surg 2001; 18:34-40.

[74] Fernandez M, Mejias M, Angermayr B, Garcia-Pagan JC, Rodes J, Bosch J. Inhibition of VEGF receptor-2 decreases the development of hyperdynamic splanchnic circualtion and porta-systemic collateral vessels in portal hypertensive rats. J Hepatol 2005; 43:98-103.

[75] Angermayr B, Mejias M, Gracia-Sancho J, Garcia-Pagan JC, Bosch J, Fernandez M. Heme-oxigenase attenuates oxidative stress and inflammation, and increases VEGF expresión in portal hypertensive rats. J Hepatol 2006; 44:1033-1039.

[76] Moon TC, St.Lauren CD, Morris KE, Marcet C, Yoshimura T, Sekar Y, *et al.* Advances in mast cell biology: new understanding of heterogeneity and function. Nat Immunol 2010; 3:111-128.

[77] Bielinska M, Narita N, Wilson DB. Distinct roles of visceral endoderm during embryonic mouse development. Int J Dev Biol 1999; 43:183-205.

[78] Oberlin E, El Hafny B, Petit-Cocault L, Souyri M. Definitive human and mouse hematopoiesis originates from the embryonic endothelium: a new class of HSCs based on VE-cadherin expression. Int J Dev Biol 2010; 54:1165-1173.

[79] Zhao S, Fu Y-M, Li X-F, Jin Z-F, Zhao R-B, Huang Q, *et al.* Alterations of bone marrow sinusoidal endothelium in rat and patients with liver cirrhosis. Dig Dis Sci 2010; 55:654-661.

[80] Sanyal AJ, Bosch J, Blei A, Arroyo V. Portal hypertension and its complications. Gastroenterology 2008; 134:1715-1728.

[81] Vollmar B, Wolf B, Siegmund S, Katsen AD, Menger MD. Lymph vessel expansion and function in the development of hepatic fibrosis and cirrhosis. Am J Pathol 1997; 151:169-175.

[82] Yamauchi Y, Ikeda R, Michitaka K, Hiasa Y, Horiike N, Onji M. Morphometric analysis of lymphatic vessels in primary biliary cirrhosis. Hepatol Res 2002; 24:107-113.

[83] Alexander JS, Ganta VC, Jordan PA, Witte MH. Gastrointestinal lymphatics in health and disease. Pathophysiology 2010; 17:315-335.
[84] Ikeda R, Michitaka K, Yamauchi Y, Matsui H, Onji M. Changes in gastrointestinal lymph and blood vessels in patients with cirrhotic portal hypertension. J Gastroenterol 2001; 36: 689-695.
[85] Cardenas A, Arroyo V. Management of ascites and hepatic hydrothorax. Best Prac Res Clin Gastroenterol 2007; 21:55-75.
[86] Arroyo V, Fernandez J, Gines P. Pathogenesis and treatment of hepatorenal syndrome. Semin Liver Dis 2008; 28:81-95.
[87] Mϕller S, Henriksen JH, Bendtsen F. Pathogenetic background for treatment of ascites and hepatorenal syndrome. Hepatol Int 2008; 2:416-428.
[88] Mahmood G, Debnath CR, Mandal AK. Evaluation of 100 cases of ascites. Mymensingh Med J 2009; 18:62-66.
[89] Schrier RW, Arroyo V, Bernardi M, Epstein M, Henriksen JH, Rodes J. Peripheral arterial vasodilation hypothesis: a proposal for the initiation of renal sodium and water retention in cirrhosis. Hepatology 1988; 8:1151-1157.
[90] Kashani A, Landaverde C, Medici V, Rossaro L. Fluid retention in cirrhosis: pathophysiology and management. Q J Med 2008; 101:71-85.
[91] Salerno F, Cazzaniga M. Autonomic dysfunction: often present but usually ignored in patients with liver disease. Liver Int 2009; 29:1451-1453.
[92] Arroyo V, Gines P. Mechanism of sodium retention and ascites formation in cirrhosis. J Hepatol 1993; 17:24-28.
[93] Paulus BM, Ali S, Zia AA, Munir A, Davis Jr RC, Mansbach CM, *et al.* Causes and consequences of systemic venous hypertension. Am J Med Sci 2008; 336:489-497.
[94] Witte CL, Witte MH. Splanchnic circulatory and tissue fluid dynamics in portal hypertension. Fed Proc 1983: 42:1685-1689.
[95] Jimenez-Saenz M, Soria IC, Bernardez JR, Gutierrez JM. Renal sodium retention in portal hypertensión and hepatorenal reflex: from practice to science. Hepatology 2003; 37:1494.
[96] Hamza SM, Kaufman S. Role of spleen in integrated control of splanchnic vascular tone: physiology and pathophysiology. Can J Physiol Pharmacol 2009; 87:1-7.
[97] Cardenas A, Gines P. Portal hypertension. Curr Opin Gastroenterol 2009; 25:195-201.
[98] Riggio O, Angeloni S. Ascitic fluid analysis for diagnosis and monitoring of spontaneous bacterial peritonitis. World J Gastroenterol 2009; 15:3845-3850.
[99] Koulaouzidis A, Bhat S, Saeed AA. Spontaneous bacterial peritonitis. World J Gastroenterol 2009; 15:1042-1049.
[100] Soriano G, Castellote J, Alvarez C, Girbau A, Gordillo J, Baliellas C, *et al.* Secondary bacterial peritonitis in cirrosis: A retrospective study of clinical and analytical characteristics, diagnosis and management. J Hepatol 2010; 52:39-44.
[101] Bernardi M. Spontaneous bacterial peritonitis: from pathophysiology to prevention. Intern Emerg Med. 2010;5 (Suppl 1):S37-S44.
[102] Medzhitov R. Origin and physiological roles of inflammation. Nature 2008; 454:428-435.
[103] Eisenhut M. Changes in ion transport in inflammatory disease. J Inflamm 2006; 3:5.
[104] Häussinger D. The role of cellular hydration in the regulation of cell function. Biochem J 1996; 331:697-710.

[105] Kennett EC, Davis MJ. Degradation of matrix glycosaminoglycans by peroxynitrite/peroxynitrous acid: evidence of a hydroxyl-radical-like mechanism. Free Rad Biol Med 2007; 42:1278-1289.
[106] Jiang D, Liang J, Noble PW. Hyaluronan in tissue injury and repair. Ann Rev Cell Dev Biol 2007; 23:435-461.
[107] Ng ChP, Helm C-LE, Swartz MA. Interstitial flow differentially stimulates blood and lymphatic endothelial cell morphogenesis *in vitro*. Microvasc Res 2004; 68:258-264.
[108] Rutowski JM, Swartz MA. A driving force for change: interstitial flow as a morphoregulator. Trends Cell Biol 2006; 17:44-50.
[109] Ng CP, Hinz B, Swartz MA. Interstitial fluid flow induces myofibroblast differentiation and collagen alignement *in vitro*. J Cell Sci 2005; 118:4731-4739.
[110] Helm C-LE, Fleury ME, Zisch AH, Boschetti F, Swartz MA. Synergy between interstitial flow and VEGF directs capillary morphogenesis *in vitro* through a gradient amplification mechanism. Proc Natl Acad Sci 2005; 102:15779-15784.
[111] Ng CP, Swartz MA. Mechanisms of interstitial flow-induced remodeling of fibroblast-collagen cultures. Ann Biomed Engineering 2006; 34:446-454.
[112] Goldman J, Conley KA, Raehl A, Bondy DM, Pytowski B, Swartz MA, *et al.* Regulation of lymphatic capillary regeneration by interstitial flow in skin. Am J Physiol Heart Circ Physiol 2007; 292: H2176-H2183.
[113] Plaku KJ, Von der Weid PY. Mast cell degranulation alters lymphatic contractile activity through action of histamine. Microcirculation 2006; 13:219-227.
[114] Kvietys PR, Granger DN. Role of intestinal lymphatics in interstitial volume regulation and transmucosal water transport. Ann N Y Acad Sci 2010; 1207:E29-E43.
[115] Fanous MYZ, Phillips AJ, Windson JA. Mesenteric lymph: The bridge to future management of critical illness. JOP J Pancreas (Online) 2007; 8:374-399.
[116] Lynch PM, Deland FA, Schmid-Schönbein GW. The primary valves in the initial lymphatics during inflammation. Lymphatic Res Biol 2007; 5:3-10.
[117] Von der Weid PY, Rehal S. Lymphatic pump function in the inflamed gut. Ann N Y Acad Sci 2010; 1207:E69-E74.
[118] Kohan A, Yoder S, Tso P. Lymphatics in intestinal transport of nutrients and gastrointestinal hormones. Ann N Y Acad Sci 2010; 1207:E44-E51.
[119] Magnotti LJ, Xu D-Z, Lu, Q, Deitch EA. Gut-derived mesenteric lymph. Arch Surg 1999; 134:1333-1341.
[120] Kaiser VL, Sifri ZC, Diksan GS, Berezina T, Zaets S, Lu Q, *et al.* Trauma-hemorrhagic shock mesenteric lymph from rat contains a modified form of albumin that is implicated in endothelial cell toxicity. Shock 2005; 23:417-425.
[121] Watkins AC, Caputo FJ, Badami C, Barlos D, Xu D-Z, Lu Q, *et al.* Mesenteric lymph duct ligation attenuates lung injury and neutrophil activation after intraperitoneal injection of endotoxin in rats. J Trauma 2008; 64:126-130.
[122] Wang Y, Ghoshal S, Ward M, De Villiers W, Woodward J, Eckhardt E. Chylomicrons promote intestinal absorption and systemic dissemination of dietary antigen (ovalbumin) in mice. Plos ONE 2009; 4:e8441.
[123] Wilting J, Becker J, Buttler K, Weich HA. Lymphatics and inflammation. Curr Med Chem 2009; 16:4581-4592.
[124] Bruyere F, Noël A. Lymphangiogenesis: *in vitro* and *in vivo* models. FASEB J 2010; 24:8-21.

[125] Mouta C, Heroult M. Inflammatory triggers of lymphangiogenesis. Lymphat Res Biol 2003; 1:201-218.
[126] Baluk P, Yao L-C, Feng J, Romano T, Jung SS, Schreiter JL, *et al.* TNF-α drives remodeling of blood vessels and lymphatics in sustained airway inflammation in mice. J Clin Invest 2009; 119:2954-2964.
[127] Jurisic G, Detmar M. Lymphatic endothelium in health and disease. Cell Tissue Res 2009; 335:97-108.
[128] Nakao S, Maruyama K, Zandis S, Melhorn MI, Taher M, Noda K, *et al.* Lymphangiogenesis and angiogenesis: concurence and/or dependence? Studies in inbred mouse strains. FASEB J 2010; 24:504-513.
[129] Ji, RC. Lymph node lymphangiogenesis: a new concept for modulating tumor metastasis and inflammatory process. Histol Histopathol 2009; 24:377-384.
[130] Liersch R, Detmar M. Lymphangiogenesis in development and disease. Thromb Haemost 2007; 98:304-310.
[131] Cueni LN, Detmar M. The lymphatic system in health and disease. Lymphat Res Biol 2008; 6:109-122.
[132] Vetrano S, Borroni EM, Sarukhan A, Savino B, Bonecchi R, Correale C, *et al.* The lymphatic system controls intestinal inflammation and inflammation-associated colon cancer through the chemokine decoy receptor D6. Gut 2010;59:197-206.
[133] Alexander JS, Chaitanya GV, Grisham MB, Boktor M. Emerging roles of lymphatics in inflammatory bowel disease. Ann N Y Acad Sci 2010; 1207:E75-E85.
[134] Lai WK, Adams DH. Angiogenesis and chronic inflammation; the potencial for novel therapeutic approaches in chronic liver disease. J Hepatol 2005; 42:7-11.
[135] Shimamura K, Nakatani T, Ueda A, Sugama J, Okuwa M. relationship between lymphangiogenesis and exudates during the wound-healing process of mouse skin full-thickness wound. Wound Repair Regen 2009; 17:598-605.
[136] Thaunat O, Kerjaschki D, Nicoletti A. Is defective lymphatic drainage a trigger for lymphoid neogenesis? TRENDS Immunol 2006; 27:441-445.
[137] Kuiper JJ, Boomsma F, Van Buren H, De Man R, Danser AH, Van den Meiracker AH. Components of the renin-angiotensin-aldosterone system in plasma and ascites in hepatic cirrhosis. Eur J Clin Invest 2008; 38:939-944.
[138] Bansal S, Lindenfeld J, Schrier RW. Sodium retention in heart failure and cirrhosis: potential role of natriuretic doses of mineralocorticoid antagonist? Circ Heart Fail 2009; 2:370-376.
[139] Mayberry JC, Welker KJ, Goldman RK, Mullins RJ. Mechanism of acute ascites formation after trauma resuscitation. Arch Surg 2003; 138:773-776.
[140] Dong MH, Saab S. Complications of cirrhosis. Dis Mon 2008; 54:445-456.
[141] Beavis J, Harwood JL, Coles GA, Williams JD. Synthesis of phospholipids by human peritoneal mesothelial cells. Perit Dial Int 1994; 14:348-355.
[142] Bourbon JR, Chailley-Heu B. Surfactant protein in the digestive tract, mesentery, and other organs: evolutionary significance. Comp Biochem Physiol 2001; 129:151-161.
[143] Obradovic MM, Stojimirovic BB, Trpinac DP, Milutinovic DD, Obradovic DI, Nesic VB. Ultrastructure of peritoneal mesothelial cells. Srp Arh Celok Lek 2001; 129:175-179.
[144] Schilte MN, Celie JWAM, Ter-Wee PM, Beelen RHJ, Van der Born J. Factors contributing to peritoneal tissue remodeling in peritoneal dialysis. Perit Dial Int 2009; 29:605-617.
[145] Li MK, Crawford JM. The pathology of cholestasis. Semin Liver Dis 2004; 24:21-24.

[146] Aller MA, Mendez M, Nava MP, Lopez L, Arias JL, Arias J. The value of microsurgery in liver research. Liver Int 2009; 29:1132-1140.

[147] Aller MA, Prieto I, Cruz M, Losada M, Arias JI, Garcia-Dominguez J, *et al.* Extrahepatic cholestasis. In: Aller MA, Arias J (editors): Microsurgery in Liver Research. Ebook Bentham Scientific; 2009; pp. 137-156.

[148] Aller MA, Duran M, Ortega L, Arias JL, Nava MP, Prieto I, *et al.* Comparative study of macro- and microsurgical extrahepatic cholestasis in the rat. Microsurgery 2004; 24:442-447.

[149] Aller MA, Lorente L, Alonso S, Arias J. A model of cholestasis in the rat, using a microsurgical technique. Scand J Gastroenterol 1993; 28:10-14.

[150] Sanchez-Patan F, Anchuelo R, Corcuera MT, Casado I, Gomez-Aguado F, Aller MA, *et al.* Biliary fibrosis in microsurgical extrahepatic cholestasis in the rat. Microsurgery 2008; 28:361-366.

[151] Ramadori G, Saile B. Portal tract fibrogenesis in the liver. Lab Invest 2004; 84:153-159.

[152] Aller MA, Arias JL, Garcia-Dominguez J, Arias JI, Duran M, Arias J. Experimental obstructive cholestasis: the wound-like inflammatory liver response. Fibrogenesis Tissue Rep 2008; 1:6.

[153] Aller MA, Arias JL, Prieto I, Losada M, Arias J. Bile duct ligation: step-by-step to cholangiocyte inflammatory tumorigenesis. Eur J Gastroenterol Hepatol 2010; 22: 651-661.

[154] Garcia-Moreno LM, Aller MA, Conejo M, Gomez MA, Martin FR, Arias J, *et al.* Brain Ag-NOR activity in cholestatic rats with hepatic encephalopathy. Hepatol Res 2002; 24:275-281.

[155] Aller MA, Nava MP, Arias JL, Duran M, Prieto I, Llamas MA, *et al.* Microsurgical extrahepatic cholestasis in the rat: a long-term study. J Invest Surg 2004; 17:99-104.

[156] Pereira RM, Dos Santos RAS, Oliveira EA, Leite VHR, Dias FLC, Rezende AS, *et al.* Development of hepatorenal síndrome in bile duct ligated rats. World J Gastroenterol 2008; 28:4505-4511.

[157] Thabut D, Tazi KA, Bonnefont-Rousselot D, Aller MA, Farges O, Guimont MC *et al.* High-density lipoprotein administration attenuates liver proinflammatory response, restores liver endothelial nitric oxide synthase activity, and lowers portal pressure in cirrhotic rats. Hepatology 2007; 46:1893-1906.

[158] Assimakopoulos SF, Vagianos CE. Bile duct ligation in rats: A reliable model of hepatorenal syndrome? World J Gastroenterol 2009; 15:121-123.

[159] Wang G, Shen H, Rajaraman G, Roberts MS, Gong Y, Jiang P, *et al.* Expression and antioxidant function of liver fatty acid binding protein in normal and bile-duct ligated rats. Eur J Pharmacol 2007; 560:61-68.

[160] Portincasa P, Grattagliano I, Testini M, Caruso ML, Wang DQH, Moschetta A, *et al.* Parallel intestinal and liver injury during early cholestasis in the rat: modulation by bile salts and antioxidants. Free Rad Biol Med 2007; 42:1381-1391.

[161] Assimakopoulos SF, Vagianos CE, Patsoukis N, Georgiou C, Nikolopoulou V, Scopa CD. Evidence for intestinal oxidative stress in obstructive jaundice-induced gut barrier dysfunction in rats. Acta Physiol Scand 2004; 180:177-185.

[162] Soylu AR, Aydogtu N, Basaran UN, Altaner S, Tarcin O, Gedik N, *et al.* Antioxidants vitamins E and C attenuate hepatic fibrosis in biliary obstructed rats. World J Gastroenterol 2006; 12:6835-6841.

[163] Garcia-Dominguez J, Aller MA, Garcia C, De Vicente F, Corcuera MT, Gomez-Aguado F, *et al.* Splanchnic Th_2 and Th_1 cytokine redistribution in microsurgical cholestatic rats. J Surg Res 2010; 162: 203-212.
[164] Waynforth HB, Flecknell PA. Methods of obtaining body fluids. In: Waynforth HB, Flecknell PA (editors): Techniques in the rat. London: Elsevier Academic Press; Second Edition; 1992, pp. 68-99.
[165] Hauss D, Fogal S, Ficorilli J. Chronic collection of mesenteric lymph from conscious, tethered rats. Contemp Top Lab Anim Sci 1998; 37:56-58.
[166] Aller MA, Nava MP, Arias J. Techniques of blood, bile and lymph samples extraction. In: Aller MA, Arias J (editors): Microsurgery in Liver Reserch. Ebook Bentham Scientific; 2009, pp- 71-92.
[167] Mittal A, Middleditch M, Ruggiero K, Buchanan CM, Jullig M, Loveday B, *et al.* The proteome of rodent mesenteric lymph. Am J Physiol Gastrointest Liver Physiol 2008; 295:G895-G903.
[168] Fang JF, Shih LY, Yuan KC, Fang KY, Hwang TL, Hsieh SY. Proteomic analysis of post-hemorrhagic shock mesenteric lymph. Shock 2010; 34: 291-298.
[169] Ohtani O, Ohtani Y. Structure and function of rat lymph nodes. Arch Histol Cytol 2008; 71:69-76.
[170] Sztrymf B, Libert JM, Mougeot C, Lebrec D, Mazmanian M, Humbert M, *et al.* Cirrhotic rats with bacterial translocation have higher incidence and severity of hepatopulmonary syndrome. J Gastroenterol Hepatol 2005; 20:1538-1544.
[171] Frances R, Chiva M, Sanchez E, Gonzalez-Navajas JM, Llovet T, Zapater P, *et al.* Bacterial translocation is downregulated by anti-TNFα monoclonal antibody administration in rats with cirrhosis and ascites. J Hepatol 2007; 46:797-803.
[172] Cheatham ML. Abdominal compartment syndrome: pathophysiology and definitions. Scand J Trauma Resusc Emerg Med. 2009; 17:10.
[173] Hou W, Sanyal AJ. Ascites: diagnosis and management. Med Clin North Am 2009; 93:801-817.
[174] Kim SU, Kim DY, Lee CK, Park JY, Kim SH, Kim HM, *et al.* Ascitic fluid infection in patients with hepatitis B virus-related liver cirrhosis: Culture-negative neutrocytic ascites *versus* spontaneous bacterial peritonitis. J Gastroenterol Hepatol 2010; 25:122-128.
[175] Chan-Kyung JC, Shan SJ, Winsor EJ, Diamandis EP. Proteomics analysis of human amniotic fluid. Mol Cell Proteomics 2007; 6:1406-1415.
[176] Tong X-L, Wang L, Gao T-B, Qin Y-G, Qi Y-Q, Xu Y-P. Potential function of amniotic fluid in fetal development-Novel insights by comparing the composition of human amniotic fluid with umbilical cord and maternal serum at mid and late gestation. J Clin Med Assoc 2009; 72:368-373.
[177] Gray T, Huestis M. Bioanalytical procedures for monitoring in utero drug exposure. Anal Bioanal Chem 2007; 388:1455-1465.
[178] Schmidt W. The amniotic fluid compartment: the fetal habitat. Adv Anat Embryol Cell Biol 1992; 127:1-100.
[179] Bellini C, Boccardo F, Bonioli E, Campisi C. Lymphodynamics in the fetus and newborn. Lymphology 2006; 39:110-117.
[180] Brace R. Physiology of amniotic fluid volume regulation. Clin Obstet Gynecol 1997; 40:280-289.

[181] Koski KG, Fergusson MA. Amniotic fluid composition responds to changes in manternal dietary carbohydrate and is related to metabolic status in term fetal rats. J Nutr 1992; 122:385-392.
[182] Wagner CL, Taylor SN, Johnson D. Host factors in amniotic fluid and breast milk that contribute to gut maturation. Clin Rev Allerg Immunol 2008; 34:191-204.
[183] Moran ET. Nutrition of the developing embryo and hatchling. Poult Sci 2007; 86:1043-1049.
[184] Lopez de Torre B, Tovar JA, Uriarte S, Aldazabal P. The nutrition of the fetus with intestinal atresia: studies in the chick embryo model. J Pediatr Surg 1992; 27:1325-1328.
[185] Delo DM, De Coppi P, Bartsch G, Atala A. Amniotic fluid and placental stem cells. Meth Enzymol 2006; 419:426-438.
[186] Insausti CL, Blanquer M, Bleda P, Iniesta P, Majado MJ, Castellanos G, *et al.* The amniotic membrane as a source of stem cells. Histol Histopathol 2010; 25:91-98.
[187] Schlievert P, Johnson W, Galask RP. Isolation of a low-molecular-weight antibacterial system from human amniotic fluid. Infect Immun 1976; 14:1156-1166.
[188] Elinson RP, Beckham Y. Development in frogs with large eggs and the origin of amniotes. Zoology (Jena) 2002; 105:105-117.
[189] Blackburn DG, Flemming AF. Morphology, development and evolution of fetal membranes and placentation is squamate reptiles. J Exp Zool B Mol Dev Evol 2009; 312:579-589.
[190] Aller MA, Arias N, Prieto I, Santamaria L, de Miguel MP, Arias JL, Arias J. Portal hypertension-related inflammatory phenotypes: From a vitelline and amniotic point of view. Adv Biosci Biotechnol, 2012; 3: 881-899.

Index

A

Acidosis 26, 154
Acute phase response 281, 316
Alexis Carrel 11
Anaerobic glycolysis 154
Angiogenesis 35, 51, 214, 317
Angiogenic phenotype 169
Anti-inflammation 250
Amniotic axis 58, 134, 217
Amniotic fluid 51, 57, 129
Ascites 309, 320, 328
ATP 52

B

Bacterial translocation 34, 180
Bile-duct ligation 326
Bilirubine 30
Biliverdin 31
Biofilms 180
Bone marrow-related axis 140, 195

C

Calne 13
Cancer 214, 221
Cancer cell 236
Causalgia 69
Cell hibernation 160
Cholesterol 118,180
Clot 139
Coagulation 64, 139
Coelomic-amniotic axis 99, 195
Cohnheim 8

Jaime Arias, Maria-Angeles Aller and Jose-Ignacio Arias (Eds)

Contusion 20
Cutaneous wound healing 131

E

Ebb phase 154
Ecchymosis 18,28
Edema 18,63
Ehrlich 9
Embryo development 129
Embryonic 51
Endocrine inflammation 107
Endocrine phase 56
Endoderm 51
Endosymbiosi 181
Endothelial egg 109,114
Epithelial-mesenchymal transition 214
Eukaryotes 180
Evo-devo 277
Exocoelomic-amniotic axis 112
Exosymbiosis 181
Experimental models 309
Extraembryonic functions 111, 129, 133, 188
Extraembryonic phenotypes 115,143
Extrahepatic cholestasis 256, 309
Exudation 65

F

Fetal development 309
Fibrin 96, 103, 105
Fibroblast 70
Fibrosis 180
Flow phase 154

G

Gastrulation 51, 60, 215, 293

Gastrulation-like process 133
Gestation 99
Glucocorticoids 180
Graft *vs* host disease 250
Granulation tissue 51, 67,77,81, 233
Granuloma 66
Gut microbiome 180
Gut microbiota 182

H

Heme 28
Hemoglobin 18
Hepatic steatosis 309
Hepatic cirrhosis 325
History 4
Hydration 277, 281
Hypothermia 161
Hypercatabolism 99
Hypermetabolism 164
Hypertrophic scar 38
Hypothalamic-pituitary-adrenal axis 154
Hypoxia 18

I

Inflamacitizen 291
Inflammation 3,80,154
Inflammatory cancer cell 220,223,
Inflammatory interstitium 109
Inflammatory mesenchyma 70,73
Inflammatory pain 51,68
Inflammatory phenotypes 54
Inflammatory response 55, 155
Injury 157
Immune phase 56

Immune inflammation 104
Immunonutrition 154
Immunotolerance 214
Interstitial-lymphatic tumoral axis 214, 224
Interstitium 129
Intraembryonic mesenchyma 129
Invertebrates 85
Ischemia 281
Ischemia-reperfusion 51, 158

J

John Hunter 5
Joseph Murray 11

K

Keloids 38

L

Leukocytes 129
Leukocytic phenotype 164, 227
Lipoprotein-related metabolism 277, 286
Liver fibrosis 250
Liver wound healing reaction 143
Low-grade metabolic inflammation 296
Lymph flow 309
Lymphangiogenesis 214, 324

M

Macrophages 99
Mast cell 82,87, 198, 202, 291, 309, 318
Mesenchyma 51
Mesenchymal-epithelial transition 214
Mesenchymal stem cell 250,
Mesoderm 51

Metabolic response 154, 157
Metabolic staging 154, 172
Metaflammation 277, 289
Metamorphosis 293
Metaorganism 182
Metastasis 214
Metchnikoff 8
Microcirculation 129
Microcirculatory failure 163
Microbiome 181
Microsurgery 309
Microsurgical cholestasis 250, 327
Mineralocorticoids 180
Mini-brain 309, 313
Multiple organ dysfunction 99
Multiple organ failure 180

N

Necrosis 18,52
Nervous phase 23,55
Neuro-immune-endocrine response 99
Neurogenic inflammatory phenotype 103
Neurogenic systemic axis 138

O

Obstructive cholestasis 326
Ontogeny 57, 99, 279
Organ transplantation 250
Oxygen 42
Oxygen metabolism 18

P

Pathological axis 61
Pentraxins 289

Peritoneum 319
Photosynthesis 39
Phylogenetic evolution 99,117, 279
Polytraumatized patient 99
Portal hypertension 309, 310
Portal hypertensive syndrome 321
Postcapillary venules 180
Post-traumatic inflammatory response 18
Prehepatic portal hypertension 311
Pus 31

Q

Quorum sensing 180

R

Recapitulated functions 133
Remodeling 67
Regeneration 18,37
Regenerative medicine 250
Remodeling 51, 293, 317
Resuscitation 163
Roy York Calne 13

S

Santiago Ramón y Cajal 10, 41
Scar 326
Senescence 129
Sepsis 180
Septic axis 192
Septic response 182
Shock 154, 162
Staphylococcus *aureus* 32
Starzl 12
Sulphydril compounds 161

Suppuration 65
Surgeon 3
Surgical infections 180
Surgical inflammation 3,14,100
Surgical inflammatory phenotypes 111
Surgical sepsis 188
Systemic inflammatory response 99, 192

T

Tetrapyrroles 18,40
Tissue inflammation 22
Tissue injury 19
Thomas E. Starzl 12
Transplant 253
Trauma 154
Trophic mechanisms 54, 155
Trophoblastic-yolk sac axis 99, 112, 195
Tumor invasion 214
Tumor development 214
Type 2 diabetes 3

U

Urobilinogen 29,

V

Vascular inflammation 61
Vitelline 129
Vitelline axis 134, 217
Vitellum 191
Von Recklinghausen 7

W

Warburg effect 214, 224
Wound healing 144, 214

Wound healing reaction 129
Wound repair 51
Wound repair phenotypes 215
Wounds 53

Y

Yolk sac 51, 70
Yolk sac axis 58
Yolk sac-hematopoietic-angiogenic axis 60